PROGRESS IN RADIOPHARMACOLOGY 1985

DEVELOPMENTS IN NUCLEAR MEDICINE
Series editor Peter H. Cox

Cox, P.H. (ed.): Cholescintigraphy. 1981. ISBN 90-247-2524-0
Cox, P.H. (ed.): Progress in radiopharmacology 3. Selected Topics. 1982.
ISBN 90-247-2768-5
Jonckheer, M.H. and Deconinck, F. (eds.): X-ray fluorescent scanning of the
thyroid. 1983. ISBN 0-89838-561-X
Kristensen, K. and Nørbygaard, E. (eds.): Safety and efficacy of radiopharma-
ceuticals. 1984. ISBN 0-89838-609-8
Bossuyt, A. and Deconinck, F.: Amplitude/phase patterns in dynamic scinti-
graphic imaging. 1984. ISBN 0-89838-641-1
Hardeman, M.R. and Najean, Y. (eds.): Blood cells in nuclear medicine I. Cell
kinetics and bio-distribution. 1984. ISBN 0-89838-653-5
Fueger, G.F. (ed.): Blood cells in nuclear medicine II. Migratory blood cells.
1984. ISBN 0-89838-654-3
Biersack, H.J. and Cox, P.H. (eds.): Radioisotope studies in cardiology. 1985.
ISBN 0-89838-733-7
Cox, P.H., Limouris, G. and Woldring M.G. (eds.): Progress in radiophar-
macology 1985. 1985. ISBN 0-89838-745-0

Progress in radiopharmacology 1985

edited by

PETER H. COX

Department of Nuclear Medicine
Rotterdamsch Radio-Therapeutisch Instituut
Rotterdam

GEORGE LIMOURIS

Department of Nuclear Medicine
Health House, National Bank of Greece
Athens

MARTIN G. WOLDRING

Department of Nuclear Medicine
Groningen University Hospital
Groningen

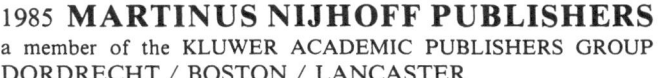

1985 **MARTINUS NIJHOFF PUBLISHERS**
a member of the KLUWER ACADEMIC PUBLISHERS GROUP
DORDRECHT / BOSTON / LANCASTER

Distributors

for the United States and Canada: Kluwer Academic Publishers, 190 Old Derby Street, Hingham, MA 02043, USA
for the UK and Ireland: Kluwer Academic Publishers, MTP Press Limited, Falcon House, Queen Square, Lancaster LA1 1RN, UK
for all other countries: Kluwer Academic Publishers Group, Distribution Center, P.O. Box 322, 3300 AH Dordrecht, The Netherlands

Library of Congress Cataloging in Publication Data

```
Main entry under title:

Progress in radiopharmacology  1985.

    (Developments in nuclear medicine)
    Based on papers given at the 4th European Symposium on
Radiopharmacology, held under the auspices of the Europe-
ean Joint Committee on Radiopharmaceuticals (ENMS/SNME.)
in Athens from March 28-31, 1984.
    Includes indexes.
    1. Radioisotopes in pharmacology.  2. Radiopharma-
ceuticals.  I. Cox, Peter H.  II. Limouris, George.
III. Woldring, Martin G.  IV. European Symposium on
Radiopharmacology (4th : 1984 : Athens, Greece)
V. European Joint Committee on Radiopharmaceuticals.
VI. Series.  [DNLM: 1. Nuclear Medicine--congresses.
2. Radioisotopes--congresses.
W1 DE998KF / WN 440 P964 1984]
RM852.P76  1985    615.8'424          85-13774
```

ISBN-13: 978-94-010-8727-8   e-ISBN-13: 978-94-009-5028-3
DOI: 10.1007/978-94-009-5028-3

Copyright

FOREWORD

This volume is based upon presentations made to the 4th European Symposium on Radiopharmacology which was held under the auspices of the European Joint Committee on Radiopharmaceuticals (ENMS / SNME) in Athens from March 28 - 31, 1984.

The Medical Insurance Foundation of the National Bank of Greece (TYPET) sponsored this meeting and the Joint Committee would like to express their gratitude to the local organising committee: G. Limouris, M. Pierroutsakou, A. Sarris, A. Tzoulis and C. Binas. A word of thanks also to Mrs. Tineke Busker who prepared the camera ready copy.

The meeting reflects the continuing and growing interest in biodistribution and factors which can influence biodistribution in the clinical situation. The choice of subjects, respiration, cerebral function, biodistribution and metabolism complement earlier volumes in this series and reflect European interests in these areas.

P.H. Cox
Rotterdam, April 1985

CONTENTS

Foreword   P.H. Cox   V

Contributors   XI

    I. THE RESPIRATORY SYSTEM

        Physiology and pathophysiology of
        the respiratory system
        J. Roth, E. Henze, W.E. Adam   3

        Generator-produced Krypton-81m in
        gas and liquid phases for medical
        applications
        M. Guillaume, N. Garzaniti, M. Zicot,
        T. Khuc, P. Bartsch   23

        Noble radionuclides for lung ventila-
        tion studies
        I. Bofilias   49

        Radioaerosols in nuclear medicine
        M. Pillay, B. Shapiro, P.H. Cox   57

        A dry aerosol of Tc^{99m}-albuminmilli-
        microspheres for lung ventilation
        scintigraphy: preparation, inhalation
        apparatus and examples of clinical
        results
        P. Angelberger, I. Zolle, A. Strigl,
        H. Köhn, A. Mostbeck, W. Fiedler   73

   II. CEREBRAL FUNCTION

        New agents for probing glucose turnover
        and receptor densities in the brain
        G. Kloster, G. Stöcklin   89

        Cerebral uptake of radioiodinated
        amphetamines - basic research and
        clinical results
        H.J. Biersack, H. Klünenberg,
        G. Friedrich, R. Knopp, R. Ledda,
        E. Doppelfeld, C. Winkler   123

        Radiolabelled Schiff bases in brain
        studies
        A.D. Varvarigou, E. Chiotellis,
        G. Evagelatos   131

III. BIODISTRIBUTION AND METABOLISM OF
RADIOPHARMACEUTICALS

Some recent progress in the development
and application of radiopharmaceuticals
labelled with ^{11}C and ^{18}F
V.W. Pike   141

Radiopharmaceuticals suitable for
cardiac emergency studies
H.W. Pabst, R. Bauer   161

The pharmacokinetics of Tc^{99m}-diethyl
ida in hyperferremic mice
C. Sawas-Dimopoulou, C. Soulpi,
N. Toubanakis   183

Subcellular distribution of Tc^{99m}-
Sn-phytate in the liver of rats
C. Dassiou   195

Treatment of thyroid disorders by
^{131}I
P. Pfannenstiel   199

IV. EXTRANEOUS FACTORS AFFECTING
BIODISTRIBUTION

Alterations in the biodistribution
of radiopharmaceuticals, caused by
extraneous influences
M.G. Woldring   219

The effects of drugs and therapeutic
procedures on the biodistribution of
skeletal reagents
P.H. Cox   231

Interaction between some disinfectants
and Tc99m-radiopharmaceuticals
A. Verbruggen, B. Cleynhens, M. Hoogmartens, M. de Roo   239

Altered uptake of Tc^{99m}-MDP, Ca^{47} and
Ga^{67} by mice osteogenic sarcoma after
administration of a cytostatic drug
R. Senekowitsch, H. Kriegel, S. Möllenstädt   251

Visualisation of gallbladder and gut
on Tc99m bone scintiscans
A. Fountos, J. Malamitsi   263

Drug-free high-quality tumour imaging
with ^{67}Ga
S.K. Shukla, I. Blotta, C. Cipriani,
G.B. Manni   271

Author index   283

Subject index   285

CONTRIBUTORS

Angelberger, P.	Chemistry Institute, Austrian Research Center Seibersdorf, Austria.
Biersack, H.J.	Institut für klinische und experimentelle Nuklearmedizin der Universität Bonn, FRG.
Bofilias, I.	Department of Medical Physics, Aristotelian University of Thessaloniki, Greece.
Cox, P.H.	Department of Nuclear Medicine, Rotterdamsch Radio-Therapeutisch Instituut, Rotterdam, The Netherlands.
Dassiou, C.	Nuclear Research Center, "Demokritos", Athens, Greece.
Fountos, A.	Naval Hospital of Athens, Greece.
Guillaume, M.	Cyclotron Research Center, University, Liege, Belgium.
Kloster, G.	Institut für Chemie 1 (Nuklearchemie) der Kernforschungsanlage Jülich, FRG.
Pabst, H.W.	Nuklearmedizinische Klinik und Poliklinik rechts der Isar der Technischen Universität, München, FRG.
Pfannenstiel, P.	Fachbereich Nuklearmedizin, Deutsche Klinik für Diagnostik, Wiesbaden, FRG.
Pike, V.W.	MRC Cyclotron Unit, Hammersmith Hospital, London, U.K.
Pillay, M.	Department of Nuclear Medicine Rotterdamsch Radio-Therapeutisch Instituut, Rotterdam, The Netherlands.
Roth, J.	Abt. Radiologie III (Nuklearmedizin) Klinikum der Universität, Ulm, FRG.

Sawas-Dimopoulou, C.

Laboratory of Radiopharmacology,
Department of Radiodiagnostic-
products and Radioisotopes,
NRC "Demokritos", Athens, Greece.

Senekowitsch, R.

Department of Nuclear Biology,
Gesellschaft für Strahlen- und
Umweltforschung, Neuherberg, FRG.

Shukla, S.K.

Istituto di Cromatografia, CNR,
Roma, Italy.

Varvarigou, A.D.

Radiopharmaceutical Laboratory
Nuclear Research Center
"Demokritos", Athens, Greece.

Verbruggen, A.

Laboratory of Nuclear Medicine and
Radiopharmacy, University Hospital
Gasthuisberg, Leuven, Belgium.

Woldring, M.G.

Department of Nuclear Medicine,
University Hospital, Groningen,
The Netherlands.

THE RESPIRATORY SYSTEM

PHYSIOLOGY AND PATHOPHYSIOLOGY OF THE RESPIRATORY SYSTEM

J. ROTH, E. HENZE, W.E. ADAM

INTRODUCTION

The application of radionuclides to study the physiology
and pathophysiology of the respiratory system comprises the
use of radioactive gases and radioactive labelled particles
for the examination of ventilation and perfusion of the lungs
as well as radioactive aerosols for the investigation of airway diseases.

Whereas conventional methods, such as whole body plethysmography and the helium single breath technique, are based
upon changes in volume and pressure and draw their final conclusions indirectly, nuclear medicine techniques "look" directly
into the lungs. One receives thus not only information about
ventilation and perfusion of the lungs as a whole but also
from individual parts of the lungs. Thus, it is possible to
receive information from the regional function of the lung as
well as its distribution with a noninvasive method.

The concentration and local distribution of gamma ray
emitting gases can be measured outside the chest after distribution within the lungs. Furthermore, dynamic processes can be
registered and analysed by functional and serial scintigrams,
respectively.

The combination of morphological - especially topographical -
and functional information allows a more detailed evaluation.
The strength of nuclear medicine diagnostic methods lies in
the presentation of an image with the potential of quantitative
analysis of regional lung function.

HISTORIC REVIEW

Although v. Hevesy had recognized the importance of radio-

nuclides in clinical diagnosis of function in the early 30's,
more than a decade passed until Mueller and Rossier (1) performed the first lung perfusion scintigraphy in 1947 using radio-
gold-charcoal-particles. The reason for the delay in applying
open radionuclides was the lack of appropriate substances. It
was only in 1963 when Taplin (2) succeeded in producing I-131
labelled macroaggregates that the decisive breakthrough in
perfusion scintigraphy with radioactive particles took place.

In the years after 1950, radioactive gases could be
produced in sufficient quantities by accelerators and Knipping
(3) was the first to use a radioactive inert gas (Xe^{133}) for
isotope-thoracography. In 1960, West and Dollery (4) examined
regional lung perfusion and ventilation using 0-15. It was in
1962, when Ball (5) used intravenously injected Xe^{133}-NaCl
for the first time to study lung perfusion and initiated the
concept of distribution for ventilation and perfusion. Following this Mioerner (6) introduced radiospirometry for measurement of breath-synchronous fluctuation of radioactivity above
the Xe^{133} filled lung in 1968.

In 1969 Loken (7) was first to use a scintillation camera
connected with a computer system for regional lung function
diagnosis where upon quantitative radiospirometry became
available as a feasible method for clinical routine use.

EVOLUTION AND FUNCTION OF THE LUNGS

The respiratory system comprises, in a wider anatomical
sense, the entire respiratory tract, the circulatory system
as well as the cellular basis membrane and enzyme systems.
Its functional importance lies in biological oxidation, in the
uptake of necessary O2, and in the disposal of the CO2 produced.
Respiration can be separated into 3 partial processes (8):
a. O2-transport from the atmosphere to the cells;
b. the biological oxidation of carbohydrates within the cells
    into H2O and CO2;
c. the transport of CO2 from the cells to the atmosphere.

The following is related to the function of the lung:
diffusion is a central process for the exchange of gases. The

entire quantitative relation is given in the first law of
diffusion of Fick by:

$$gas\ flow = D*F*(C1-C2)/d\ (9)$$

Diffusion is therefore depending on the diffusion constant D,
the surface F, the difference of concentration (C1-C2) and the
diffusion distance d.

   An effective exchange by diffusion requires a large surface
and a short distance. In consequence, only small organisms
with a diameter of less than 1mm have a sufficient exchange of
gases through the surface of their bodies. The evolutionary
development of larger organisms necessitated enlarging the
surface and diminishing the distance. The result of evolution
is remarkable: whereas the body surface of an adult man is only
1.73 sqm, the alveolar membranes have an extension of about
100 sqm and whilst the human skin can be of considerable thickness the thickness of the alveolar membrane is only scarcely
1 um.

   Parallel to this evolution there was the development of
2 convective systems for the fast transport of gases over long
distances:
a.   the bellows-like system between respiratory tract and
     thorax connecting lungs and atmosphere by ventilation;
b.   the cardiovascular system for the transport from the lung
     alveoli to cells and vice versa.

The absolute quantities of ventilation, diffusion and perfusion are not the only standards to evaluate the efficiency of
lung function, but they are essential in their relationship to
one another. This is expressed by the quotient ventilation/
perfusion, which ranges from 0.9 - 1.0 in a healthy lung.

   RADIOSPIROMETRY METHODS
   Radiopharmaceuticals. Radioactive gases used for radiospirometry can be subdivided into gases with a good or poor
affinity to or solubility in blood (10), respectively.

a. good affinity: 0-15, C11 (in form of C11 CO);
b. poor solubility: Kr^{85}, Kr^{77}, Xe^{127}, Xe^{133}.

0-15 and C11 are positron emitters. Their high energy radiation
does not permit the use of conventional scintillation camera's.
Furthermore, the short half life of most of the positron emitting isotopes limits their use to institutes within the proximity
of a cyclotron.

The inert gases Kr and Xe are poorly soluble in blood. Kr
would be the ideal substance due to its low solubility in blood.
However, there is no suitable radioisotope for routine clinical
use. Kr^{77} has too short a half-life, of 1.2 h, and Kr^{85} has a
gamma radiation of only 0.7% efficiency. Xe, in contrast to Kr,
shows a higher solubility in blood. However, it has a disturbing affinity to fat and nerve tissue. Matthews and Dollery (11)
discovered the following disturbancing factors in ventilation
and perfusion studies using a multicompartment model:

a. radioactivity in the chest wall;
b. inflow from other organs into the lungs;
c. removal by the blood during continuous expiration.

These advantages restrict the value of these gases for examinations, where very accurate measurements are required, even
though mathematical methods to correct for these disturbing
factors have been described (12). Xe^{127}, a pure gamma emitter,
with an energy range from 170 to 203 keV has suitable physical
properties. There are, however, considerable difficulties in
production, thereby limiting its clinical application at
present.

In consequence, Xe^{133} having a favourable half life of
5.2d and a gamma peak of 81 keV suitable for gamma camera's is
the most frequently used radioactive gas nowaday.

Technical equipment. For radiospirometry, gamma camera
systems with an integrated computer are mainly used (13).
Both lungs can be observed simultaneously with a large field
of view camera equipped with a parallel hole collimator.
Serial scintigrams allow registration of fast changes in radioactivity in space and time. The computer aids not only in

establishing time activity curves over the whole lung but also from variable regions of interest.

Performance and Radiospirometry. Radiospirometry usually starts with the measurement of lung perfusion (14). 5 mCi Xe^{133} dissolved in physiological NaCl-solution are injected into a cubital vein. The patient sits in front of the gamma camera withholding breath for 10-15 sec. Because of its low solubility in blood, Xe^{133} diffuses quantitatively into the perfusing air within the alveoli. Activity measured over the lungs then shows the volume of the lungs containing air (fig 1). The length of Q gives a measure of relative perfusion. Subsequently, the patients breath out via the Xenon trap. During the following 3 min, the wash-out is registered. The slope of the decrease of radioactivity and the elimination constant are indices of ventilation. Measurements of ventilation and volume then follow. The patient breathes a defined Helium-0-2-air mixture in a closed spirometer system. After definition of the functional residual capacity (FRC) for He with an on-line computer, 30 mCi Xe^{133} are blown into the system. As soon as equilibration between spirometer and lung is achieved, the camera-computer system is started again.

The average value in steady-state-registered count rates corresponds closely to the FRC. The residual volume (RV) is received upon complete exhalation. Then, the patient inhales to maximum and the volume obtained is equivalent to the total lung capacity (TLC). Finally, definition of ventilation follows. The patient inhales air and exhales over the Xenon trap. The elimination constant and half life are derived from this wash-out phase. Fully automated computer programs guarantee a rational and observer independent evaluation. The method provides 48 data from 6 lung regions in total and allows a detailed evaluation of lung function. Fig 2 shows the data from 24 healthy subjects. At the bottom, the results of whole body plethysmography, blood gas analysis and lung catheterization are shown.

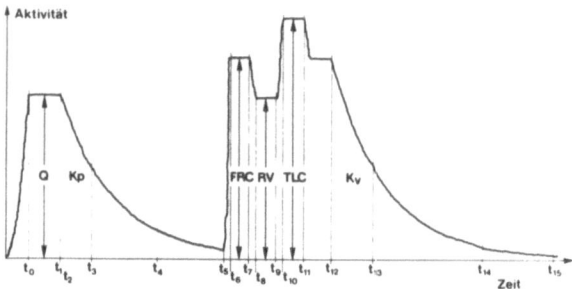

AKTIVITATSVERLAUF ÜBER DER LUNGE
WÄHREND DER PERFUSIONS-UND VENTILATIONSSTUDIE MIT Xe-133

Fig. 1. Schematic presentation of radiospirometry using Xe[133] (details see 4.3).

Normalpersonen
(n = 24, Alter = 37,4)

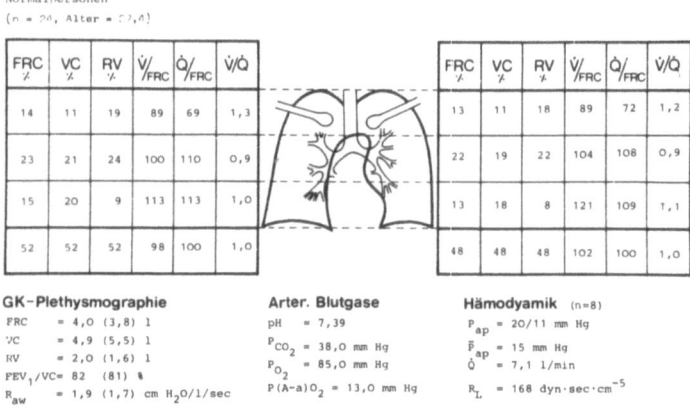

FRC %	VC %	RV %	$\dot{V}/_{FRC}$	$\dot{Q}/_{FRC}$	$\dot{V}/\dot{Q}$		FRC %	VC %	RV %	$\dot{V}/_{FRC}$	$\dot{Q}/_{FRC}$	$\dot{V}/\dot{Q}$
14	11	19	89	69	1,3		13	11	18	89	72	1,2
23	21	24	100	110	0,9		22	19	22	104	108	0,9
15	20	9	113	113	1,0		13	18	8	121	109	1,1
52	52	52	98	100	1,0		48	48	48	102	100	1,0

GK-Plethysmographie
FRC = 4,0 (3,8) l
VC = 4,9 (5,5) l
RV = 2,0 (1,6) l
FEV_1/VC= 82 (81) %
R_{aw} = 1,9 (1,7) cm H_2O/l/sec

Arter. Blutgase
pH = 7,39
P_{CO_2} = 38,0 mm Hg
P_{O_2} = 85,0 mm Hg
$P(A-a)O_2$ = 13,0 mm Hg

Hämodyamik (n=8)
P_{ap} = 20/11 mm Hg
$\bar{P}_{ap}$ = 15 mm Hg
$\dot{Q}$ = 7,1 l/min
R_L = 168 dyn·sec·cm^{-5}

Fig. 2. Standard values obtained by radiospirometry in 24 normal volunteers.

PHYSIOLOGY OF REGIONAL LUNG FUNCTION

The physiology of the lung depends on the influence of gravity (15). With the supine body, there is a homogeneous distribution of volume in all lung parts. In the upright position, however, the relative alveolar size is larger in the upper parts of the lungs than in basal parts (16). This is caused by the weight of the lungs: The pleural pressure is more negative in the apex of the lungs than in the vicinity of the diaphragm. Thus, the transpulmonary pressure responsible for the expansion of the lungs is decreasing from apex to base. As a result, there is a larger RV in the upper parts than in the lower parts of the lungs. Simultaneously, the share of VC in TLC is smaller in the upper parts.

To demonstrate the dynamic parameter of ventilation the definition of "compliance" is of importance. The latter means the quotient of inspired volume and the concomitant change of intrathoracic pressure (17). This is a measure of the elasticity of the lungs. The compliance does not follow a linear but rather an S-shaped relation which explains regional differences in ventilation. The apical lung regions work in the upper, flat part of the curve. Accordingly, a cranio-caudal ventilation gradient is recorded (18). The law of gravity also explains the phenomenon of the "closing volume", which means that lung volume with small airways (<2mm) are closed while exhaling.

For examination, 2 mCi Xe^{133} are "shot" as a bolus into the mouth of the patient. The patient inhales slowly and stops breathing at maximum inspiration for some seconds and then exhales again slowly. Fig 3 shows the activity curve measured over the lungs. The bend in this curve shows the closing volume of the basal lung regions (19). The bend is caused by the collapse of the small airways which again is caused by the gravity-dependent transmural pressure exceeding the intra-alveolar pressure while exhaling. The gas is trapped in the alveoli, therefore called "trapped air". The closing volume increased with the age and exceeds FRC from the middle of the 6th decade of life (20).

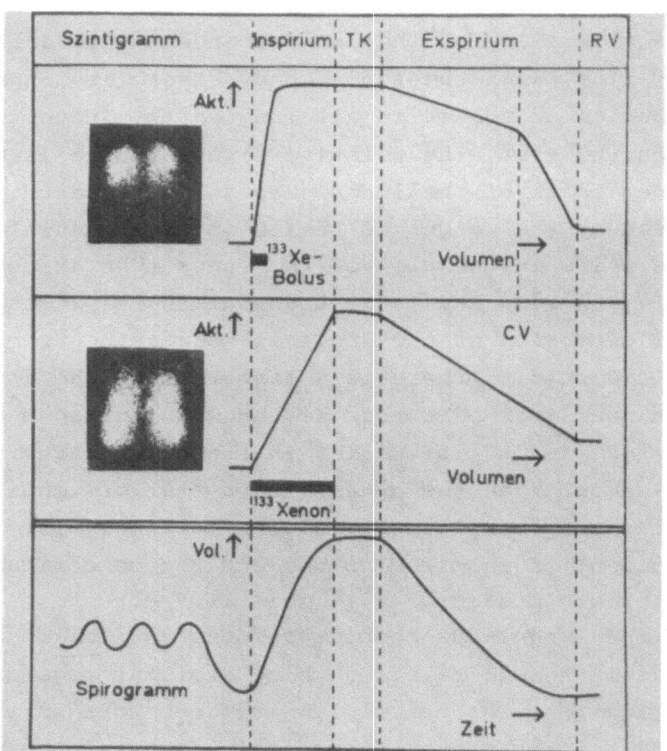

Fig. 3. Présentation of Xe bolus technique: The volume, at which the bend in the curve occurs while exhaling, corresponds the closing volume (CV) of the lower parts of the lungs.

The principle of "first in - last out" is based upon the closing volume and finally upon the law of gravity (21). Inhalation is not a Dirac function. During inspiration, the first part of the breathing volume predominantly flows into the apical parts of the lungs. Vice versa, the gas leaves the lung apex only at the end of exhalation. The moment, at which the discharge of the apical parties occurs, corresponds to the closing of the small airways in the basal lung regions. Gravity plays a similiarly important role in the regional distribution of perfusion. Three pressures and their relationships are decisive for the perfusion: The alveolar pressure P (A) is equal in all pulmonary regions. The arterial P (a) and the venous P (v) increase from cranial to caudal by the

11

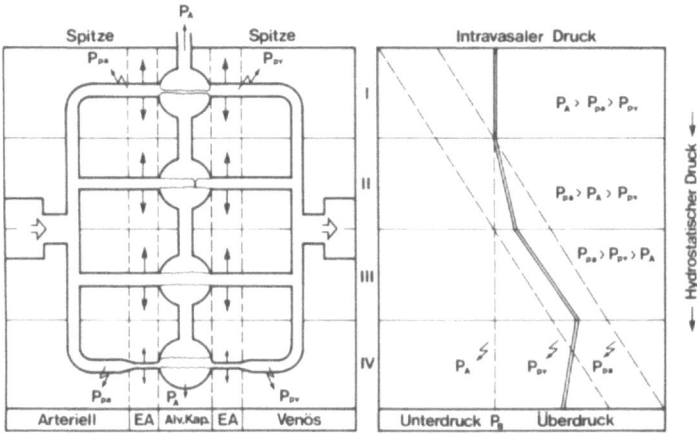

Fig. 4. Zone model of lung perfusion: Perfusion depends on the pressures in the pulmonary artery P (a), in the alveoli P (A) and in the pulmonary vein P (v).

magnitude of the hydrostatic component (22,23).

Accordingly, West (24) found 3 zones of perfusion in tests with isolated lungs (fig 4). There is no perfusion in zone 1, because P (A) > P (a). Zone 2 covers the largest part of the lung, where P (a) > P (A). As a result, perfusion is determined by the transmural pressure gradient. The difference between arterial and venous pressure at last is decisive for the quantity of perfusion in zone 3. In total, there is an increase in perfusion towards the caudal direction.

PATHOPHYSIOLOGY OF REGIONAL LUNG FUNCTION

Two mechanisms are of importance in understanding region-al pathophysiology of the lungs. They can change the distribu-tion pattern caused by gravity of ventilation and perfusion:

    a. alveolar-vascular mechanism (25)
    b. alveolar-bronchial mechanism (26)

In cases of alveolar hypoxia, the alveolar-vascular mechanism leads to throttling of perfusion in the corresponding pulmonary artery. Ubiquitous hypoxia can lead to a general vasoconstriction with consecutive increase of pulmonary artery pressure. The pulmonary hypertension due to high altitude hypoxia may be quoted as an example (27).

The alveolar-bronchial mechanism leads to bronchoconstriction in case of alveolar hypocapnia in the corresponding region of the lungs and, thus to throttling of ventilation. Generalized hypocapnia results in an increase of airway resistance even in healthy subjects. Both mechanisms together enable the adaptation of ventilation and perfusion to each other necessary for pulmonary function (28). The external ventilation-perfusion quotient registered by Xe^{133} complies with the average value of an alveolar population as "seen" by the gamma camera. In extreme cases, not perfused but ventilated alveoli and also not ventilated but perfused alveoli are simultaneously used for determination of the V/Q-quotient. The mean value is mathematically correct, physiologically, however, without any sense. Under these aspects the following pattern of regional disturbances of function are seen.

Localized processes. The pathophysiology of regional lung function can be separated in the following basic pattern:

a.   airway obstruction with or without blood shunting;
b.   changes in lung tissue with increased or decreased
     compliance;
c.   obstruction of lung vessels.

a.   Obstruction of airways. A complete obstruction of an airway (for example, caused by a foreign body or a tumour) leads to a substantial reduction of all static volumes. Ventilation is essentially cut off. Perfusion is distinctly reduced because of the alveolar-vascular effect. However, perfusion is normal or even slightly increased in relation to the still remaining volume.

Fig 5 shows an example of a 62 year old man with a

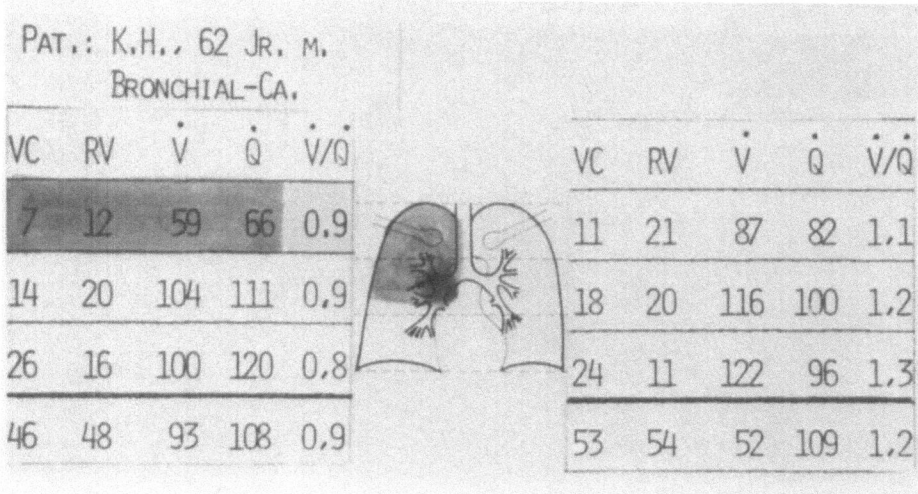

PAT.: K.H., 62 JR. M.
BRONCHIAL-CA.

VC	RV	V̇	Q̇	V̇/Q̇
7	12	59	66	0.9
14	20	104	111	0.9
26	16	100	120	0.8
46	48	93	108	0.9

VC	RV	V̇	Q̇	V̇/Q̇
11	21	87	82	1.1
18	20	116	100	1.2
24	11	122	96	1.3
53	54	52	109	1.2

Fig. 5. Complete bronchial obstruction without blood shunting: The alveolar-vascular mechanism leads to a complete adaptation of ventilation and perfusion, resulting in a normal V/Q quotient.

PAT.: L.J., 55 JR. M. DIAGN.: BRONCHIAL-CA. LI. HAUPTBRONCHUS

VC	RV	V̇	Q̇	V̇/Q̇
19	38	230	70	1.8
36	27	172	98	1.7
49	20	201	109	1.8
92	85	203	92	2.2

VC	RV	V̇	Q̇	V̇/Q̇
2	6	21	120	0.18
4	6	16	115	0.14
2	3	13	125	0.11
8	15	17	120	0.15

Fig. 6. Complete bronchial obstruction with blood shunting: The insufficient adaptation of ventilation and perfusion, resulting in a decreased V/Q quotient, leads to a blood shunting.

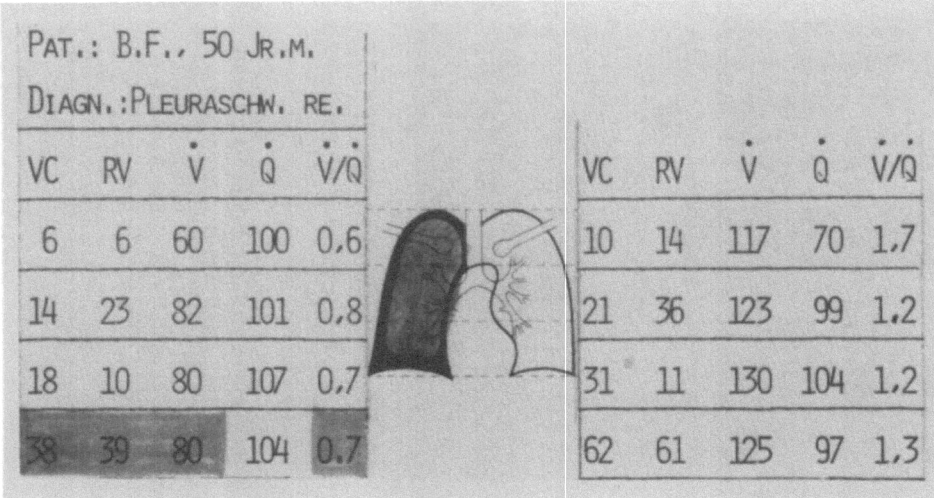

Fig. 7. Decreased compliance: The pleura scar on the right side "chains" the lung. The reduced V/Q quotient corresponds to a blood shunting.

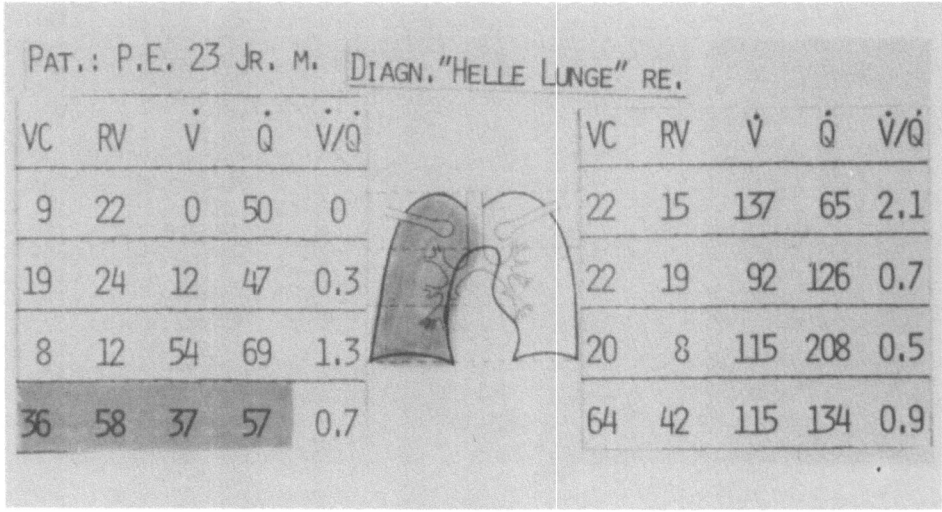

Fig. 8. Increased compliance: A markedly reduced ventilation and an incomplete adapted perfusion results in a blood shunting in the upper two thirds of the right lung.

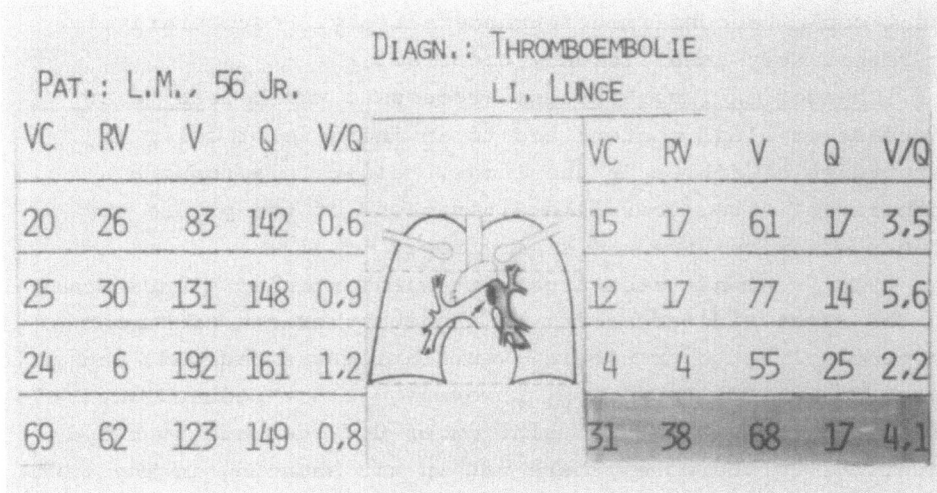

Fig. 9. Complete lung vessel obstruction: The alveolar-bronchial mechanism leads only to an incomplete adaptation of ventilation and perfusion, resulting in a distinct blood shunting.

central bronchial carcinoma. A complete obstruction of the right upper lobe bronchus demonstrates the effect on regional lung function. Ventilation is heavily reduced, the alveolar-vascular mechanism leads to a similiarly evident decrease in perfusion. The resulting normal regional V/Q quotient corresponds to the complete adaptation of ventilation and perfusion. There is no blood shunting.

In contrast, the following case shows a complete obstruction of airways along with blood shunting (fig 6). In a 55 year old man suffering from a central bronchial carcinoma a complete obstruction of the left main bronchus could be diagnosed by bronchoscopy. The ventilation of the left lung was almost negligible. Relative perfusion is related to FRC. However, it showed a value of approximately 120 in radiospirometry. The V/Q quotient of the left lung was 0.15, corresponding to a distinct blood shunting. The static volume and VC were markedly reduced. There were signs of trapped air accounting for the difference between the methods of whole body plethysmography and Helium defined FRC. Together with global examinations of pulmonary functions radiospirometry proved, that the left side was functionally pneumonectomized. Indeed, the predicted blood shunt could be confirmed intraoperatively. Postoperatively, no respiratory insufficiency occurred.

b. <u>Changes in lung tissues</u>. Processes, which lead to an increase of fluid content and to an increase of cells or structures of fibres in the lungs, result in a reduced compliance. Also, scar-like alterations of the pleura and pleura effusion have the same effect.

Fig 7 demonstrates a patient with extended pleura scars on the right side secondary to a pneumothoracic treatment of cavernous lung tuberculosis. Ventilation was reduced, and so were VC and TLC. Perfusion, however, was not reduced when measuring the V/Q with a relation of 0.7 adequate to blood shunting. Furthermore, there was an air shunting in the left lung with a V/Q of 1.3. The still maintained cranio-caudal perfusion gradient complied with the still normal hemodynamic values in lung circulation.

On the other hand, processes with a lack of lung tissues (emphysema) lead to an enlarged compliance. The pathophysiological consequences of increased compliance are primarily evident in pulmonary volumes. Fig 8 shows the pulmonary function values of a 23 year old man with a radiologically one sided lucent lung. Radiospirometry showed an increased RV and a markedly diminished ventilation of the upper part of the left lung. Perfusion was not completely adapted. In consequence, a reduced V/Q quotient was calculated, caused by blood shunting.

c. <u>Lung vessel obstruction</u>. The cause of obstruction in the pulmonary artery tract derives from inside the lumen in most cases (for example by embolism). Rarely, the lumen is blocked from outside impact (for example by tumour compression). Whole body plethysmography revealed no sign of any disturbance of pulmonary function with a 56 year old women suffering from repeated hemoptoe. X-ray of the chest showed only a left sided lucent lung and a prominent pulmonary segment, also on the left side. In fig 9 the functional data of radiospirometry are listed. There is a complete loss of perfusion of the left lung. The static volumes and ventilation were slightly reduced.

The high V/Q quotient of 4.1 over the left lung proved an
extended primary disturbance of perfusion without any doubt.
Pulmonary angiography showed a complete block of the left
pulmonary artery and thus confirmed the diagnosis. The high
V/Q quotient shows that the alveolar-bronchial mechanisms is
considerably less effective than the alveolar-vascular one.

CONCLUSIONS AND FUTURE ASPECTS

Radionuclides have considerably contributed to our knowledge and understanding of physiology and pathophysiology of
the lung. With radioactive inert gases, a detailed analysis
of the regional lung function became possible. Washin, steady
state and washout deliver exact information about ventilation,
perfusion and volume of parts of the lungs. Radiospirometry
with gases, however, applied in clinical routine requires
considerable investment in time and equipment. In short form,
it has recently been replaced by examination with radioactive
aerosols. The deposition pattern of inhaled radioactive
particles is - in addition to ventilation - depending on a
large number of different factors. In addition to the physical
properties of the aerosol (size, electrical charge, density of
aerosol), morphological aspects of the airways (stenosis,
bending, disortion) play a role (29).

To achieve results by particle inhalation scintigraphy
comparable to those of radiospirometry, a substance is needed,
which is able to reach the alveoli and, thus, allows an assessment of ventilation. This requires a highly homogenous size of
particles below 1 μm in diameter (30,31). Tc^{99m} - or In^{111m} -
aerosols with an average diameter of 2-3 μm and a range from
0.5-10 μm in size produced by nozzle or ultrasound atomizing
only partially meet the requirements (32).

Accordingly, examinations with Tc^{99m} particles,(even in
healthy subjects) deviated considerably from the results
obtained by radiospirometry using inert gases. In patients
suffering from lung diseases there was essentially no correlation between aerosol and gas inhalation scintigraphy. Examination of ventilation using these aerosols are not accurate.

They did deliver, on the other hand, important and new information of non-respiratory pulmonary function, especially of the
mucociliary cleansing system. Foreign particles inhaled and
deposited distal the glottis are removed from the respiratory
tract with the help of two cleansing systems (33).

a.   Alveolar macrophages take this task on the alveolar
     level. Upon phagocytosis of the particles, they are
     withdrawn from the alveolar cells and are transported
     through an epithelial layer. For this reason, they
     are called "free cells of the lungs" (34).

b.   The cylinder epithelium layer of the airways is
     coated with a mucociliar film and is responsible
     for transportation towards the pharynx (35).

Foreign particles are transported by this "escalator" to the
glottis from where they may be removed by coughing. Inhaled
Tc^{99m} particles show a deposition pattern depending on airway
resistance. Serial scintigraphy after inhalation assesses
disturbances of alveolar and mucociliar cleasing function.
Chronic bronchitis leads to obstruction of the airways via
bronchospasm and thickening of the mucous membrane. Inhalation
scintigrams with aerosols show a central deposition within the
large airways (36). The importance of this escalator mechanism
is evidently shown by serial scintigrams 30 min and 120 min
after the inhalation, respectively. Recent examination under-
score the value of the qualitative and quantitative inhalation
scintigraphy with radioactive aerosols for the study of the
cleansing system as an appropriate measure in diagnosing airway diseases (37). Most problems of the application of radioactive gases for the study of respiratory lung function have
been solved satisfactorily. Inhalation scintigraphy with
radioactive aerosols used in the diagnosis of disturbances of
mucociliary cleansing function have made considerable progress.
     Future efforts should mainly focus on ventilation studies
applying aerosols. Modern technology enables the production
of nearly monodispersed particles in range of nm (38,39). In

the near future, reliable ventilation measurements could be possible even with patients suffering from airway diseases. Studies comparing ventilation with Kr^{81} and radioactive aerosols showed nearly identical results in healthy subjects. In cases of obstructive airways diseases, zones of minor aerosol penetration corresponded with regions of diminished activity in the Kr^{81}-scan (40,41). The future development will provide the impact of particle inhalation scintigraphy in the diagnosis of disturbances in respiratory pulmonary functions.

20

REFERENCES

1. Müller J, Rossier P, De l'emploi d'isotopes radioactifs artificiels, dans le but d'exercer un effect radiobiologique localise. Experientia 3:75, 1947.

2. Taplin GV, Dore EK, Johnson DE, Lung photoscans with macroaggregates of human serum radioalbumin. Hlth. Phys. 10:1219, 1964.

3. Knipping HW, Bolt W, Venrath H, Eine neue Methode zur Prüfung der Herz- und Lungenfunktion. Die regionale Funktionsanalyse in der Lungen- und Herzklinik mit Hilfe des radioaktiven Edelgases Xe-133 (Isotopen-Thorakographie). Dtsch. med. Wschr. 80:1146, 1955.

4. West J, Dollery CT, Distribution of blood flow and ventilation-perfusion ratio in the lung, measured with radioactive CO-2. J. appl. Physiol. 15:405, 1960.

5. Ball WC, Stewart PB, Newsham LG, Regional pulmonary function studies with Xe-133. J. clin. Invest. 41:519, 1962.

6. Mioerner G, Xe-133-Radiospirometry. Scand. J. Resp. Dis. Suppl. 64, 1968.

7. Loken MK, Medina JR, Regional pulmonary function evaluation using Xe-133, a scintillation camera and a computer. Radiology 93:1261, 1969.

8. Bartels H, Gaswechsel. Lehrbuch der Physiologie. Keidel W, (ed), Thieme Verlag, Stuttgart, pp 4.1-4.16, 1975.

9. Thews G, Lungenatmung. Physiologie des Menschen. Thews G, Schmidt T, (eds), Springer Verlag, Berlin, Heidelberg, New York, 1976.

10. Radiological handbook. US Dept. of Health, Education and Welfare. Washington 25 DC, 1960.

11. Matthews CH, Dollery CT, Interpretation of Xe-133 lung wash-in and wash-out curves using an analogue computer. Clin. Sci. 28:573, 1965.

12. Bitter F, Konietzko N, Kampmann H, Adam WE, Lungenfunktionsdiagnostik mit Xe-133. Biomed. Technik 21:194, 1976.

13. Burdine JA, Murphy PH, Alagarsamy V, Rider LA, Carr WN, Functional pulmonary imaging. J. nucl. Med. 13:933, 1972.

14. Lütgemeier J, Kampmann H, Konietzko N, Adam WE, Lungendiagnostik mit Radionukliden. Gustav Fischer Verlag, Stuttgart, 1977.

15. Milic-Emili J, Henderson JAM, Dolovich MB, Regional distribution of inspired gas in the lung. J. appl. Physiol. 21:749, 1966.

16. Glazier JB, Hugh-Jones M, Maloney JE, Vertical gradient of alveolar size in lungs of dogs frozen intact. J. appl. Physiol. 23:694, 1967.

17. Rahn H, Otis AB, Chadwick LE, The pressure volume diagram of the thorax and lung. Amer. J. Physiol. 146:161, 1946.

18. Bühlmann AA, Rosier PH, Klinische pathophysiologie der Atmung. Springer Verlag, Berlin, Heidelberg, New York, 1970.

19. Dollfuss RE, Milic-Emili J, Bates DV, Regional ventilation of the lung studied with boluses of Xe-133. Resp. Physiol. 2:234, 1967.

20. Leblanc P, Ruff F, Milic-Emili J, Effects of age and body position on "airway closure" in man. J. appl. Physiol. 28:448, 1970.

21. Macklem PT, Obstruction in small airways: a challenge to medicine. Amer. J. Med. 52:721, 1972.

22. Bannister J, Torrance RW, The effect of tracheal pressure upon flow: pressure relations in the vascular bed of isolated lungs. Q. J. exp. Physiol. 45:352, 1960.

23. Permutt S, Bromberger-Barnea B, Bane HN, Alveolar pressure, pulmonary venous pressure and the vascular waterfall. Med. Thor. 19:239, 1962.

24. West JB, Dollery CT, Naimark A, Distribution of blood flow in isolated lungs, relation to vascular and alveolar pressures. J. appl. Physiol. 19:713, 1964.

25. v. Euler US, Liljestrand G, Observations on the pulmonary arterial blood pressure in the cat. Acta Physiol. scand. 12:31, 1946.

26. Newhouse MT, Bechlage MR, Effect of alterations in end tidal CO-2 tension on flow resistance. J. appl. Physiol. 19:745, 1964.

27. Hultgren HN, Grover RF, Circulatory adaption to high altitude. Amer. Rev. Med. 19:119, 1968.

28. Sterling GM, The mechanism of bronchoconstriction due to hypocapnia in man. Clin. Sci. 34:277, 1968.

29. Henning K, Woller P, Perfusion- und Inhalationsszintigraphie mit Partikeln. Handbuch der Radiologie. Springer Verlag, Berlin, Heidelberg, New York, pp 265-334, 1978.

30. Heyder J, Mechanisms of aerosol particle deposition. Chest 80:820, suppl.

31. Hayes M, Taplin GV, Chopra SW, Knox DE, Elam D, Improved radioaerosol administration system for routine inhalation lung imaging. Radiology 131:256, 1979.

32. Herzog H, Georg R, Fridrich R, Die Beurteilung verschiedener Technieken des Aerosoltherapie durch Aktivitätsmessungen über den Lungen nach Applikation radioaktiver Kolloide. Med. Klin. 66:948, 1972.

33. Green GM, Alveolar transport mechanism. Arch. intern. Med. 131:109, 1973.

34. Morrow PE, Alveolar clearance of aerosols. Arch. intern. Med. 131:101, 1973.

35. Gosselin RE, Physiologic regulation of ciliary motion. Amer. Rev. Resp. Dis. 93:41, 1966.

36. Thomson ML, Short MD, Mucociliary function in health, chronic obstructive airway disease and asbestosis. J. appl. Physiol. 26:535, 1969.

37. Weiss T, Dorow P, Felix R, Continuous aerosol inhalation scintigraphy in the evaluation of early and advanced airway obstruction. Eur. J. Nucl. Med. 9:62, 1984.

38. Arborelius Jr, M, Generation of microaerosol suitable for deposition in the peripheral airway. Eur. J. Resp. Dis. (suppl. 119), 63:19, 1982.

39. Newman SP, Agnew JE, Pavia D, Inhaled aerosols: Lung deposition and clinical applications. Clin. Phys. Physiol. 3:1, 1982.

40. Short MD, Dowsett DJ, Head PJD, Pavia D, A comparison between monodisperse Tc-99m-labelled aerosol particles and Kr-81m for the assess-

ment of lung function. J. nucl. Med. 20:194, 1979.

41. Hayes M, Lung imaging with radioaerosols for the assessment of airway diseases. Sem. Nucl. Med. 10:243,1980.

GENERATOR-PRODUCED KRYPTON-81m IN GAS AND LIQUID PHASES
FOR MEDICAL APPLICATIONS

M. GUILLAUME, N. GARZANITI, M. ZICOT, T. KHUC, P. BARTSCH

INTRODUCTION

A great deal of work has been dedicated in the last three
years, in our center, to the short-lived generator-produced
radionuclides (1-3).

The strategy stems, for a not-negligible part, from a
fundamental observation made by Ter Pogossian in 1966 who
said:

"The degree of spation resolution we can achieve with
external counting is, most of the time, too low mostly
because of the statistical fluctuations in counting rate
resulting from the limits imposed on the total amount of
activity that can be injected without radiation damage
for the patient".

It is clear that this situation improves considerably with
the short-lived nuclides. Of course, the optimisation of a
given in vivo measurement requires the matching of the half-
life of the nuclide with the phenomenon to be studied. Besides
this single limitation, the short-lived generator-produced
nuclide has to be considered as the most attractive tracer of
experimental value provided its availability is no longer
limited to institutions operating a cyclotron.

One knows that the success of the nuclear medicine is so
far mostly due to a medium-lived generator-produced nuclide
on which rely to-day most hospitals throughout the world
namely the popular cow-system $Mo^{99}-Tc^{99m}$.

The number of suitable cow-systems is necessarily limited
and we believe that cyclotrons are the most suitable facilities
to cover fully the increased demand for short-lived isotopes,
anticipated in the near future.

Table 1.

Generator-produced radionuclides prepared or
under study at Liege Cyclotron Center (CRC).

Nuclear pair	Half-live	Main radiation of daughter (KeV-%)	Chemical form	Useful activity (mCi)	Target organ
^{81}Rb-^{81m}Kr	4.6h-13s	$\gamma(190-65)$	gas sol	3 - 50 3 - 50	Lung heart, angi
^{82}Sr-^{82}Rb	25d-80s	$\beta^{+}\gamma(511-192)$	Rb^{+}	50 - 100	heart
^{195m}Hg-^{195m}Au	41h-30.5s	$\gamma(262-77)$	$(Au\ Cl_4)$	20 - 50	vascular
^{68}Ge-^{68}Ga	280d-68m	$\beta^{+}\gamma(511-176)$	Ga^{+++}	20 - 50	non speci
^{62}Zn-^{62}Cu	9.2d-9.8m	$\beta^{+}\gamma(511-195)$	Cu^{++}	under study	angiology
^{191}Os-^{191m}Ir	15.4d-4.9s	$\gamma(129-0.26)$	$IrCl_6^{2-}$	under study	angiology

Table 1 lists the potential nuclear pairs which have been
or are presently under investigation in our center to yield a
medically useful generator.

Full priority has been given to this very attractive field
of interest with the constant objective to develop simple and
reliable methods of production of the parent-nuclide and of
separation of the daughter-element.

The first parameter to be considered first of all is the
nuclear reaction of production of the parent nuclide. This
reaction has to be compatible with a low energy cyclotron.

The ideal solution consists in a gazeous target which
makes it easy to handle and automate the chemical separation
of the produced radionuclide from the target nuclei.

The second part of the research to be done will proceed

as follows:

- an efficient method has to be found for separation of the parent and daughter elements mostly based on a large difference between their distribution coefficients on a specific exchanger. The inorganic exchanger will be preferably choosen instead of the organic material for reasons of radiation resistance;
- a constant and efficient useful elution yield of the daughter has to be managed with an eluant which can be injected into the blood-circulation without any secondary effect;
- the radiochemical and radionuclide purity of the eluted daughter have to be as high as possible with respect with the dosimetric data. In other words, the rate of loss of the precursor adsorbed on the column has to be kept as low as possible but always inferior to 10^{-4}/ml;
- the operational properties of the generator have to be as constant as possible during the working life of the generator and therefore independent if possible on the high radiation dose due to the precursor activity fixed on the top of the column.

All of these requirements are scarcely encountered in a generator.

Kr^{81m} GENERATOR, PHYSICAL ASPECTS

Choice of a nuclear reaction. A realistic example will be taken with the Rb-Kr pair for which the great deal of research done since 1979 permitted to develop an optimal method for routine production of Kr generators on a very large scale commercially exploited now with our compact cyclotron.

The following figures allow to review the main steps of our work. Fig 1 recalls the basic properties of the Rb-Kr nuclear pair. Rb^{81} precursor has an half-life of 4.58 hour and decays by E.C. and positron emission into the 13 sec half-life Kr^{81m}. The latter decays by I.T. emitting 65% of unconverted 190 KeV γ rays to stable Kr^{81}.
A Kr generator is based on the physical separation of the

26

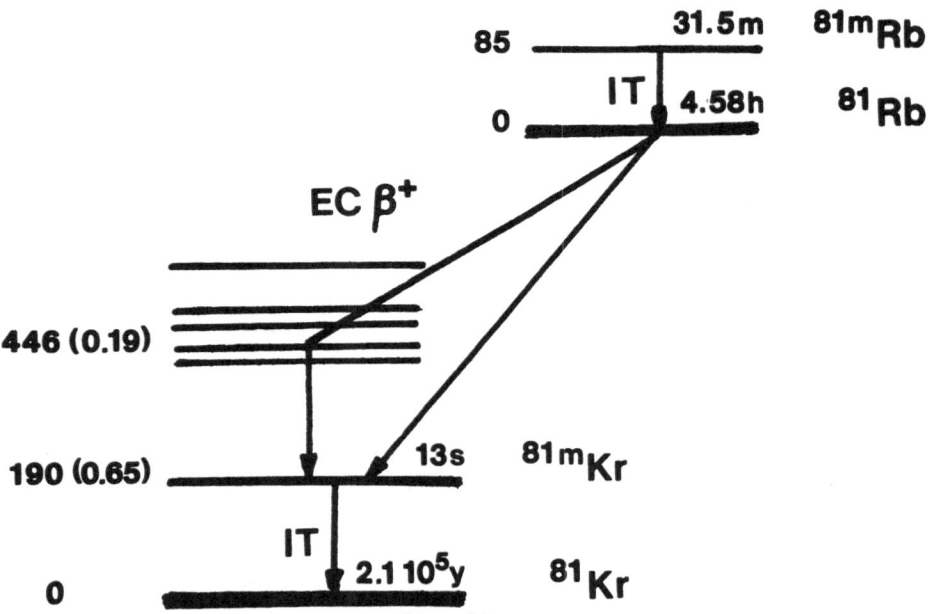

Fig. 1. Decay scheme of the Kr^{81}–Kr^{81m} pair.

Table 2.

Litterature data on nuclear reactions producing ^{81}Rb.

N°	Nuclear reaction producing ^{81}Rb	Projectile energy (MeV)	^{81}Rb production at AOB (mCi/µA.h).	
1	^{79}Br (α,2n)	30-35	2,5	(4)
2	^{81}Br (α,4n)	50	3,0	(5)
3	^{79}Br (^{3}He,n)	21	0.030	(6)
4	^{82}Kr (p,2n)	-	-	
5	^{80}Kr (d,n)	11	3.2	(7)
6	^{82}Kr (d,3n)	52	15	(8)
7	^{80}Kr (^{3}He,pn)	20	0.225	(9)

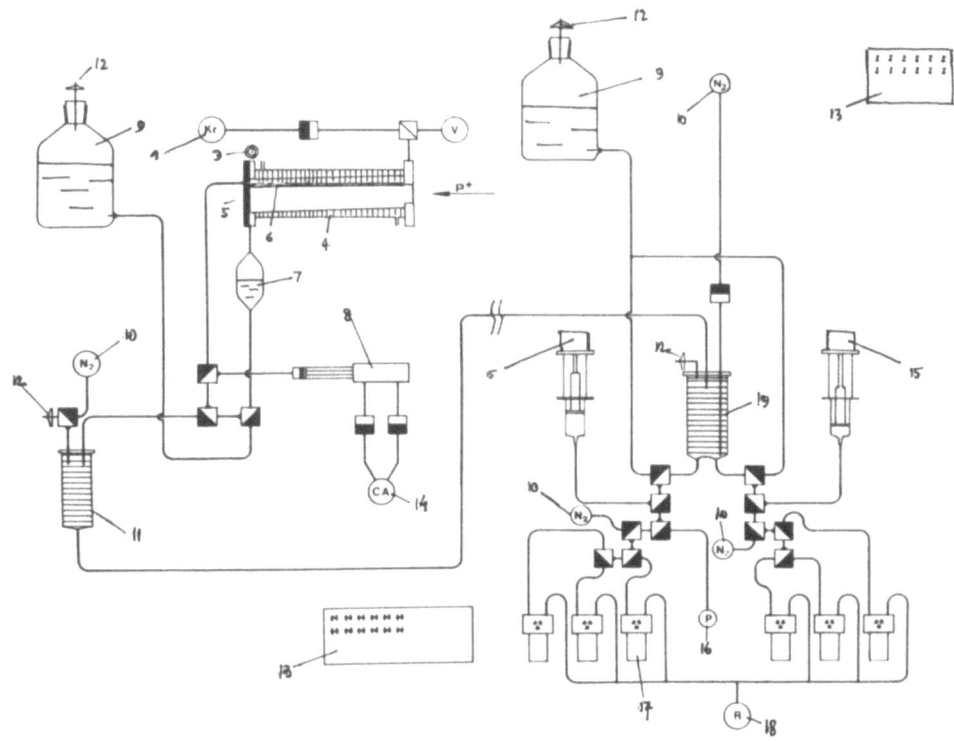

Fig. 2. Production and loading-full assembly flow diagram.

1. Natural Kr stock
2. Vacuum pump
3. Manometer
4. Stainless steel water jacketed target
5. Isolated backing degrader
6. Sprinckler
7. Buffer vessel
8. Air operated piston-pump
9. Sterile water reservoir
10. Nitrogen pressure
11. Transfer vessel
12. Millipore filter
13. Power and control interface
14. Pressurisedair
15. Piston pump with stepping motor
16. Sampling
17. Generator in loading step
18. Waste output
19. Second recuperation reservoir

radionuclides. This separation is made possible by two conditions:

- a strong and irreversible fixation of the Rb^{81} parent on a cationic exchanger;
- a lack of affinity of the Kr^{81} daughter for the exchanger, allowing a maximum extraction of the Kr by elution in a gas phase or with an injectable solution.

After considering the different possible nuclear reactions for the production of Rb^{81} with a compact cyclotron (see table 2), the following reaction

$$^{nat}Kr \ (p,2n) Rb^{81}$$

has been selected.

Production methodology. The entire production system developed in Liege is schematically shown in fig 2. This system consists of two different parts:

The first one concerns the production of the precursor and its continuous solubilization in water during bombardment. During bombardment electromagnetic valves determine a closed loop which allows, by means of a seringe operated by a speed controlled pneumatic jack, a permanent washing of the inner walls of the stainless steel cylinder. The result is the quantitative solubilization of the Rb^{81} produced in the course of the bombardment.

The second part (located in a hot controlled area 25 m distant from the bombardment-room) concerns the dispensing system which is used for the generator loading. This loading requires the transfer of the radioactive Rb^{81} solution into this main receiver where it will be distributed, according to the total produced activity, into a series of preconditioned shielded generators ready to-be loaded.

The production and loading steps are fully automated under the control of an Apple 2 microcomputer. The total working time for both steps has been drastically reduced as well as the health hazards faced by the chemists in charge of the routine work.

Table 3.

Main parameters of Liege production procedure of ^{81m}Kr generators.	
Nuclear reaction	^{nat}Kr (p,2n)
Proton energy	23 MeV
Production yield	
. from nat kr	3.5 ± 0.3 mCi/μA.h
. from 25 % enrich. Kr	6.5 ± 0.5 mCi/μA.h
Relative amounts of contaminants :	
. from nat. Kr	^{82m}Rb (6.3h) 1.28
	^{83}Rb (83 d) 0.021
	^{84}Rb (33 d) 0.024
	^{86}Rb (18,8 d) 0.008

Generators characteristics

	Ventilation	Perfusion
. Typical loading calibrated at 9 am	12 mCi	20 mCi
. Mass of dowex exchanger	200 mg	50 mg
. Kr extraction yield	95-98 %	85-90 %
. Extraction flowrate	250 ml/min	15 ml/min
. Brea kthrough	not detected	10^{-9}/ ml.

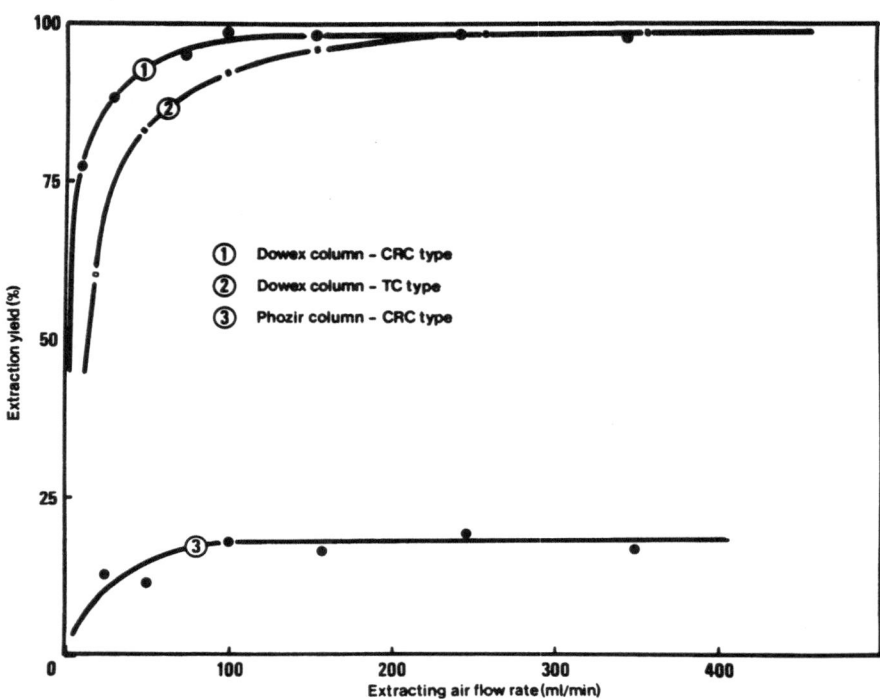

Fig. 3. Gaseous Kr^{81m} extraction yield as a function of air flow-rate
and for different types of column and exchanger.

Table 3 summarizes the main production parameters of the
Liege procedure. The two fundamental parameters which have to
be optimized for any generator are the elution yield and the
parent breakthrough.

Characteristics. Fig 3 refers to the Kr^{81m} ventilation
generator. It shows that the gas-eluted Kr activity increases
exponentially with the flow-rate of the gaseous eluant, in
this case normal medical air. We observe that a minimum flow-
rate of 250 ml/min is required to get a quantitative elution
yield in the gaseous form.

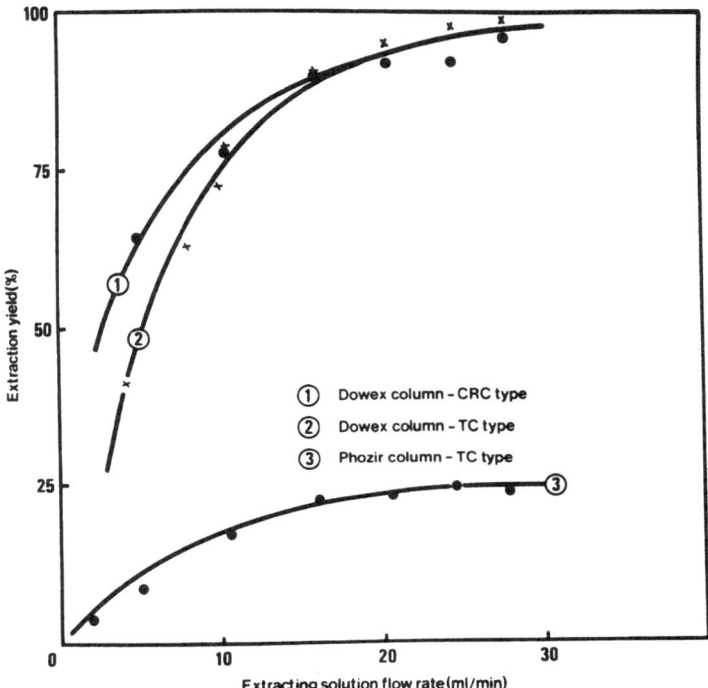

Fig. 4. Solubilized Kr^{81m} extraction yield as a function of 5%-glucose flow-rate.

Fig 4 refers to the perfusion generator. It shows that the elution yield of Kr^{81m} in solution depends on:
- the nature of the exchanger (strong cationic exchanger looks much better than inorganic packing);
- the dimensions of the column (a miniaturized column allows the reduction of the dead volumes and the attainment of high elution yields - specially at flow-rates higher than 15 ml/min).

Fig 5 shows a scale picture of both generator columns giving the previous characteristics.

^{81m}Kr perfusion generator
CRC-IRE model

CRC type
for ventilation

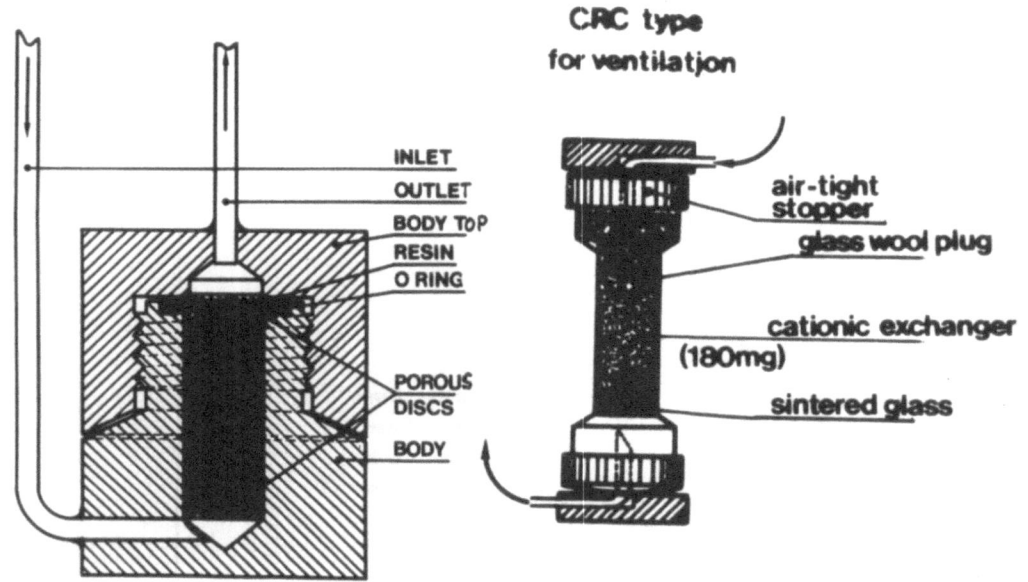

INLET
OUTLET
BODY TOP
RESIN
O RING
POROUS DISCS
BODY

air-tight stopper
glass wool plug
cationic exchanger (180mg)
sintered glass

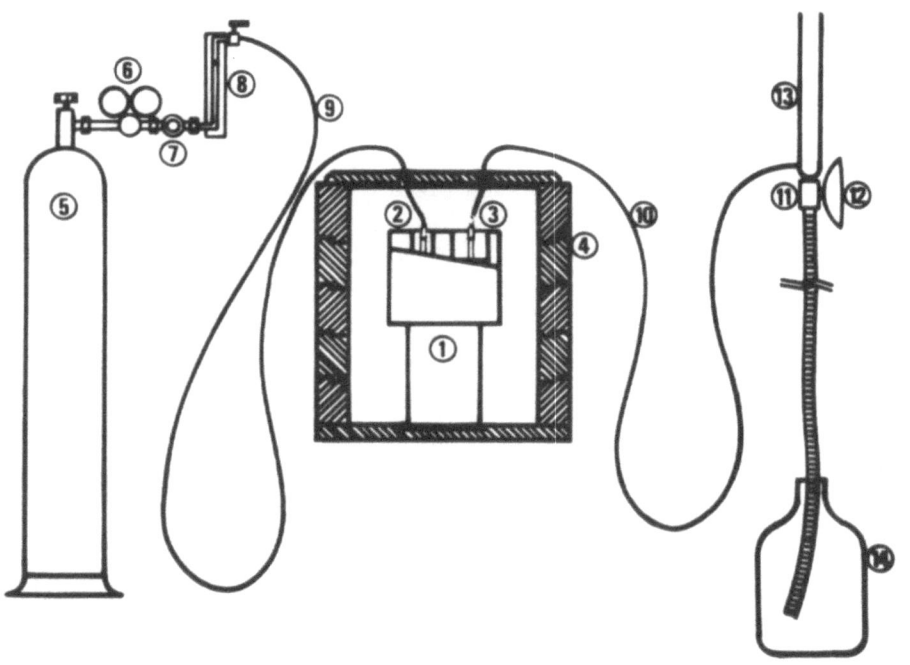

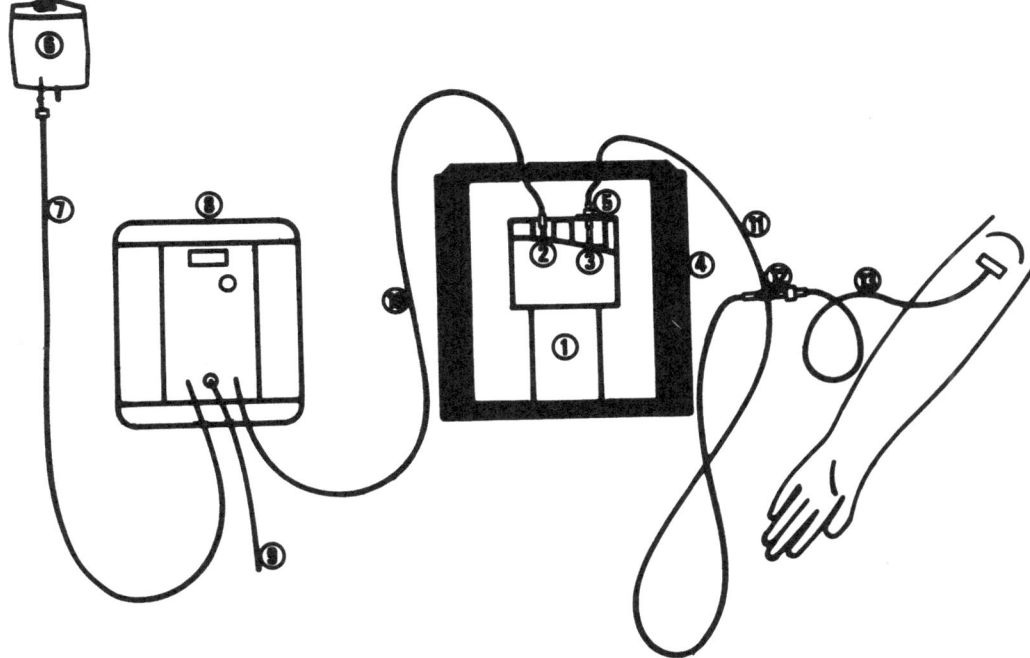

Legend of fig 5:
Colums used for either type of generator.

Legend of fig 6:
Kr^{81m} generator line used for ventilation studies.

1. Generator
2. Inlet
3. Outlet
4. Shielding (Pb 5 cm)
5. Pressurized medical air
6. High and low pressure
   manometer

7. Flow regulator
8. Flow meter
9-10. Soft tubing ($\emptyset_i$ 1mm; 1=2 m)
11. Ruben non rebreathing valve
12. Anaesthetic mask (Hegelback 5)
13. Kr reservoir (10 ml)
14. Waste gas reservoir

Legend of fig 7:
Kr^{81m} generator used for perfusion studies.

1. Generator
2. Luer inlet
3. Luer outlet
4. Shielding (Pb 5cm)
5. Millipore filter (0.22)
6. Viaflex-500 ml- 5% glucose sol
7-10. Soft tubing ($\emptyset$: 2 mm)

8. Pulsation free perfusion pump
   DURAMAT D1
9. Purging
11. Vygon catheter ($\emptyset$: 1 cm-1= 1mm)
12. One-way stop clock
13. Perfusion microcatheter
   "butterfly"

34

Table 4.

Total absorbed dose (mRad) during a 100 ml perfusion of ^{81m}Kr 200 K counts, breakthrough 510^{-7}/ml			
Target organ	^{81m}Kr dose	Rb dose	Total dose.
Heart-walls	55	38	59
Lungs	9	0.4	9.5
Liver	4	0.05	4
Pancreas	5	0.08	5
Adrenals	5	0.06	5
Total body	2.5	0.03	2.5

Clinical methodology. The very simple medical use of the generator, either for ventilation or perfusion studies is very well demonstrated by the figs 6 and 7. For lung studies the supply of medical air is delivered at a constant flow-rate via a high quality manometer equipped with a pressure regulator and a flow-meter.

In the perfusion system, the supply of 5% glucose sterile solution is transferred by means of a very reliable perfusion pump through the column into the patient by continuous i.v. or bolus injection. For the medical and paramedical personnel as well as for the patient, it is clear that the Kr^{81m} is not only a very attractive diagnostic tool but also a very safe radionuclide in comparison with the conventional nuclear medicine procedures.

Table 4 shows indeed how safe a generator with a standard breakthrough of 10^{-7}/ml is, but also how dangerous it could be if the Rb were extracted with an ionic solution such as physiological 9°/°° NaCl solution.

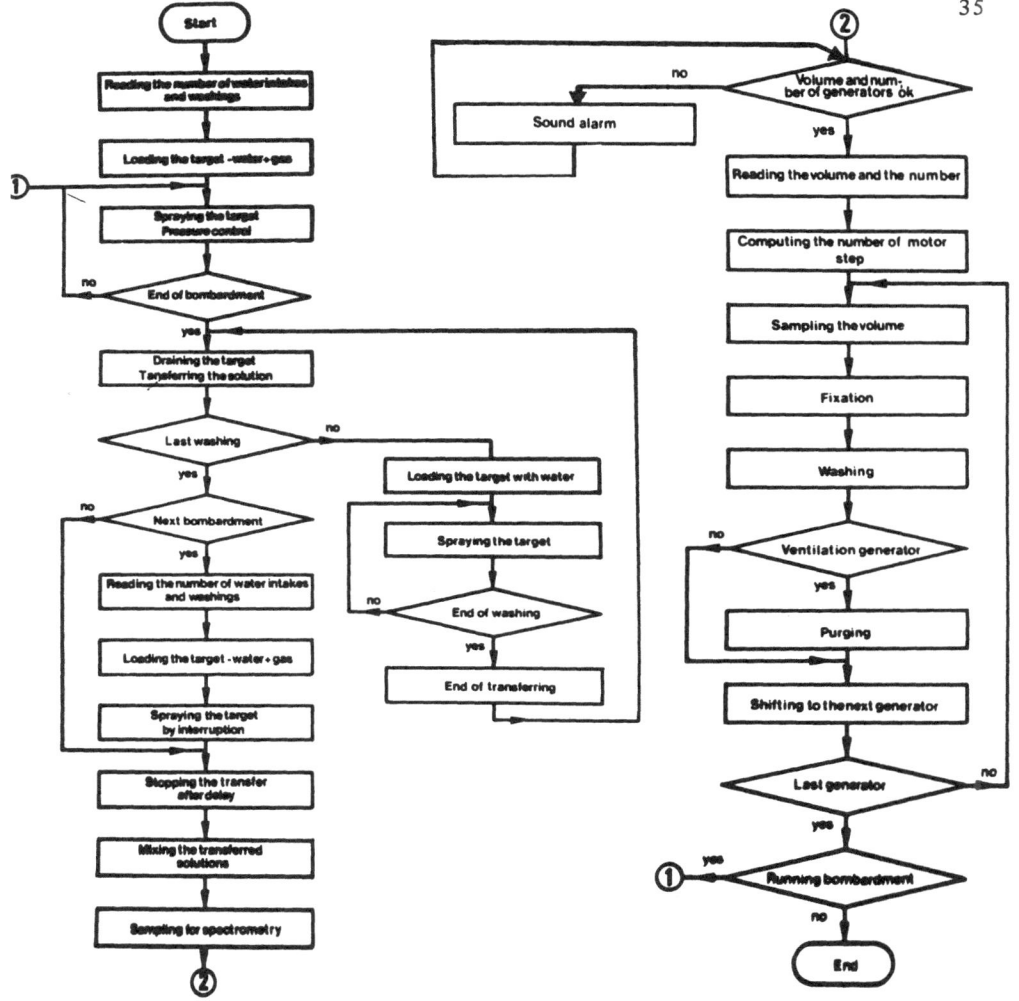

Fig. 8. Software diagram.

Availability. "Unless the Kr generators were made more
widely available to routine nuclear medicine centers they
would, probably remain an elegant curiosity".

To challenge such criticism, different solutions have
been given to the severe problem of continuous, reliable and
early daily availability.

The perfection of our entirely automated production system
controlled by a microprocessor according a very versatile

software is shown by fig 8. This program of the different
sequential functions of the complete production and loading
phases requires the following data for each production batch:
- the water volume to be injected into the target cylinder;
- the number of target washings;
- the number of generators to be prepared;
- the total volume of available radioactive Rb mother solution.

Such an automated system results mainly in:
- the total absence of manual intervention;
- the simultaneous management of the production and the
  loading operations and the time saving this entails;
- the reproductibility of the operating conditions and the
  resulting high quality generator.

A second solution the the availability problem was the
early morning production followed by rapid distribution to the
medical centres either by car or by plane. Such a logistics
of production and distribution needs careful planning followed
by delay-free execution. It allows now a wide spread and regular use of ventilation and perfusion generators prepared by the
Liege Cyclotron Center and supplied in a minimum of time on
the European market.

MEDICAL APPLICATIONS

If the production logistic aspects have been thoroughly
studied, considerable efforts have been spent to develop new
approaches of clinical investigation with Kr^{81m} (4-11). The
main lines where significant results have been collected and
are still in progress in our center are:
- dynamic regional lung function studies and
- the isotopic arteriography and venography.

The respective methodologies used for both topics are
described as well as some typical results recently obtained.

Regional lung function. The use of Kr for routine imaging
of regional lung function is one of the most important advances
in radionuclide clinical investigation of recent years.

The compartmental model of Kr in the lungs during the continuous respiration is given by the following equations. When the steady state is obtained, the arrival in the alveolar compartment equals the removal by the ventilatory wash-out and radioactive decay:

$$\overset{\circ}{V}_A C = \overset{\circ}{V} C_A + \lambda N_A$$

$$\text{if} \quad C_A = N_A / V_A$$

$$N_A = \frac{\overset{\circ}{V}_A \, C_i}{\overset{\circ}{V}_A / V_A + \lambda}$$

$$\lambda = 3.2 \, \text{min}^{-1}$$

$$\overset{\circ}{V}_A / V_A \cong 1 \, \text{min}^{-1} \quad \text{in physiological conditions}$$

$\overset{\circ}{V}_A$ means the alveolar ventilatory rate in 1/min;

C_i the concentration of Kr in the inspired gas;

C_A the concentration of Kr in the alveolar compartment;

N_A the number of radioactive Kr atoms in the alveolar compartment.

As the denominator is dominated by the high value for the constant λ, the measured radioactivity (total or regional) is mostly correlated with V_A. Kr can therefore be considered as a specific tracer for the study of the regional distribution of flow into the lung and by extrapolation in any organ.

The fundamental advantages of Kr as polyvalent flow tracer are summarized in the following items:
- chemically-biologically inert gas;
- solution in plasma freely diffusible;
- non fat soluble;
- very short half-life in relation with physiological range

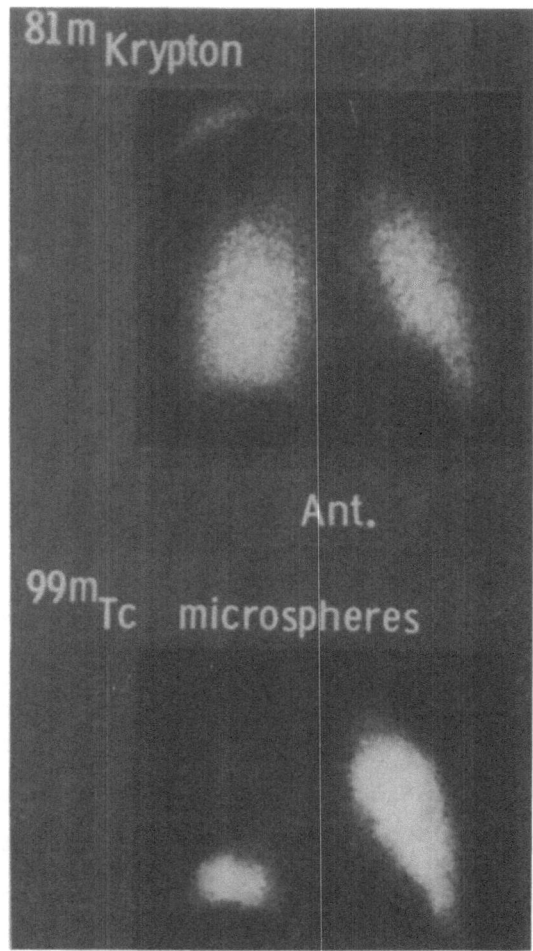

Fig. 9. Dismatching Kr^{81m} and Tc^{99m} lung images. Typical embolism.

-   quick equilibration;
-   only right heart tracer from i.v. injection.

The methodology consists in four successive views of 250 K counts taken with a high resolution collimator during continuous inhalation of krypton through a respiratory mask. After injection of Tc^{99m} microspheres, the perfusion scintigraphy is performed on the patient in the same positions (see fig 9).

The image interpretation is based on the general following rules:

- absence of decrease of ventilation matching with absence or decrease of perfusion means emphysema, pneunomia, bronchectasy or obstructive aspecific lung disease;
- intact ventilation associated with absence or decrease of perfusion usually means embolism.

As conclusion, it can be certified that the now conventional method based on the coupled Kr ventilation and Tc perfusion scintigraphies is:

- very simple, fast, accurate and non invasive;
- it leads to an easy diagnosis of embolism;
- we and others have shown that the detection of bronchial cancer and emphysema can be improved as well as the evaluation of extension of other pathological processes.

It gives therefore very useful information for presurgical evaluation.

Besides these previous qualitative lung studies, the development of a quantitative approach of the regional ventilation and its dynamic parameters has been considered. Instead of cumulated views, list mode acquisition is used at equilibrium during 2 min of tidal breathing. After reconstruction of the respiratory cycles, a specific software selects all cycles of same frequency and creates one resulting sum-cycle made of 16 sequential images. Three equivalent regions of interest are considered for each lung and the curves of amplitude and automatically phased histograms are respectively calculated and automatically displayed. This study yields an approximation of the regional functional residual capacity (FRC), of the regional amplitude which represents the regional tidal volume and of the corresponding peak of phase.

The following step under study is the correlation of these regional ventilation data with the perfusion ones in order to evaluate the parallelism of regional impairment in function of the lung pathology and to obtain a quantitation of the regional V/Q values.

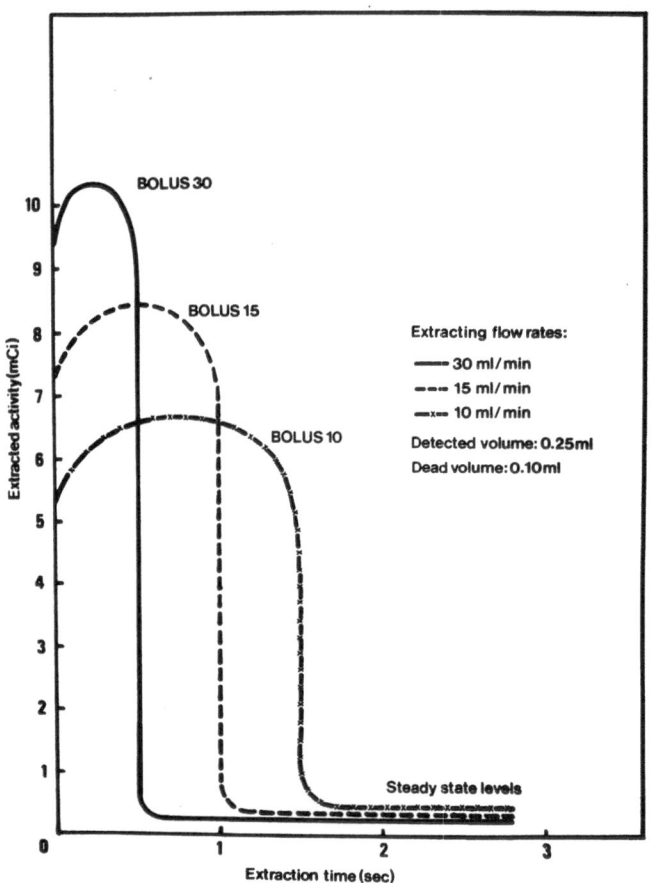

Fig. 10. Activity-time profiles at the output of a 10 mCi perfusion generator for different extracting flow-rates.

Angiology studies. Krypton-81m generators for infusion
studies have been developed at Liege for use in routine clinical investigations. Their widespread application is now only
dependant on the originality and usefulness of the clinical
data supplied by the 13 sec half-life radionuclide.

Delivery of Kr^{81m} in the liquid phase has been recently
optimized. It is mainly dependent on the improved quality
eluant, the pulsation-free infusion pump and the miniaturi-
zation of the generator column and catheter system.

Two possible methodologies can be applied: firstly the
bolus injection technique and secondly the continuous infusion
technique. These two methods are very well illustrated by the
time-activity profiles measured at a perfusion generator's
output extracted at different flow-rates, as shown in fig 10.
Both methods have their own and specific characteristics.
Continuous or bolus infusion through 0.3 mm inside diameter,
150 mm long catheter at a flow-rate ranging from 5 to 60 ml/
min permits access to virtually all organs and regions of the
body.

With the continuous technique, a steady state is obtained
in less than 20 sec in virtually all instances. The Kr^{81m}
gives a heterogeneous image reflecting blood-flow and time of
interval into the region of interest. Moment to moment changes
in the steady state pattern as influenced by pathophysiological,
pharmacological or physical stimuli may be easily ascertained.

The bolus injection enables multiple first pass studies at
short time intervals, with exceedingly high photon activity
contained in a very small injected volume. Time-activity
curves can be easily obtained which finally allow more accurate
measurements of hemodynamic parameters regarding arteriography, venography or oesophagial transit studies.

Intravenous infusion. The most promising application of
intravascular Kr^{81m} infusion has been infusion via the intravenous route. This approach was mainly explored in our center
for right heart dynamic studies and evaluation of blood-flow
in the venous blood-return.

Assessment of the right ventricular ejection fraction

(RVEF) can be successfully carried out with Kr^{81m} by means of
the bolus technique. In such an application, Kr is an ideal
tracer for the following reasons:

- it has a very low solubility in tissues and when i.v.
  perfused, it is exhaled very rapidly by the lungs and does
  not return to the left heart. A selective imaging of the
  right heart without contributions from left heart activity is therefore possible;

- a great number of heart cycles can be available for the
  analysis and provide count densities considerably above
  those attained with Tc^{99m} using the first pass technique.
  Automatic edge definition techniques could be easily
  applied for the calculation of the ejection fraction.

In normal subjects, a RVEF of 50 ± 2% has been measured.
In patients with cardiomyopathy, the RVEF drops down to 20-30%.
The RVEF is also sensitively decreased in patients with pul-
monary perfusion defects.

Dynamic studies of the right heart, otherwise difficult
to investigate with the conventional methods is therefore one
of the main potentialities of soluble Kr^{81m}. Fast changes can
be observed by rapid sequential studies, offering a considerable potential for the control of drug effects.

A recent application of the Kr perfusion generator developed in Liege is the detection studies of deep vein thrombosis.

Advantage can indeed be taken of the interesting characteristics of the liquid Kr to analyse the venous blood-return in
the lower limbs of patients suffering from chronic venous
obstructions. The method is very simply.

The generator is flushed by a constant flow-rate of about
15 ml/min of a glucose solution and connected to a small gauge
butterfly needle inserted into a superficial vein of the foot.
The γ camera is successively focused on the three fields
necessary to cover the whole lower limb. Dynamic and static
data are recorded by the computer.

Kr^{81m} may follow different routes related to the injection
site and the relative resistance of the different pathways
(superficial or deep). If the superficial route is preferential-
ly used while the deep system is partially or totally open, it

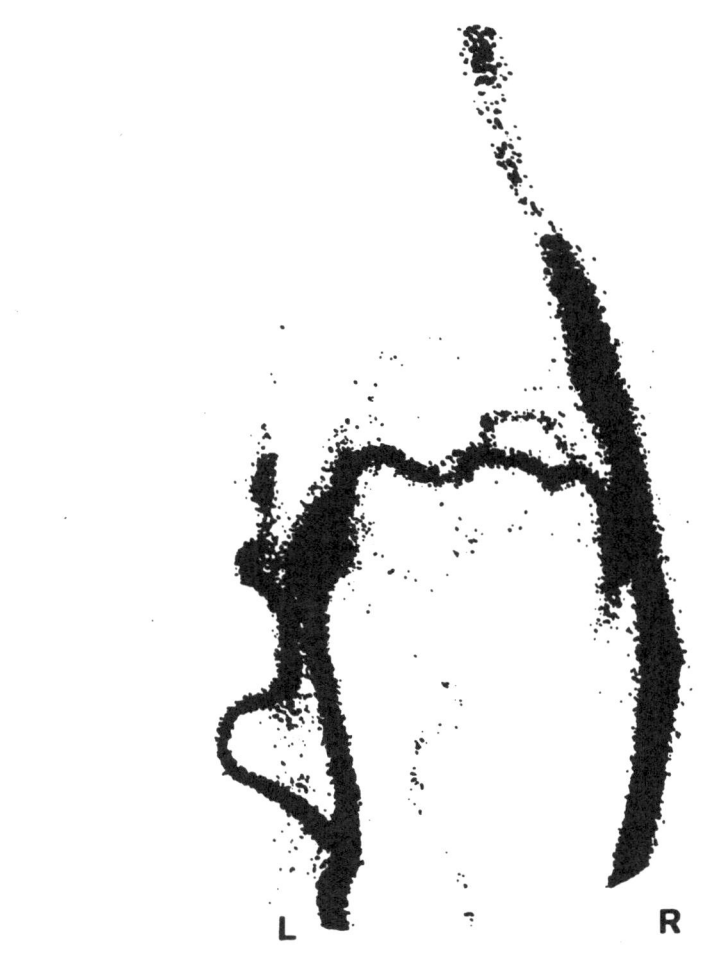

Fig. 11. Obstruction of the left iliac and femoral weins.

44

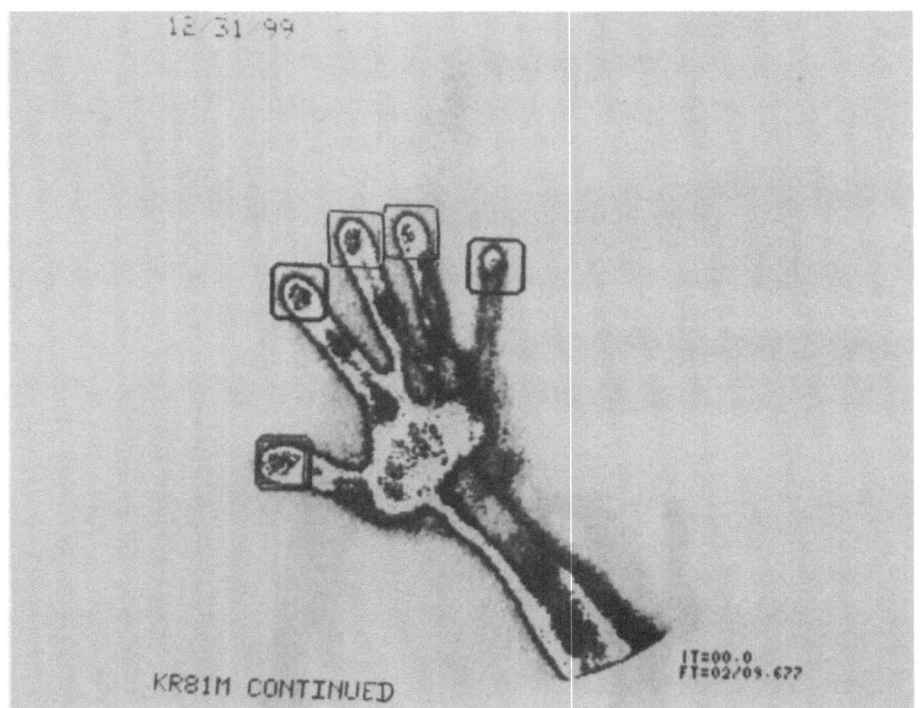

Fig. 12. Normal hand under Kr^{81m} continuous perfusion. Regions of interest on tips.

is generally possible to secondarilly force the labelled plasma into the deep veins. This requires the application of suitable tourniquets. Such a method allows the evaluation of the switching of the radioactive flow from one way to the other by means of iterative or prolonged perfusions. The definition of the popliteal, superficial femoral veins as well as the common femoral vein and the iliocaval system is of very good diagnostic quality.

Fig 11 shows a typical obstruction of the left femoral vein. The flow is derived by the great saphenous vein on the left. The study of the pelvic veins is particularly rewarding. There is no superposition of the opaque bone images as it is in contrast phlebograms. The definition is of high quality and does not require proximal injection. In addition the method can be considered as perfectly atraumatic.

Intra-arterial infusion. Regional cerebral blood-flow
(rCBF) measurement has been the first clinical application of
intravascular Kr^{81m} via the arterial route. It can be assessed
by intracarotid injection. The procedure described by Fazio
(12) can be summarized as follows:

The eluted Kr^{81m} is infused via a small polyethylene
canulla into the internal carotid artery with the head of the
patient positioned in front of the γ camera until 300 K counts
are collected. This is usually achieved in 30-60 sec. Due to
the rapid decay of Kr^{81m}, the procedure can be repeated many
times.

The continuous infusion technique proved to delineate
successfully areas of reduced perfusion and to follow rapid
changes of regional distribution of blood-flow induced by
hyperventilation or other chemical stimuli. It appears as an
unique technique for investigating the size and shape of in-
farcted areas as well as the loss of autoregulation of damaged
braintissue.

A very late application of krypton intra-arterial infusion
concerns the study of blood-vascularization in patients with
re-implanted fingers or limbs after a severe injury.

The method consists of a continuous perfusion of the intra-
humeral artery with liquid eluted Kr and to measure with the
computer-assisted γ camera the dynamic transit of the radioactivity into the different regions of the hand and especially
in the most distal territories, the finger tips or pulps.

It has been observed that this steady-state activity is
quantitatively dependant upon the quality of permeation of
the finger arteries and more upstream blood-vessels, and is
therefore a very useful indication of the efficiency of micro-
surgery (see fig 12).

A final objective is to find out about a possible correlation between the rapidity of the restoration of the sensory
nerves of the finger or the hand and the blood-flow restoration performed by surgery.

CONCLUSION

The major drawback with Kr^{81m} generators is their availability on a routine basis for clinical use. At the Cyclotron Research Center at the University of Liege, this disadvantage has been surmounted by the development of a fully automated production and generator loading system. With an experience of more than 5000 krypton generators behind us, we have reached a very high level of production and distribution at the Liege CRC. This has involved all three phases of the krypton cycle: process control, target development and distribution management.

Process control: A third generation of automatic process-control equipment has been recently developed in our center. Well designed hardware and reliable remote manipulation systems eliminate any contact between the highly radioactive mother solution and the production operator. A particular flexible software package has been perfected, allowing the operator's intervention whenever necessary to insure consistant radio-pharmaceutical quality matching the practician's needs.

Target development has also reached the third generation. Our most recent thick gaseous target has been perfected to allow a low loss risk use of Kr^{82} enriched gaseous krypton, with the advantages offered by this target substrate. These advantages are twofold. Firstly the production yield is increased. This allows a decrease in cyclotron time, an important factor in a multiple isotope research center, and increased clinical availability, because the generators can leave the production center earlier, thereby allowing for longer transport times and distances, and better, earlier service for the clinics within our distribution network. Secondly, the radio-isotopic purity of the rubidium production is increased, due to the decrease of cross-reactions producing rubidium-83 and -82m, and radiobromines. Therefore, the radiopharmaceutical delivered is of a much higher grade, and the surface dose rate delivered by the generator is much lower than with a naturel krypton target.

Our distribution network is extremely flexible and geared

to the needs of the clinician. The generators are available
on any day of the work week, on one day's notice. The practician needs only telephone and order the type of generator
and the loading activity the day before his scheduled examinations. A small clinic can order a 3 millicurie generator at a
low cost for a few patients or for an emergency diagnosis,
while a large city hospital can order a generator of up to
20 mCi and screen more than 30 patients in a single day. An
efficient interactive surface and air transportation network
ensures early delivery to over 35 different medical centers
in Holland, Germany, Belgium and Austria.

While krypton ventilation studies have become a classic
tool for the pulmonary diagnostician, perfusion Kr^{81m} generators are avaliable at a convenient cost on a routine basis.
This tried and proven perfusion generator's utility is limited
only by the practician's imagination. Numerous scintigraphic
studies taking advantages of the physical properties of Kr^{81m}
(gaseous solubility, short half-live, lack of preferential
fixation, rapid repeatability of examinations) have been performed.

This generator combines high elution yield with a physiological eluant, optimum photon energy (190 KeV, and a phenomenal-
ly low parent radionuclide breakthrough (less than 10^{-9}/ml).
An additional bonus of this perfusion generator, with important economic considerations, is that after having been used,
eluted with a 5% glucose solution, as a perfusion generator,
it can then be eluted with air as a ventilation generator.
This double usage, perfusion studies followed by pulmonary
examinations can, in a well organized clinical infrastructure,
result in substantial savings for a hospital's radiopharmaceutical budget.

Notwithstanding the widespread availability of thousands
of krypton generators over a 5 year period the multiple
possibilities offered by ventilation and perfusion generators
are barely tapped. In the near future, imaginative clinicians
can develop new examination techniques based on a proven radioisotope with guaranteed availability.

REFERENCES

1. Guillaume M, Czichosz R, Richard P, Fagard E, Krypton-81m generator
   for ventilation and perfusion. Dosimetry, routine production, methodologies for medical applications. Bull. Soc. roy. Sci, Liege, tome LII,
   fasc. 3,4, 1983.

2. Brihaye Cl, Guillaume M, Lavi N, Cogneau M, Development of a reliable
   195mHg-125mAu generator for the production of 195mAu, a short-lived
   nuclide for vascular imaging. J. nucl. Med. 23:1114, 1982.

3. Guillaume M, Brihaye Cl, The short-lived radionuclide generator.
   Physical characteristics, assessment and conditions for optimal clinical use. ACS Symp. Series 241:185, 1983.

4. Clark JC, Buckingham PD, Short-lived radioactive gases for clinical
   use. Butterworth, 1975.

5. Yano Y, Mac Rae J, Anger HO, Lung function studies using short-lived
   81mKr and the scintillation camera. J. nucl. Med. 11:674, 1970.

6. Guillaume MA, Krypton-81m generator production with a small cyclotron.
   Brit. J. Radiol. Special Report no.15:16, 1978.

7. Hichma RD, Daube ME, Nickles RJ, Small scale targetry for the production of 81Rb and 51Mn. 3rd Int. Symp. Radiopharm. St. Louis, 1980.

8. Kernert N, Peters TW, Sheikh SA et al, Status of 81Rb production at
   the Karlsruhe cyclotron. KFK Annual Report, Oct. 1980. Kernforschungs-
   zentrum Karlsruhe, p 98.

9. Rich B, Lembares N, Harper PC et al, Radiopharmaceuticals. Soc. Nucl.
   Medicine Inc. New York, p 174, 1974.

10. Linsmaux D, Rigo P, Merchie G, Guillaume M, La scintigraphie pulmonaire
    au 81mKr. Revue Medic. Liege, vol. XXXIV, no. 9, p 30, 1979.

11. Ham H, Vandevivere Y, Guillaume M, Niethammer T, Radionuclide veno-
    graphy using continuous 81mKr infusion. Clin. Nucl. Med. 6:481, 1981.

12. Fazio F, Nardini M, Fieschi C, Forli C, Assessment of regional cerebral
    blood-flow by continuous infusion of Krypton-81m. J. nucl. Med. 18:962,
    1977.

NOBLE RADIONUCLIDES FOR LUNG VENTILATION STUDIES

I. BOFILIAS

INTRODUCTION

Among the various radiopharmaceuticals which serve as a measure of "in vivo" metabolism, there exist two noble radioactive gases, Xe^{133} and Kr^{81m} which fulfil the most of the requirements to examine lung dysfunction. Of course, these two radionuclides can not entirely substitute the vital behaviour of the short lived positron emitters as O^{15}, N^{13} and C^{11}. But Xe/Kr-ventilation examinations do not need sophisticated systems for radionuclide production such as cyclotrons sited close to the patient. Only a γ-camera, a spirometer and a suitable free programmable, interactive computer system are necessary.

By performing both Xe^{133} and Kr^{81m} ventilation scintigraphy in the same group of patients we observed different lung ventilation patterns. This is due to: 1. application technique and 2. the nature of lung diseases.

METHOD

The Xe^{133} inhalation technique. This technique combined with the 3P-BIS (single breath (SB), equilibrium (E) and washout (WO)), is a technique which was developed in the Clinic of Nuclear Medicine of the Technical University of Munich (1). The patient breaths the Xe-activity at residual lung volume by bolus inhalation. It follows the equilibrium phase with activity distribution also to the hypoventilated departments of the lung. Two min after inhalation begins the well known wash-out phase (2). One of the benefits of the 3P-BIS lies in the registration of the SB-Phase in absence of background activity.

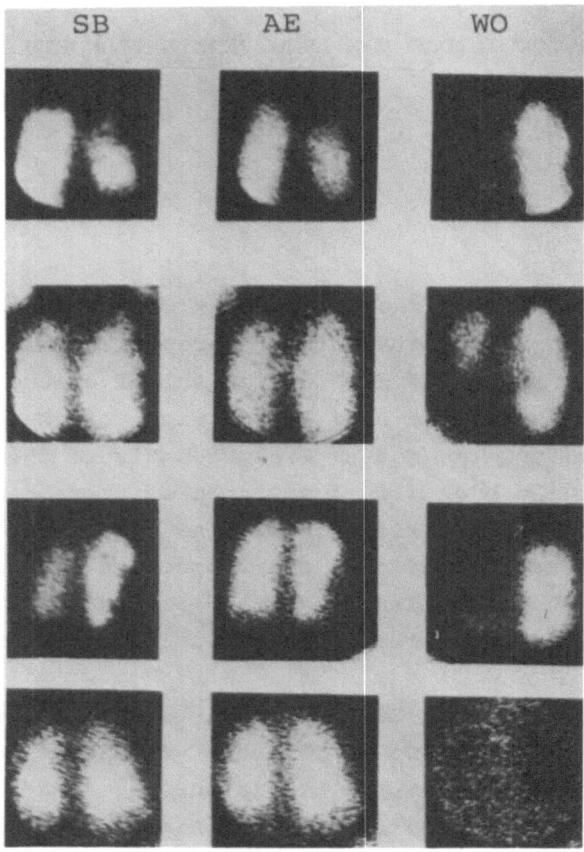

Fig. 1. 3P-BIS technique. 1st row: Restrictive ventilation abnormality accompanied by Xe-trapping. 2nd row: Xe-trapping by homogeneous activity distribution in SB and WO-phases. 3rd row: Overt inflation and Xe-trapping at same lung side. Homogeneous distribution in the AE-phase. 4th row: Normal lung ventilation in all three phases.

The Kr^{81m} ventilation technique. Krypton is continuously delivered by the Rb^{81}/Kr^{81m} generator. The method is the same as published by Fazio et al (3). A gas flow-rate of 250 ml per sec generates count rates of 100.000 c/min. This permits preparation of scans in 4 projections with an optimal signal-to-noise-ratio. Because of its very short half-life mobilizing volumes as VC can not be obtained by sequential or function scintigraphy.

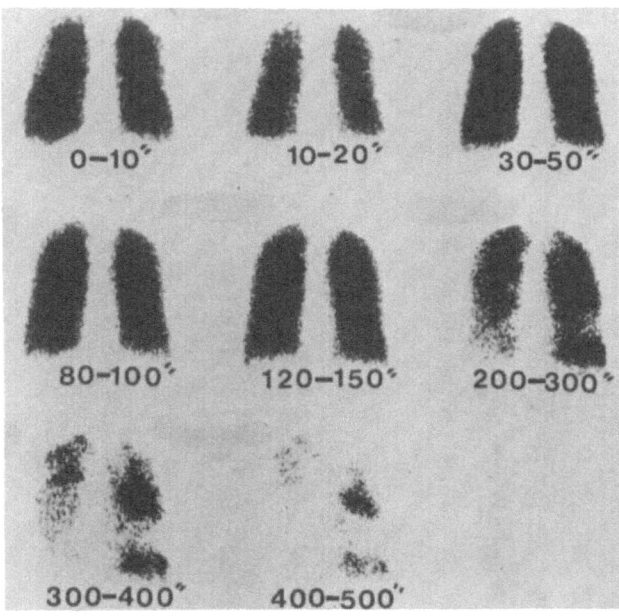

Fig. 2. Completely 3P-BIS by emphysema, Xe-trapping during WO, by homogeneous activity distribution in SB and AE-phases.

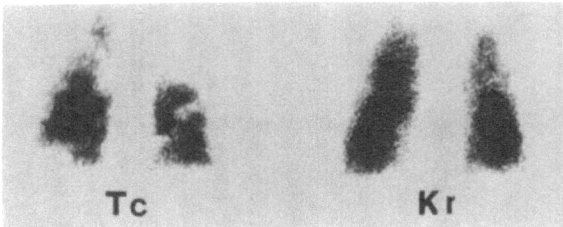

Fig. 3. Focal defect in the right upper lung segment in Tc^{99m} aggregate
scan (left). Kr^{81m} homogeneous activity distribution, posterior view.

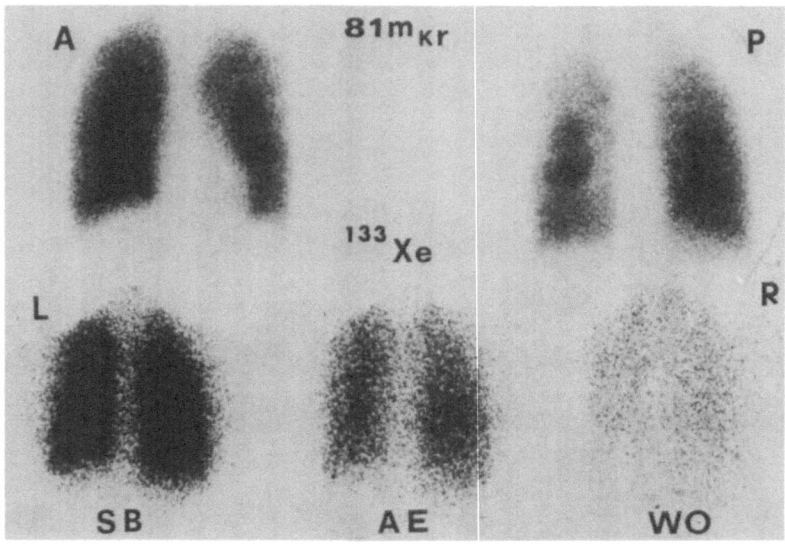

Fig. 4. 1st row: Increased Kr^{81m} activity distribution at the middle of the right lung (posterior view, P). 2nd row: 3P-BIS unsuspicious.

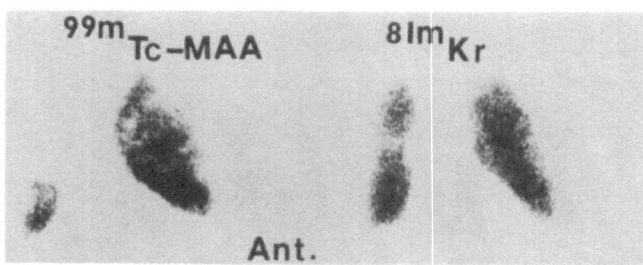

Fig. 5. Focal defect on the right upper lung segment by Tc^{99m}-MAA perfusion scan, Kr^{81m} ventilation is unsuspicious (anterior view).

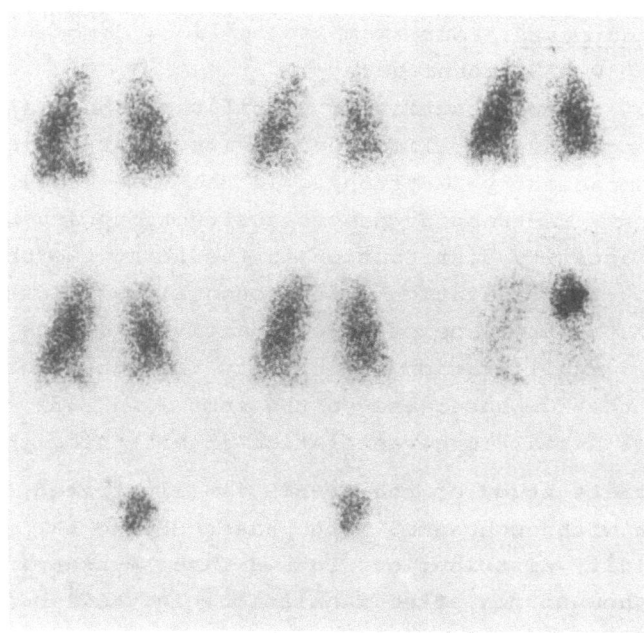

Fig. 6. Completely 3P-BIS in case of lung cancer. Focal Xe-trapping in WO phase, (same case as in fig 5).

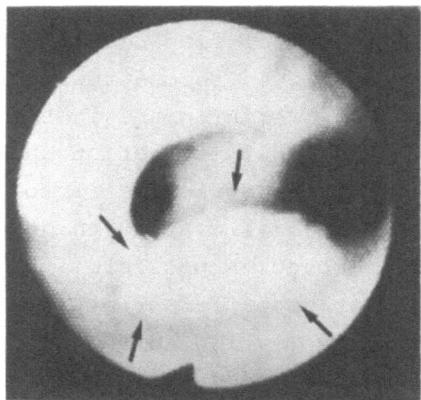

Fig. 7. Lung tumour, lens shape, 5 mm diameter (between the 4 files), endoscopically observed by Laser irradiation (plate epithelial carcinoma).

RESULTS

Bullae and cysts. Four examples in fig 1 demonstrate the
value of the 3P-BIS technique.

First row: Shows restrictive ventilation abnormality in
the right lung caused by limited activity distribution during
VC-test accompanied by Xe-trapping in the same lung.

Second row: Xe-trapping due to obstruction with nearly
homogeneous activity distribution in the first two phases.

Third row: Overinflation with bronchial wall instability,
indicated by the presence of more Xe-activity in the SB-phase
(right lung), equilibration of activity in both lungs and Xe-
trapping in the WO-phase also on the same lung side.

Last row: Normal lung ventilation in all three phases.

The complete study of the 3P-BIS is illustrated in fig 2
in a patient with emphysema. Both phases SB and AE present
uniform activity distribution. But we have Xe-trapping in the
WO clearly shown 5 min after inhalation. In whole body plethysmography we found increased RV and FRC.

In contrast, Kr^{81m} shows, in fig 3, homogeneous activity
distribution in the posterior view. In fact, the Tc^{99m}-macro-
aggregate perfusion scan indicates a focal defect in the upper
lung segment. In the case of a 17 years old patient with hyper-
transradiancy as radiological finding, all three phases in Xe-
scintigram are normal (fig 4, second row). The increased activity distribution in Kr^{81m} scintigrams in the middle of the
right lung (fig 4, first row), posterior and anterior view,
indicates distortion of the effective alveolar ventilation.
After operation two bronchial cysts with good connection to
bronchial tree were removed. A possible explanation for these
different lung ventilation patterns between Xe^{133} and Kr^{81m}
ventilation scintigraphy may lie in the differences in pathophysiology between bullae and cysts. Bullae consist of the
same alveolar epithelial as normal lung but they never have a
good connection to the bronchial system, while cysts show all
the characteristics of the bronchial wall musculature but with
different wall elasticity. They present malformations of the
lung. In cases of bullae the amplitude of VC is decreased and

Table 1. Results of the 3P-BIS and Kr^{81m} ventilation scintigraphy by N=30 patients. The Xe^{133} shows better sensitivity.

	3P-BIS (xe-133)	kr-81m	Σ
Pos.	10	6	16
Neg.	7	7	14
Σ	17	13	30

generally all three phases of 3P-BIS may shown abnormal ventilation. Cysts with a good communication to the bronchial tree do not always show abnormal ventilation in Xe-scinti-graphy. But as Krypton measures the amplitude of the tidal volume corresponding to the "effective" alveolar ventilation, cysts with only small different elasticity of bronchial wall be better observed in Kr-scintigraphy.

Lung cancer. In case of lung cancer, even relative small tumours may evoke abnormal ventilation. The ischaemic areas may be larger than the abnormalities in the radiograph. Fig 5 demonstrates this situation. While a focal defect in the upper right segment in Tc^{99m} scan exists, no such indication may be seen in Kr^{81m} scintigram. Furthermore, in radiographs no radiological abnormalities could be observed. The 3P-BIS shows clearly in the wash-out phase a focal Xe-trapping (fig 6). A tumour has been observed endoscopically by Laser-irradiation. It has the shape of small lens with a diameter of 5 mm, shown in fig 7, between the 4 files. The histology was positive for plaveiselcell-epithelial carcinoma.

In 30 cases with combined Xe/Kr scintigraphy we have obtained 16 positives (table 1). Ten of them due only to 3P-BIS and only six to Kr^{81m} scintigraphy, while seven negatives were registered in both studies. This demonstrates better sensitivity of the 3P-BIS and of course its value is of major clinical importance, while Kr^{81m} scintigraphy affecting dysfunction of effective alveolar lung ventilation is unavoidable.

CONCLUSION

Both 3P-BIS and Kr^{81m} may serve for detecting abnormal ventilation patterns due to restrictive ventilation abnormalities, actual lung volume, obstructive airway diseases (3P-BIS) and effective alveolar ventilation (Kr^{81m}).

REFERENCES

1. Bofilias I, Systemanalytische Signalverarbeitung in der Nuklearmedizin. Habilitationsschrift, TU München, 1981.

2. Bofilias I, Ascherl R, Buttermann G, Androulakis G, Blümel, Pabst HW, Anwendung organisomerpher Prinzipien zur Quantifizierung von induzierten Funktionsänderungen. Med. Physik. Bunde E (ed), pp 665-670, 1981.

3. Fazio F, Jones T, Assessment of regional ventilation by continuous inhalation of radioactive Krypton-81m. Brit. med. J. 3:673, 1975.

RADIOAEROSOLS IN NUCLEAR MEDICINE

M. PILLAY, B. SHAPIRO, P.H. COX

INTRODUCTION

The increasing interest in the use of radioaerosols as a
diagnostic tool in nuclear medicine warrants the standardiza-
tion of nomenclature, protocol and materials used, to avoid
ultimate misconceptions which may prevail.

The purpose of this article is to introduce the fundamental theory of particle distribution in the respiratory tract,
a brief protocol description, and the possible choice of
radiopharmaceuticals.

AIRWAY MODEL

The respiratory tract may be described as a continuously
branching system of tubes such as the model proposed by Weibel
(1,2) (fig 1). A particle in such a system will follow a
tortuous path, complicated by its own physical properties and
extraneous influences upon it. However, this model of airways
allows us to make certain theoretical predictions of particle
behaviour in the lungs. The model proposes that the airways
be divided into 24 generations so that the generation number
will be proportional to the airway volume and inversely
proportional to the airway diameter (table 1).

Dependant on the particle size, one or more of these
processes may dominate. The trapping process becomes significant only with particle size orders of magnitude larger than
is useful in diagnosis, and for this reason may be omitted
from further discussion. Of the remaining three, impaction
and sedimentation are considered to be the most important for
our purposes.

Impaction is the result of turbulent airflow, occuring

58

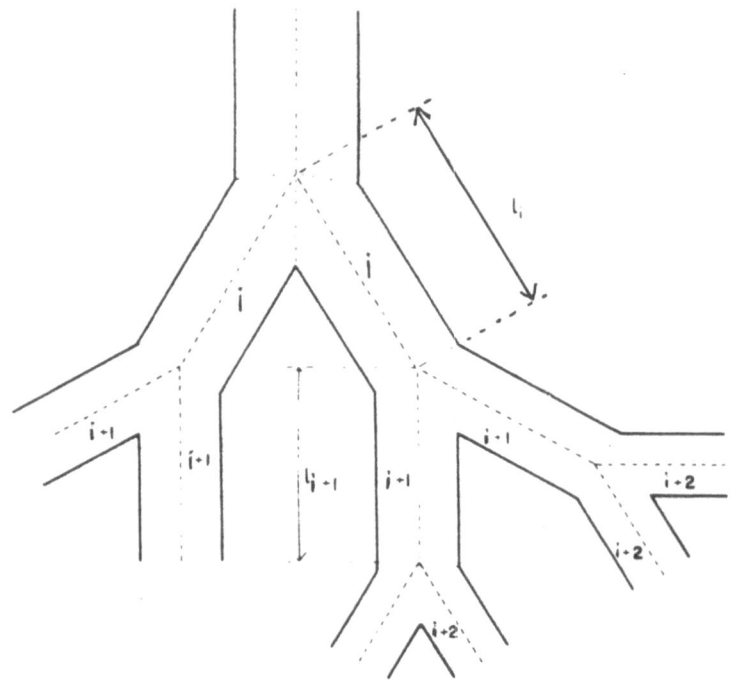

Fig. 1. Symmetrical lung model of Weibel (2).

primarily at the airway bifurcations. The deposition of particles become directly impacted on the inner walls and at the
obstructing bifurcations (3). Impaction is proportional to the
airflow (air velocity), solution density, particle surface
area, and is inversely proportional to the airway diameter and
viscosity of air (4). Due to the reduction of air velocity
towards the lung periphery, turbulence and hence, impaction
deposition is largely limited to the ciliary or larger airways. In terms of the lung model this will probably be the
first 16 generations!

Sedimentation of particles results from the effect of
gravitation so that deposition will be dependant primarily on
the body orientation. Sedimentation of particles is proportional to, the solution density, particle surface area, and is
inversely proportional to the viscosity of air-assuming zero
air velocity (5). Particle sedimentation dominates at the
lung periphery due to the very low air velocity experienced

Table 1. Airway generations of Weibel (2)				
Generation no.	No. of airways	Airway diameter (cm)	Airway length (cm)	Airway volume (cm^3)
0	1	1.800	12.000	30.50
1	2	1.220	4.760	11.25
2	4	0.830	1.900	3.97
3	8	0.560	0.760	1.52
4	16	0.450	1.270	3.46
5	32	0.350	1.070	3.30
6	64	0.280	0.900	3.53
7	128	0.230	0.760	3.85
8	256	0.186	0.640	4.45
9	512	0.154	0.540	5.17
10	1024	0.130	0.460	6.21
11	2048	0.109	0.390	7.56
12	4096	0.095	0.330	9.82
13	8192	0.082	0.270	12.45
14	16384	0.074	0.230	16.40
15	32768	0.066	0.200	21.70
16	65536	0.060	0.165	29.70
17	131072	0.054	0.141	41.80
18	262144	0.050	0.117	61.10
19	524288	0.047	0.099	93.20
20	1048576	0.045	0.083	139.50
21	2097152	0.043	0.070	224.30
22	4194304	0.041	0.059	350.00
23	8388608	0.041	0.050	591.00

there. Because of the physical limitations of respiration (tidal volume) during the ventilation investigation, the turbulent airflow and its progress to an area of "stagnation" at the periphery should be considered as given parameters. Since particle impaction and sedimentation are both proportional to the square of the particle diameter, the optimal particle sizes for these processes was estimated to be 2 - 5μ and 0.5 - 2μ respectively (6-8). Particles of size smaller than 0.2μ are diffused into the smaller airways where they will finally be deposited by sedimentation. Particle deposition in the respiratory tract as a function of particle size is shown in fig 2. Since particle deposition will predominate on inspiration, the total number of particles in the airways at the beginning of expiration will be insignificantly small and could for practical purposes be ignored.

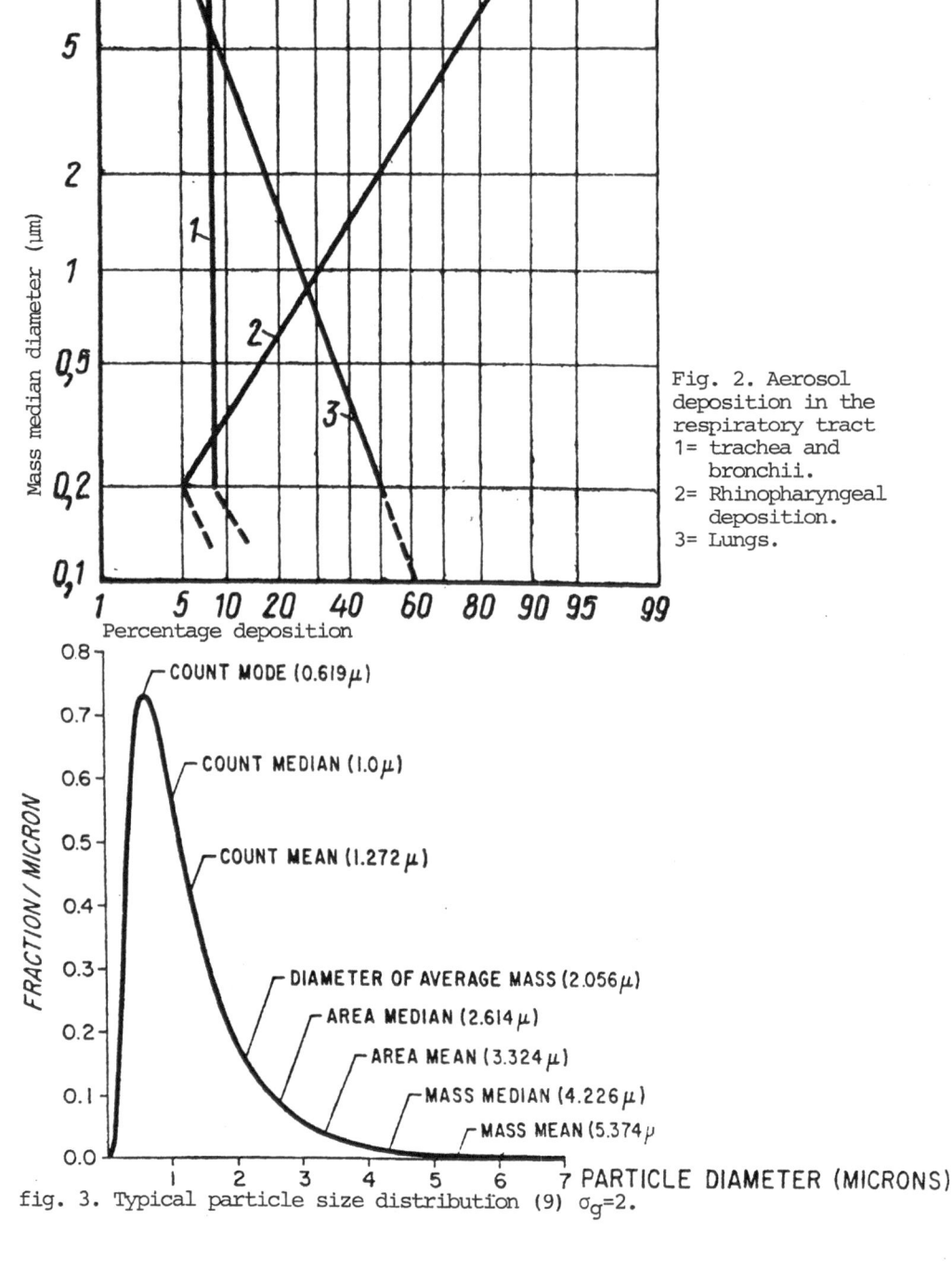

Fig. 2. Aerosol deposition in the respiratory tract
1= trachea and bronchii.
2= Rhinopharyngeal deposition.
3= Lungs.

fig. 3. Typical particle size distribution (9) σ_g=2.

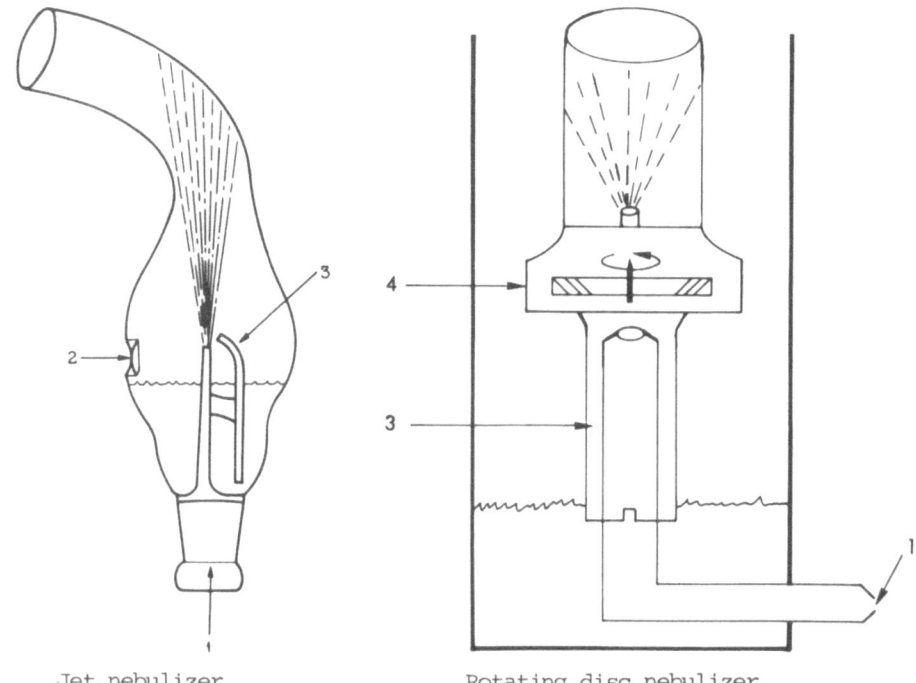

Jet nebulizer   Rotating disc nebulizer

Fig. 4. Jet- en rotating disc nebulizers. 1= Air flow under pressure.
2= Optional window. 3= Fluid feed channel. 4= Rotating disc.

The use of hygroscopic substances (e.g. powders) introduce
additional problems of particle growth during its transit and
on settling in the humid airways, and could result in agglomera-
tion of particles in certain areas of the lung.

CHARACTERIZATION OF PARTICLE SIZE
Nebulization produces a particle distribution which is
best described by the distribution as plotted on semi-loga-
ritmic co-ordinates (fig 3).
It is practically most convenient to describe the particle
size distribution in terms of its mass, hence the terms Mass
Median Diameter (MMD) and Geometric Standard Deviation (σg) as
characteristic parameters. The MMD is the measure of particle
size and the σg, of particle size distribution describing its
monodespersity. A higher degree of monodespersity implies a

Table 2. Comparison of jet- and rotating disc- type nebulizers

	System	
Parameter	Jet - type	Rotating disc- type
MMD (5 mg/ml DTPA)	0,7 μm	0,5 μm
σ_g (5 mg/ml DTPA)	1,6	2,0
system efficiency*	>10%	± 2%
airflow	10-12 L/min	8-10 L/min
solution volume	3-4 ml	3 ml
dose (Tc^{99m})	25-35 mCi	30-45 mCi
breathing time**	3-5 min	15-24 min
bacterial/radioactive contamination	filter trapping	filter trapping
shielding (Tc^{99m})	adequate	adequate
design	easy to use	easy to use

* - Relative activity deposited in the respiratory tract
** - 300.000 Counts obtained with LFOV gamma camera fitted with LEAP collimator

better reproducibility of a given particle size, which may ultimately influence the homogeneity of distribution in the lung fields.

MATERIAL AND METHODS
Nebulizer systems. Aerosols in radiodiagnoses are produced by nebulizers of which a number are commercially available. Two of the most widely used types are the jet- and rotating disc systems (fig 4).

Table 2 shows the most important differences of the jet-

and rotating disc systems with respect to their particle size
and systems efficiency. The efficiency was defined as the
amount of radioactivity in the lungs at the end of inspiration
in relation to that introduced into the nebulizer.

The jet nebulizing system proved to be more efficient at
the cost of its NMD, while the rotating disc system produced
smaller particles. It would, therefore, be expected that the
rotating disc system be used to approaximate gas distribution
at the periphery and less suitable to investigate mucociliary
transport.

In conclusion, the higher efficiency of the jet nebulizer
makes it more attractive as a general purpose nebulizer with
which the larger airways may equally well be outlined, it also
scores where difficult patients are encountered so that the
minimum breathing time on the apparatus will suffice.

Choice of radiopharmaceutical. It is recommended that the
radiopharmaceutical for aerosol lung investigations have a
relatively short biological half-life and that they be highly
soluble. Sulphur colloids tend to irritate the lung muscus
membranes and therefore, should be used only with extreme
caution. The blood-clearance of the pharmaceutical should be
fast to avoid superimposition of the blood-background on the
airway image. Taking these factors into consideration, the
most reasonable choice for a pharmaceutical will be among those
cleared by the renal or hepato-biliary systems. It is therefore, understandable that the most commonly used radiopharmaceutical for this purpose at the present time is the renal
agent, Dimethyl-Triamine-Panteacetic Acid (Tc^{99m} DTPA), which
has a high extraction and excreted by the kidneys. Another
possible candidate for this type of investigation would be the
hepato-biliary agent HIDA which is extracted from the blood by
the hepatocytes and excreted via the gastro-intestinal tract.

Study protocol. The study protocol for radioaerosol investigations may be divided into ventilation image as may be
required where lung emboli is suspected, or into a slightly
more complicated study of the alveolar- and mucociliary clearance. In both cases, however, the patient has to breathe through

64

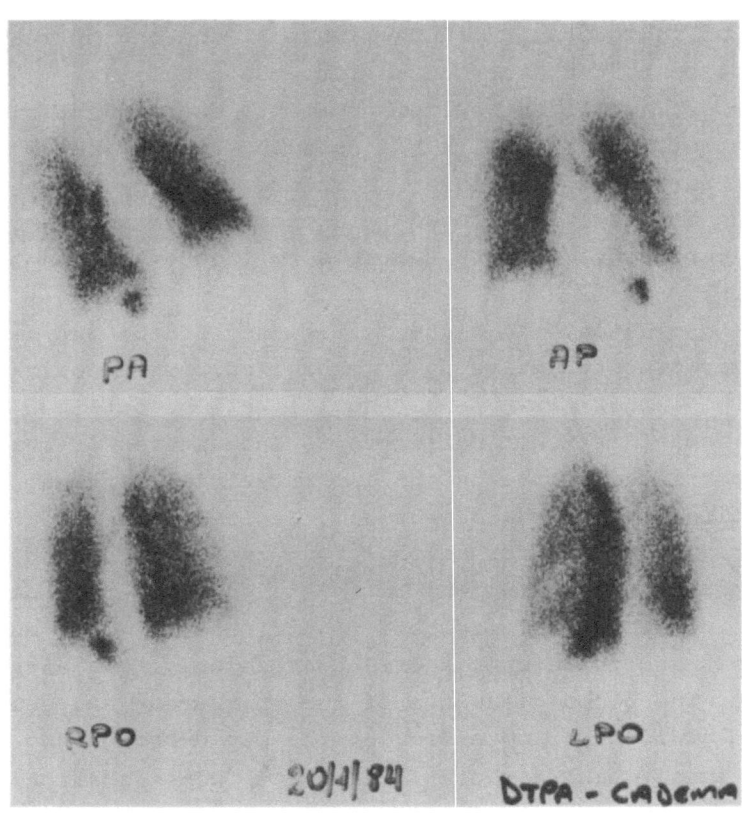

Fig. 5a. Normal ventilation images obtained with Tc^{99m} DTPA jet nebulizer.

the nebulizing apparatus until sufficient radioactivity has
been deposited in the lungs. For the ventilation images, the
patient is then positioned in front of the camera in the
required orientations. Because Tc^{99m} will be used in both the
perfusion and ventilation studies, a significant difference in
count densities between the two radiopharmaceuticals must be
achieved when imaging at the same sitting. It is suggested that
the ventilation images be done first with a total activity in
the lungs of approximately 1 mCi, followed by the perfusion
image with 3 to 4 times the activity of the ventilation image.
Fig. 5a and 5b show the normal ventilation images obtained

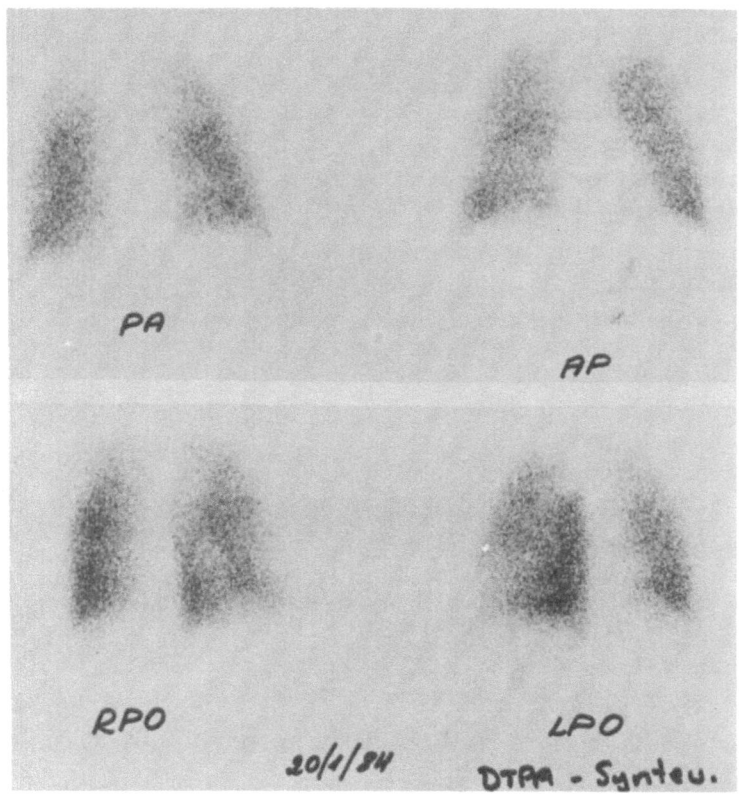

Fig. ⌐⌐. Normal ventilation images obtained with Tc^{99m} DTPA rotating disc nebulizer.

with radioaerosols produced by the two nebulizing systems. This combination has proven to yield good results and stays within the radiation dose limits recommended by the ICRP.

The clearance studies in general will not warrant an additional perfusion investigation, and for this reason, the activity nebulized may be increased to 2-3 mCi to improve the counting statistics. The subject is positioned in the posterior so that the maximal lung fields are in view and sequential counting performed with the aid of a computer for the following 45 - 60 min. For completeness, the other orientations are also acquired as static images. The data processing of the

66

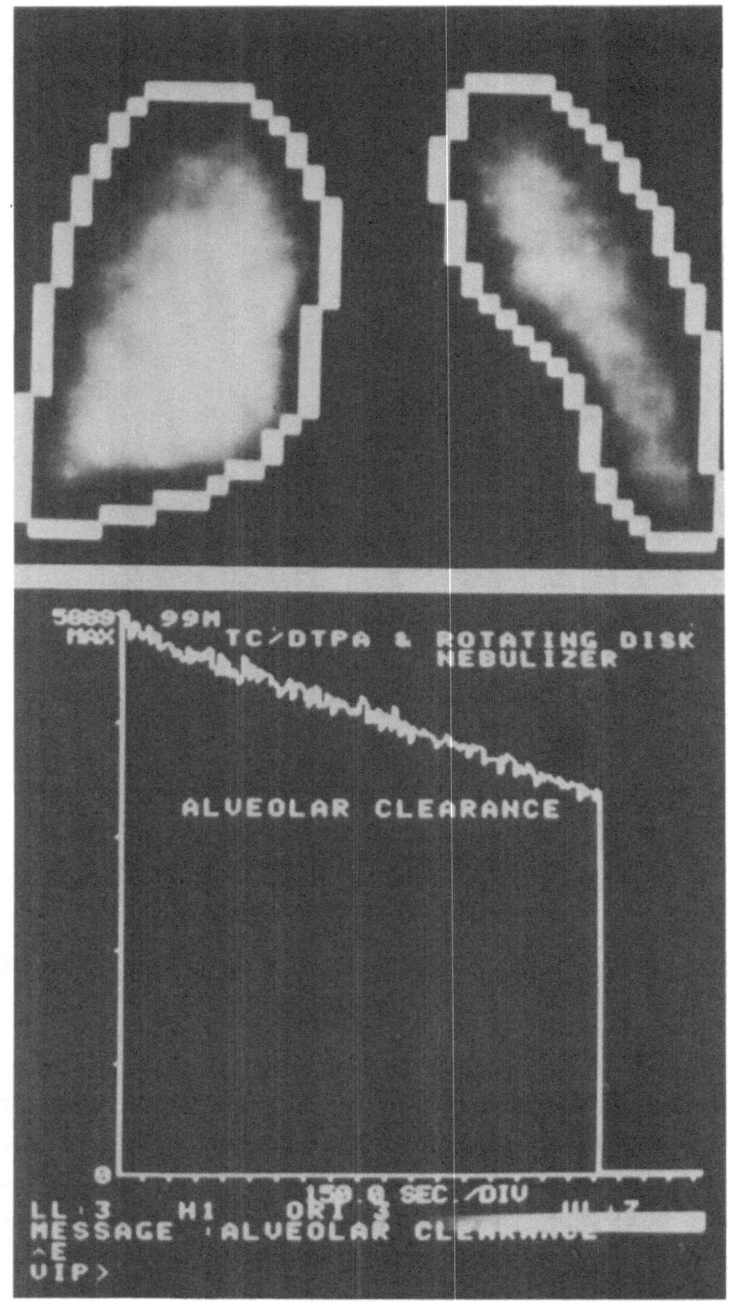

Fig. 6. Alveolar clearance patterns with Tc^{99m} DTPA.

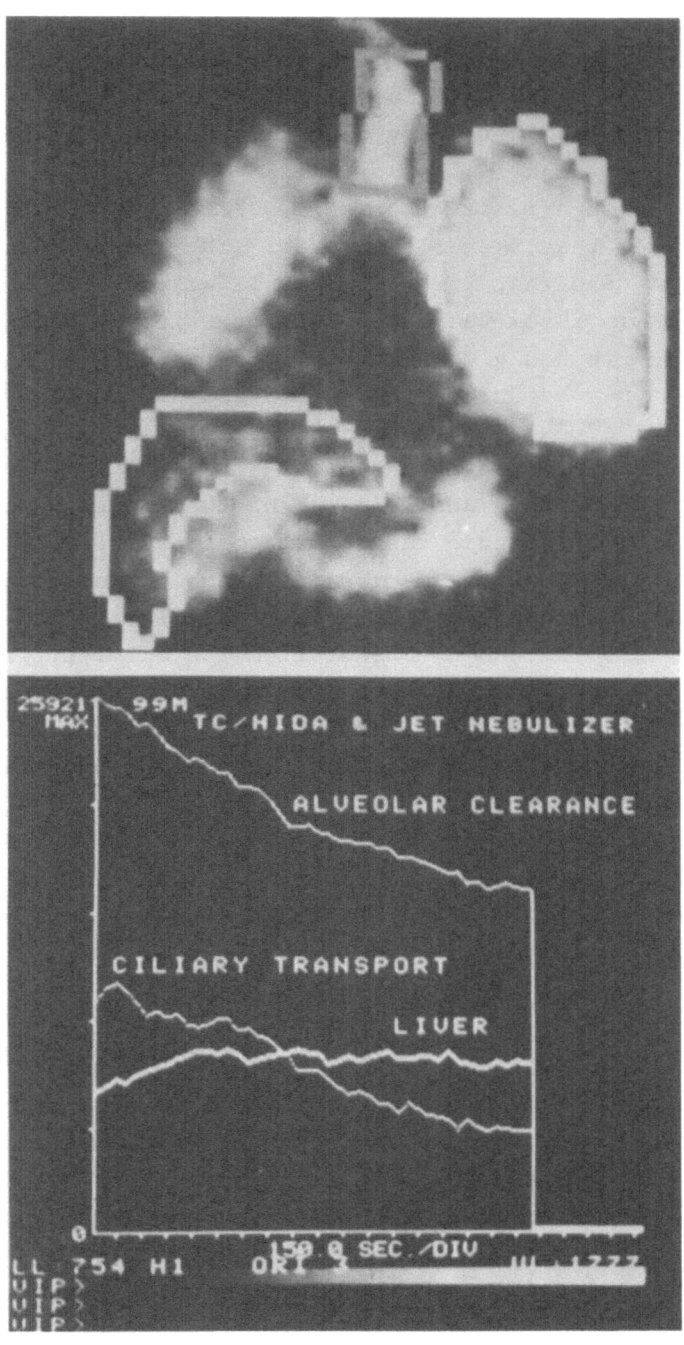

Fig. 6. Alveolar clearance patterns with Tc^{99m} HIDA.

acquired information involves curve generation over the whole
lung and may extend to regional areas of interest (fig 6).
It is expected that the alveolar clearance for the different
lobes of the lung will vary according to their blood-supply
and possible pathology.

Our own experience with Tc^{99m} DTPA and Tc^{99m} HIDA has
demonstrated that the half-time for DTPA clearance approximated
50 - 60 min and that for HIDA was slightly faster averaging
around 45 min. From the curves in fig 6 it can be seen that
the DTPA curve has a more linear appearance than that of the
HIDA. This may be due to the lypophylic and complex nature of
the HIDA as opposed to that of DTPA. An additional use for
the radioaerosol study with Tc^{99m} HIDA could be the detection
of right sub-phrenic abscesses since the lungs and liver could
be imaged with a single radiopharmaceutical.

Patient dosimetry. The radiation dose is dependant on the
pharmaceutical, nuclide, particle size distribution (nebulizer
type), deposition and clearance from the airways. The estimation by the MIRD method is not optimal because of the imhomo-
geneity of particle distribution and lung tissue. Hence, the
calculations were carried out assuming homogenous distribution
of the nuclide (10).

Table 3 displays the dosimetric values of the jet- and
rotating disc type systems using Tc^{99m} DTPA. The values obtained are comparable to that obtained in earlier studies with
^{133}Xe.

DISCUSSION
The high diffusion capacity of the radioactive gases allows
it to trace most of the airways through to the periphery and
to some extent also partakes in the alveolar gas exchange.
However, the presently available radioactive noble gases, ^{133}Xe
and Kr^{81m}, both have inherent disadvantages. The 81.0 KeV of
^{133}Xe is less optimal than the 190.3 KeV of Kr^{81m} for imaging.
The most significant limiting factor for Kr^{81m}, is the short
half-life of the parent nuclide ($t_{\frac{1}{2}}$=4.58 hours. The short $t_{\frac{1}{2}}$
of Kr^{81m} ($t_{\frac{1}{2}}$=13.3 sec) makes it possible to record different
projections consecutively with virtually no interference of

Table 3. Patient dose estimates with Tc^{99m} DTPA (11,12)

| | Dose mrad / mCi | |
Organ	Jet-type	Rotating disc-type
Lungs	50	65
Kidneys	42	39
Urinary bladder	555	632
Testes	16	19
Ovaries	19	31
Total body	16	10

blood-background activity. Finally, the cost and limited delivery of the radioactive noble gases makes it difficult and sometimes impossible to carry out ventilation studies irregularly.

The present nebulizer technology makes it possible to produce ventilation images with radioaerosols. The optimal particle size which mimics the gas distribution can be described as particles with a MMD= 0.2µm and σ_g= 1.22. It has been shown that a smaller particle size does not improve the peripheral deposition significantly (3). The nebulizer efficiency is another important parameter and determines the total radioactivity used and the breathing time on the apparatus. The introduction of radioaerosols has resulted in detailed studies of comparison with the radioactive gases, and has emerged as a valuable alternative in the clinical routine (13-16).

The investigation of alveolar and mucociliary clearance has been more widespread among environmental hygienists and somewhat rather neglected by the diagnosticians. The mucus transport in the large airways was observed at 5 mm/min (17). Eventual extension of the lung investigation with radioaerosols will undoubtedly lead to more optimal design of nebulizer systems, and the development of radiopharmaceuticals for this specific purpose. The use of short-lived radionuclides may aid in the investigation of respiratory distress and possibly asthma, where repeated studies could be performed.

CONCLUSION

1. The radioactive gases will remain superior to radioaerosols especially where chronic lung pathology affect the airway patency.
2. Lung studies with radioaerosols offer a valuable alternative for ventilation imaging with the possible advantage of determining the alveolar and/or mucus clearance.
3. The combination of ventilation and perfusion images with Tc^{99m} will significantly increase the specificity of comparison of the two types of images.
4. Tomography with radioaerosols is dependant on the nebulizer efficiency which is at present too low.

ACKNOWLEDGEMENTS

We wish to thank Solco and Cadema Medical Products for supplying the nebulizer systems.

LITERATURE

1. Weibel ER, Morphometry of the human lung. Springer Verlag, Berlin, 1963.

2. Ferron GA, On the deopsition of aerosols in the human airways. Thesis, University Press, Delft, 1976.

3. Thomas RL, Deposition and initial translocation of inhaled particles in small laboratory animals. Hlth. Phys. 16:417, 1969.

4. Mercer TT, Aerosol technology in hazard evaluation. Acad. Press, New York, 1973.

5. Davies CN, Aylward M, Impingement of dust from air jets. AMA. Arch. Med. Ind. Occup. Med. 4:354, 1951.

6. Aspin N, Wong JW, Yeates DB, Levison H, Mucociliary clearance in cystic fibrosis. Modern Problems in Paediatrics, 19:199, 1977.

7. Lippman M, Yeates DB, Albert RE, Deposition, retention and clearance of inhaled particles. Brit. J. industr. Med. 37:337, 1980.

8. Lourenco RV, Cotromanes E, Clinical aerosols. Arch. intern. Med. 142: 2163, 1980.

9. Task group on lung dynamics: Deposition and retention models for internal dosimetry of human respiratory tract. Hlth. Phys. 12:173, 1966.

10. Prato FS, Vinitski S, Radiation dose calculations for inhalation of Tc-99m sulfur colloid radioaerosol. J. nucl. Med. 24:816, 1983.

11. Taplin GV, Atlas for lung imaging using radioaerosols. Univ. Calif. Press, L.A., 1979.

12. Synaco Inc. SynteVent aerosol delivery system. Catalogus, 1983.

13. Taplin GV, Poe ND, A dual lung scanning technique for evaluation of pulmonary function. Radiology 85:365, 1965.

14. Taplin GV, Poe ND, Greenburg A, Lung scanning following radioaerosol inhalation. J. nucl. Med. 7:77, 1966.

15. Arborelius M, Generation of a microaerosol suitable for deposition on peripheral airways. Eur. J. Resp. Dis. Suppl. 119, 63:19, 1982.

16. Pavia D, Thomson ML, Clarke SW, Shannon HS, Effect of lung function and mode of inhalation on penetration of aerosol into the human lung. Thorax, 32:194, 1977.

17. Yeates DB, Aspin N, Levison H, Jones MT, Bryan AC, Mucociliary tracheal transport rates in man. J. appl. Physiol. 39:487, 1975.

A DRY AEROSOL OF Tc^{99m} - ALBUMINMILLIMICROSPHERES FOR LUNG VENTILATION SCINTIGRAPHY: PREPARATION, INHALATION APPARATUS AND EXAMPLES OF CLINICAL RESULTS

P. ANGELBERGER, I. ZOLLE, A. STRIGL, H. KÖHN, A. MOSTBECK, W. FIEDLER

INTRODUCTION

The diagnostic applicability of regional lung ventilation could be greatly extended if a suitable radioactive aerosol were readily available. The radioactive gases in use for ventilation studies, Kr^{81m} and Xe^{127}, are both expensive and not available on a daily basis, aerosol preparations on the other hand so far suffered from polydisperse size-distribution, aggregation and inadequate application procedures.

The measurement of regional aerosol deposition was introduced in 1965 by Taplin (1) and, independently, Pircher (2). Several aerosol generator-delivery systems have been developed for the use of a monodisperse aerosol. In most cases an aqueous solution or suspension of a Tc^{99m}-compound, such as pertechnetate, sulfur-colloid, DTPA, human serum albumin HSA-milli-Microspheres (HAmM), was nebulized thus generating the aerosol droplets and delivering this wet aerosol to the patient. A persistent problem with such wet aerosols is the subsequent formation of larger particles which cause aerosol deposition in the posterior pharynx, trachea and major bronchi ("central deposition"). Therefore more recent systems use separating devices to remove the larger aerosol particles (3-5). In addition the delivery efficiency to the lung is low, typically only about 1% of the radioactivity loaded into the nebulizer (6). Other investigators have prepared dry aerosols from wet aerosols by heating (7,8) or, recently, by using a suspension of HAmM in ethanol for nebulization (9). Dry aerosols achieved a considerable improvement in delivery efficiency to the lung, namely 15-40% of activity loaded into the nebulizer (7,9). Since particle size is the principal parameter for aerosol deposition in the lung, optimum control of particle size should be the main consideration. For this reason we chose to work on a dry aerosol consisting of preformed presized HAmM.

MATERIALS AND METHODS

HAmM preparation. HAmM were prepared by a modification of the method developed by Zolle (10) by making a very fine emulsion of 0.5 ml 20% HSA in 40 ml cottonseed oil, first by means of glass-sphere sliding in a glass-cylinder followed by repeated passage through a mechanical homogenizer. The tiny HSA-droplets were then denatured by heating to 170°C and isolated from the oil by repeated suspension and centrifugation in ether.

Sizing was performed in ethanol suspension first by differential centrifugation (the centrifuge conditions having been established with standard 1 µm Latex microspheres) to sediment out HAmM larger than 1 µm and followed by repeated ultrasonic suspension/settling/decantation to remove the majority of HAmM smaller than 0.2 µm.

HAmM size distribution was evaluated by Scanning Electron Microscopy (SEM) and determined quantitatively by Transmission Electron Microscopy (TEM). A HAmM sample was taken in ethanolic suspension, the ethanol evaporated and HAmM were coated with gold vapor.

A projection image of HAmM was obtained by TEM, the projection diameters were measured with a circular gauge and counted, followed by statistical analysis of data.

Tc^{99m} labelling of HAmM was performed by electrolytic generation of Sn^{++} ions using a Sn-anode and a Pt-cathode in a standard 10 ml vial. A precision constant current supply and electronic timer allowed passage of an accurate number of milli-Coulomb and corresponding liberation of µg-amounts of Sn^{++} (fig 1). To 1 mg HAmM in 0.5 ml suspension of water with 5% ethanol and 0.2% Tween 80 was added the required activity of Tc^{99m}-TcO_4^- in saline and adjusted to p_H 1,7. Electrolytic generation of 6 µg Sn^{++}/ml was followed by 10 min reaction period in an ultrasonic bath. Labelled HAmM were isolated by

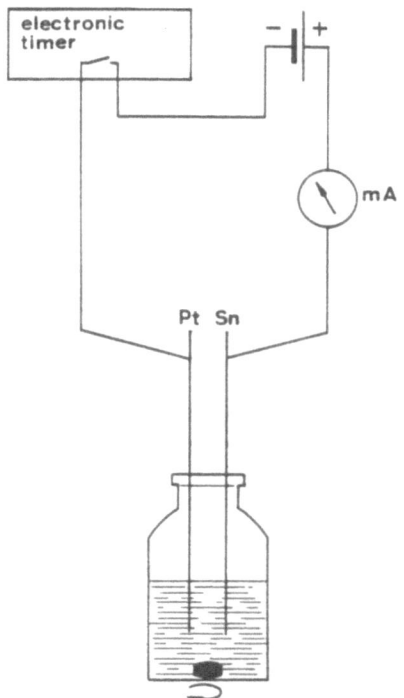

TcO$_4^-$ reduction by electrolytic generation of Sn^{++} ions

Fig. 1. Scheme for electrolytic Tc^{99m}-labelling.

centrifugation or Nuclepore filtration, then washed free of
unbound Tc and water with ethanol and finally resuspended in
0,3 ml ethanol per patient dose.

Aerosol inhalator. An apparatus was constructed for preparation and inhalation of a dry aerosol from labelled HAmH as
shown in fig 2: nebulization of 0.3 ml ethanol suspension of
Tc^{99m}-HAmM is effected by compressed air in the jet-nebulizer
(nr. 3 in fig 2) leading to evaporation of ethanol and formation of a dry aerosol composed of labelled HAmH in the airtight
chamber (nr. 1). Depending on position of valves (nr. 5 and 6)
the patient breathes via the mouthpiece (nr. 4) first room air
(to get used to the inhalator and breathing instructions), then
labelled aerosol from the chamber. During the latter process
the sliding bellows (nr. 7 expands, keeping pressure and

HAmM AEROSOL INHALATOR

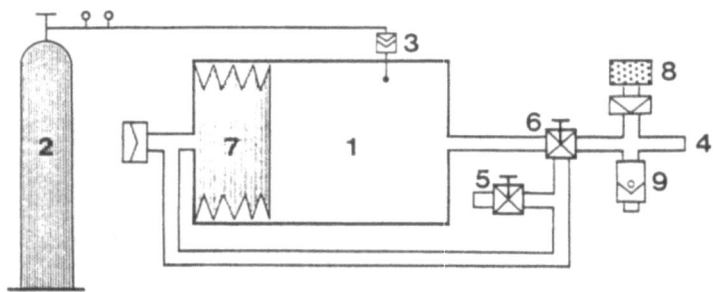

1	airtight chamber	5, 6	valves
2	pressurized air	7	sliding bellows
3	nebulizer	8	exhalation filter
4	mouthpiece	9	low pressure valve

Fig. 2. Scheme of aerosol inhalator.

aerosol concentration in the chamber constant. Exhaled air is passed through an activity retaining filter (nr. 8). A low pressure valve (nr. 9), high pressure limit and electronic control of valve positions provide complete safety even in case of false handling.

Clinical studies comprised 48 patients with chronic obstructive airway disease (COAD) who were classified according to usual spirometric data and 24 patients with suspected pulmonary embolism (PE). Patients were instructed to breathe slowly and to achieve large tidal depths with inspiratory stops during the inhalation period of 3-5 min. Aerosol scintigrams were compared with Kr^{81m} or Xe^{127} ventilation studies in the same patient. Penetration to the lung periphery of the aerosol was compared with that of Kr^{81m}: a penetration index was defined as ratio of pixelnormalized counts in a central over a peripheral lung region.

To evaluate the significance of aerosol hot spots for the

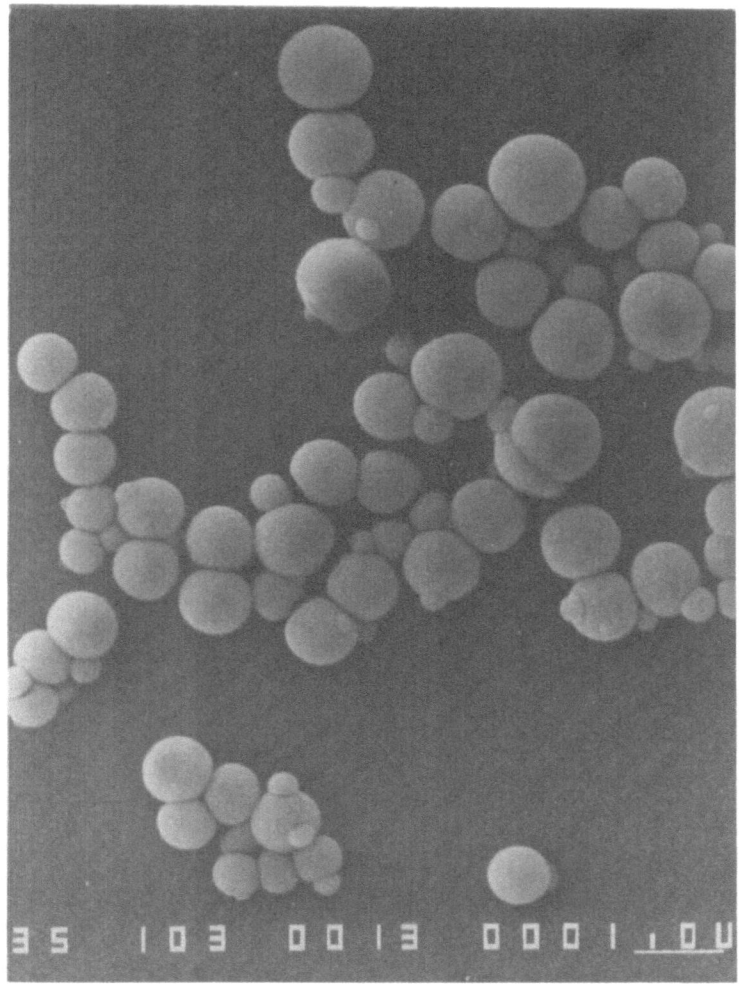

Fig. 3. Scanning electron microscope picture of human-albumin-milli-microspheres.

degree of obstruction a "hot spot score" was defined as number of hot spots in the aerosol scintigram and plotted against the Forced Expiratory Volume per second (FEV_1).

RESULTS

The emulsification and sizing process decribed yielded regular shaped microspheres of fairly uniform size as shown by SEM (fig 3).

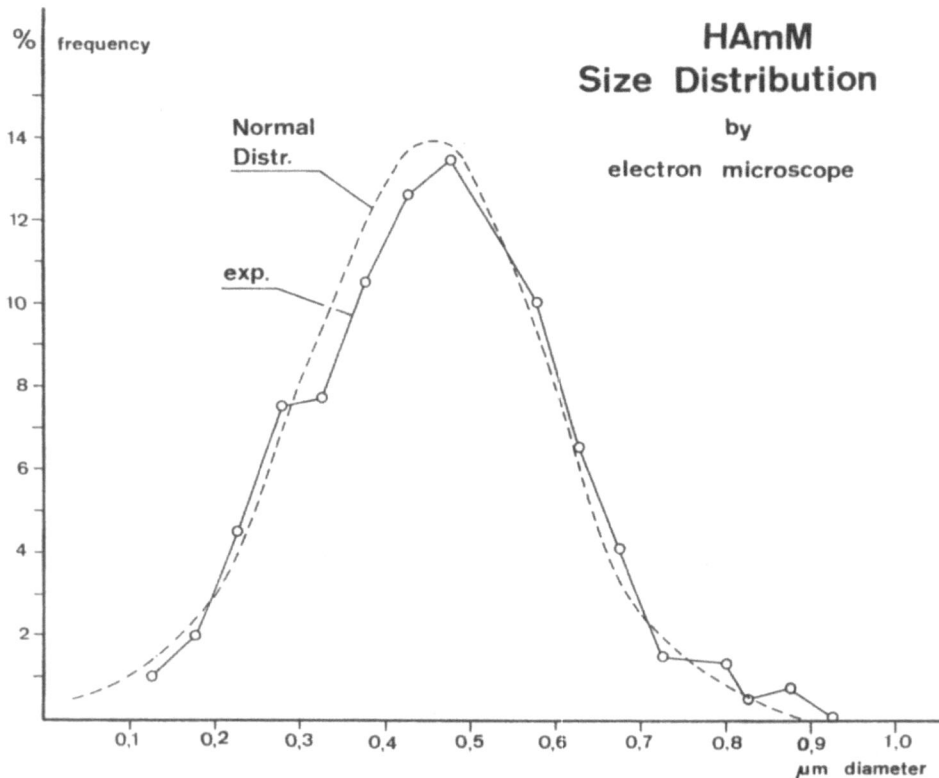

Fig. 4. Human-albumin-milli-microspheres size distribution by transmission electron microscope.

The resulting size-distribution (frequency vs diameter) as measured by TEM is shown in fig 4. Experimental points are connected by straight full lines, whereas for comparison a normal (Gauss) distribution is indicated by the dashed curve. The maximum of the size-distribution i.e. the most frequently occuring diameter of this HAmM batch was between 0,45 and 0,50 µm. HAmM with diameters above 0,8 µm have been almost complete-ly removed while some smaller than 0,2 µm remain which are how-ever not detrimental in ventilation studies. The separation of these small HAmM could be improved by Nuclepore filtration which is however technically difficult.

Results from statistical analysis are contained in fig 5: summed frequencies plotted against diameters on single-log paper yield a straight line thus corresponding to a normal

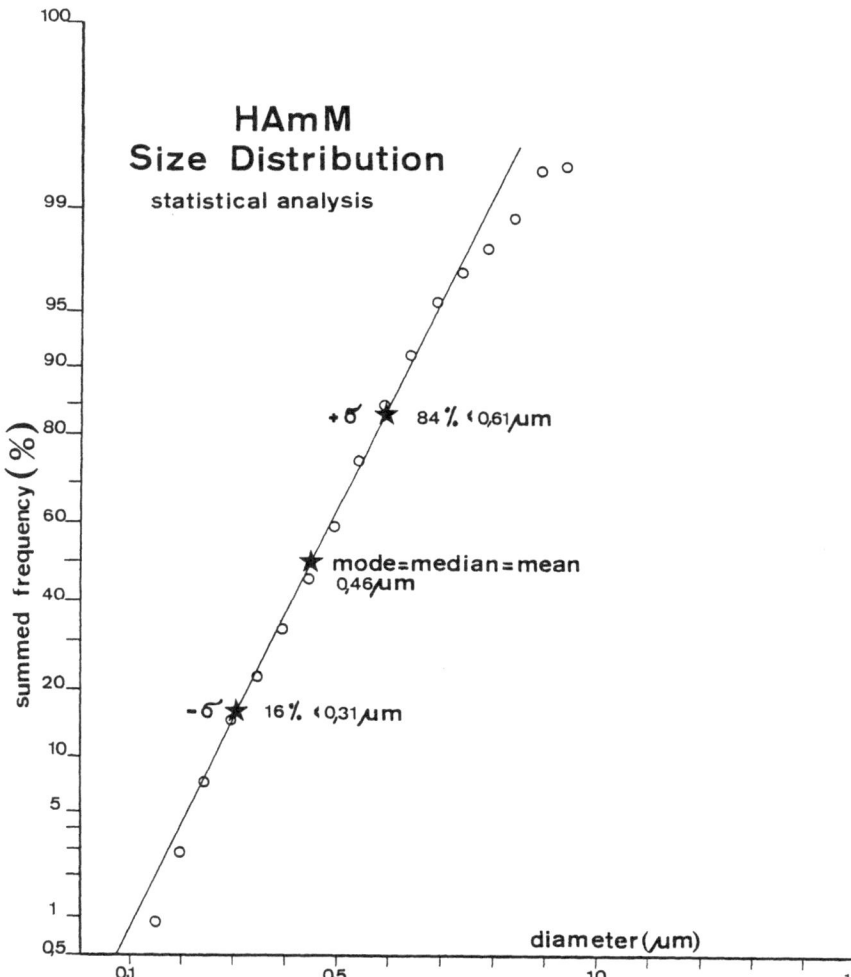

Fig. 5. Statistical analysis (probability net) of size distribution.

(Gauss) distribution. Mean, median and mode of such a distribution are identical: $\mu \pm \sigma = 0,46 \pm 0,15$ µm diameter for this HAmM batch, i.e. 16% are smaller than 0,31 µm and 84% smaller than 0,61 µm.

When the Tc^{99m}-labelling procedure was performed batchwise with about 90 mCi TcO_4^- the yield (mean ± sd) of final product after washing ready for aerosol formation was 64 ± 10% (n = 10) but increased to 87 ± 4% (n = 7) when only about 5 mCi were used. Considering the ready availability and low cost of Tc^{99m}-

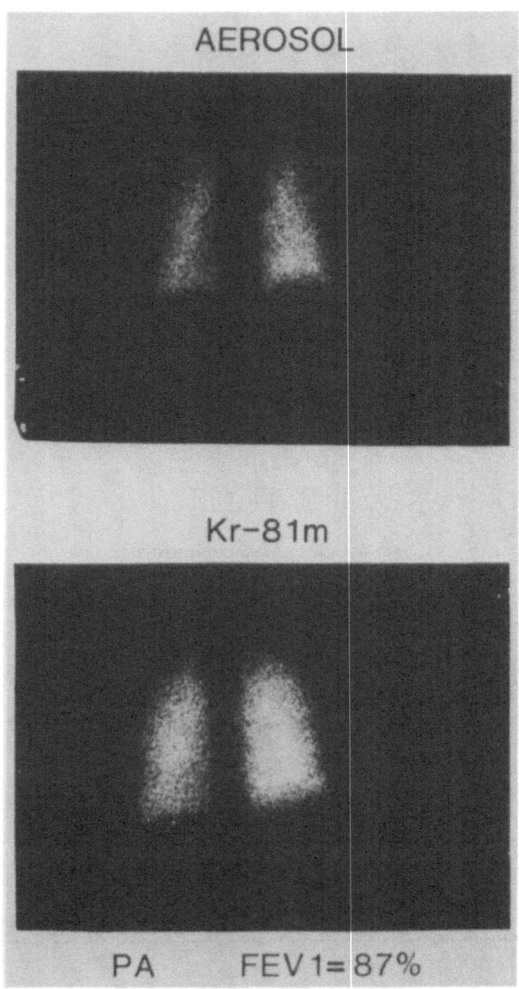

AEROSOL

Kr-81m

PA   FEV1=87%

Fig. 6. Normal aerosol ventilation scintigram (pattern 1) with Kr^{81m} ventilation scintigram for comparison.

TcO_4^- as well as complete removal of unbound Tc^{99m} this yield was found satisfactory.

Inhalator activity balance. If the Tc^{99m}-HAmM activity injected into the nebulizer is taken as 100% then patients inhaled 40 ± 9% (n = 3) while about 60% remained in the inhalator mainly on the surface of the chamber and bellows. Of the 40% inhaled about 18% were recovered in the exhalation filter while 22 ± 4% (n = 3) were actually deposited in the lungs, i.e. about 5 mCi

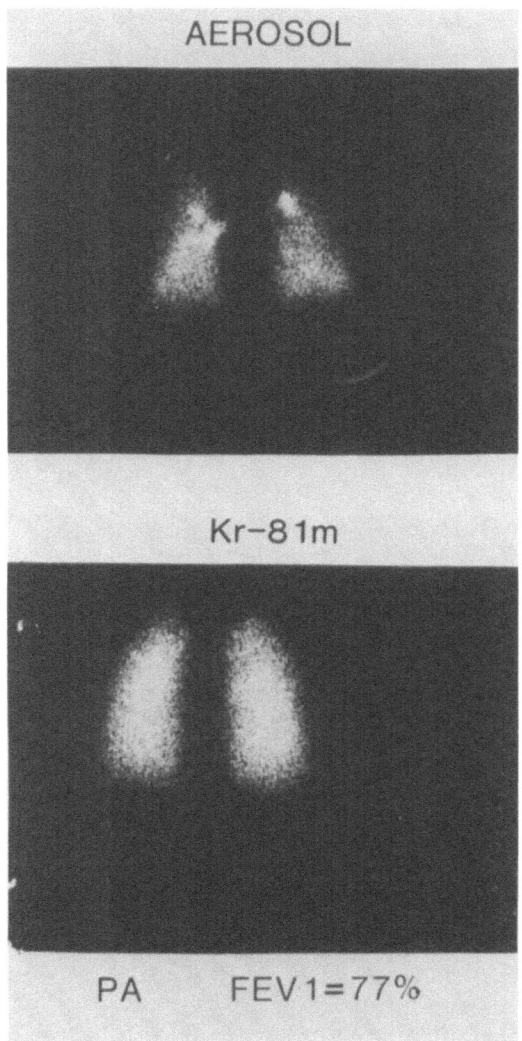

Fig. 7. Aerosol ventilation scintigram with singular central hot spots (pattern 2) and Kr^{81m} for comparison.

Tc^{99m}-HAmM must be nebulized to achieve 1 mCi lung activity. This is a much higher efficiency than obtained with wet aero-sols and could possibly be improved further by better separa-tion of HAmM <0,2 μm which would decrease the filter and in-crease lung activity.

Clinical studies. After inhalation of Tc^{99m}-HAmM aerosol. 4 different characteristic patterns of ventilation scintigrams

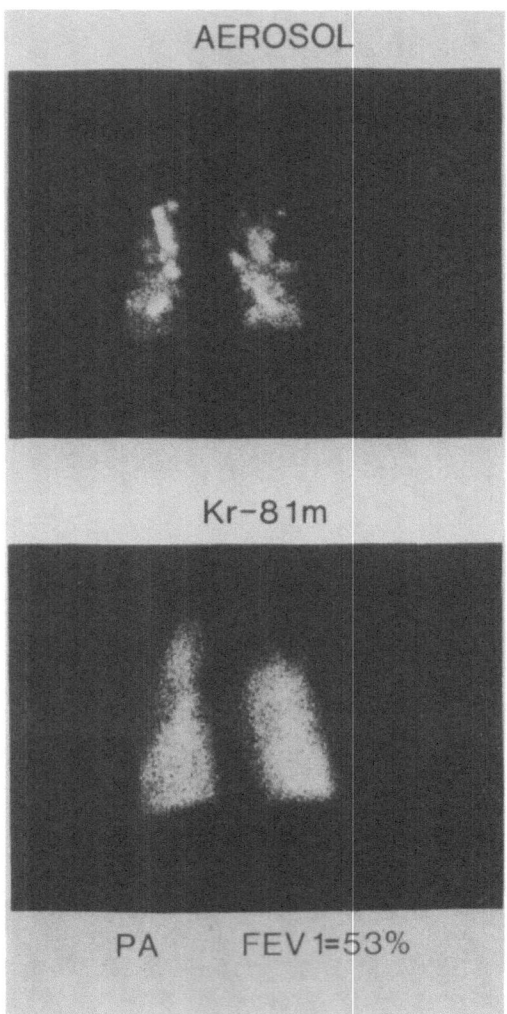

Fig. 8. Aerosol ventilation scintigram with multiple hot spots in COAD (pattern 3) and Kr81m for comparison.

were observed:

1. a normal homogeneous activity distribution with good penetration into the lung periphery comparable to Kr^{81m} (fig 6) was found in patients with normal lung function.

2. a homogeneous deposition with occurence of singular central "hot spots" (sharply defined small areas of increased activity)(fig 7) was found in patients without COAD displaying a normal Kr^{81m} ventilation scintigram.

83

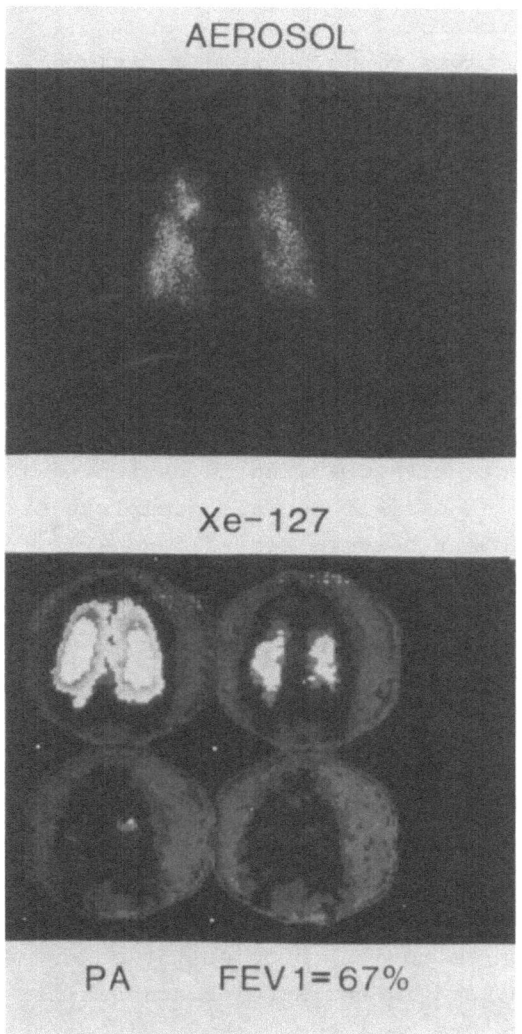

Fig. 9. Aerosol ventilation scintigram with multiple deposition defects (pattern 4) and Xe127 washout.

3. multiple hot spots in areas with inhomogeneous activity deposition (accumulation defects) indicate obstruction in patients with chronic bronchitis and/or emphysema (fig 8). The Kr^{81m} images displayed ventilation defects as well.

4. a "spotty" deposition pattern with multiple small defects but without hot spots (fig 9) was rare and correlated with prolonged Xe^{127} washout and gas-trapping indicative of

airway obstruction.

No difference was found between scintigrams acquired in smokers compared to non-smokers up to at least 1 hour after aerosol inhalation.

The penetration index (p.i.) calculated for the Tc^{99m}-HAmM aerosol correlated highly significant with the p.i. for Kr^{81m} (r = 0,86, p <0,001) demonstrating penetration of aerosol to the lung periphery to be comparable with Kr^{81m}.

A good correlation was also found between FEV_1 and the aerosol "hot spot score" (r = -0,77, p <0,001) which thus gave reliable information about the severity of airway obstruction in patients with COAD.

In 48 patients with COAD and 24 patients with suspected PE, qualitative assessment revealed complete or predominant diagnostic agreement between aerosol and Kr^{81m} or Xe^{127} ventilation studies.

DISCUSSION

Aerosol deposition in the lung is influenced by the physical properties of the aerosol, primarily particle size, and the breathing pattern. The primary mechanism of deposition for particles larger than about 2 µm and with high velocity is impaction by inertia in the major conducting airways. For slow moving particles with diameters in the range 1-2 µm it is mainly sedimentation while for those smaller than about 1 µm diffusion (Brownian motion) becomes the major mechanism (11).

84% of HAmM used in our studies are smaller than 0,6 µm and it can therefore be assumed that this aerosol reaches the lung periphery mainly by diffusion. While penetration to the lung periphery is highest with particles below 0,5 µm diameter, retention in the lungs is maximal with aerosol particles in the range 1-2 µm (8). This is demonstrated by the equally good penetration of our aerosol compared to Kr^{81m} while, due to HAmM smaller than 0,3 µm, about 18% of the inhaled aerosol is exhaled and trapped in the exhalation filter. This fraction might be reduced with simultaneous increase of lung retention by a better separation of HAmM smaller than 0,3 µm.

The formation of an aerosol from HAmM provides considerable advantages over wet aerosols where a radioactive solution is nebulized into droplets of widely varying size. Large droplets will contain a much higher proportion of activity than corresponding to their frequency in the size-distribution because the volume of a spherical droplet is proportional to its (radius)^3. This is one reason for the low delivery efficiency of wet aerosols using separating devices for removal of large droplets.

On the contrary we use preformed microspheres of controlled size which can be labelled and then transformed into a dry aerosol in the inhalation apparatus. Its function is merely nebulization of an ethanolic HAmM suspension leading to a dry aerosol without problems of droplet aggregation. The overall delivery efficiency to the lung of about 22% deposits about 1 mCi activity in the lung available for scintigraphy within a few minutes breathing time from only 4-5 mCi loaded into the inhalation apparatus.

The radiation dose associated with the deposition of Tc^{99m}-HAmM-aerosol in the lung is influenced by large variations in the clearance rates with the type and severity of airway disease. For a Tc^{99m}-HSA aerosol with mass median diameter of 0,46 µm a lung clearance half-time of 19,6 hours was measured in anesthetized dogs (12). Thus it may be assumed that radiation dose to the lung is mainly affected by the physical half-life of the radionuclide. For the entire lung an average of 0,37 rads for a total activity of 1 mCi uniformly deposited in the lung was calculated for a 1-2 µm Tc^{99m}-sulfur colloid aerosol (13) in good agreement with 0,4 rads/mCi for uniformly distributed Tc^{99m}-macro-aggregated albumin (9).

The clinical studies suggest that, for routine examination of regional ventilation in patients with suspected PE or with COAD, Kr^{81m} and Xe^{127} gas may be replaced by the described aerosol. For the diagnosis of COAD the aerosol is more sensitive than Kr^{81m}: it is assumed that airway obstruction causes turbulence which appears as hot spot in the aerosol scintigram, a special diagnostic criterion not seen with Kr^{81m} and correlated with the degree of obstruction.

86

REFERENCES

1. Taplin GV, Poe ND, A dual lung scanning technique for evaluation of pulmonary function. Radiology 85:365, 1965.

2. Pircher FJ, Lerner SR, Cooper PH et al, Distribution of pulmonary ventilation determined by radioisotope scanning. Amer. J. Roentgenol. 94:807, 1965.

3. Hayes M, Taplin GV et al, Improved radioaerosol administration system for routine inhalation lung imaging. Radiology 131:256, 1979.

4. Greening AP, Miniati M, Fazio F, Regional deposition of aerosols in health and in airways obstruction: A comparison with Krypton-81m ventilation scanning. Bull. Eur. Physiopath. Resp. 16:287, 1980.

5. Suzuki T, Swift DL, Wagner HN et al, A new apparatus for generating hygroscopic radioactive aerosols for inhalation studies. Eur. J. Nucl. Med. 7:474, 1982.

6. Spitz J, Berlad T, Erste klinische Erfahrungen mit einem neuen Aerosol-Dosiergerät zur Lungenventilationsscintigraphie. In: Radioaktive Isotope in Klinik und Forschung 16 (1). Höfer R, Bergmann H (eds), Egermann, Wien, pp 61-69, 1984.

7. Kotrappa P, Raghunath B et al, Scintiphotography of lungs with dry aerosol-generation and delivery system. J. nucl. Med. 18:1082, 1977.

8. Arborelius M, Generation of microaerosol suitable for deposition in the peripheral airways. Eur. J. Resp. Dis. (Suppl. 119), 63:19, 1982.

9. Hannan WJ, Emmet PC et al, Effective penetration of the lung periphery using radioactive aerosols. J. nucl. Med. 23:872, 1982.

10. Zolle I, Hosain F, Rhodes BA et al, Human serum albumin millimicrospheres for studies of the reticuloendothelial system. J. nucl. Med. 11:379 ff, 1970.

11. Brain JD, Valberg PA, Deposition of aerosol in the respiratory tract. Amer. Rev. resp. Dis. 120:1325, 1979.

12. Suzuki T, Watanabe S, Wagner HN et al, Imaging alveolar capillary permeability in experimental respiratory distress syndrome. In: Proc. of 3rd World Congr. of Nucl. Med. and Biology. Raynaud C (ed), Pergamon Press, Paris, pp 2537-2541, 1982.

13. Prato FS, Vinitski S, Radiation dose calculations for inhalation of Tc^{99m} sulfur colloid radioaerosol. J. nucl. Med. 24:816, 1983.

CEREBRAL FUNCTION

NEW AGENTS FOR PROBING GLUCOSE TURNOVER AND RECEPTOR DENSITIES IN THE BRAIN

G. KLOSTER, G. STÖCKLIN

INTRODUCTION

In vivo functional imaging of the brain has, in contrast to that of other organs like heart or liver, only developed in the last decade. This is mainly due to a special feature of brain physiology, namely the blood-brain-barrier (BBB). BBB selectively restricts the access to the brain of most non-lipophilic substances borne in blood; only a relatively small number of vital substrates are transported into the brain by specialized carrier system. Thus, most of the radio-pharmaceuticals available in the early days of nuclear medicine were excluded from the brain. Only in areas with a destroyed BBB (some tumours etc) was it possible to observe measurable concentrations e.g. of Tc^{99m}-compounds (1). This situation has dramatically changed recently with the application of metabolic tracers or analogs labelled with short-lived "organic" radionuclides. These radionuclides that form stable covalent binds to carbon, either the positron emitters ^{11}C ($T_{\frac{1}{2}}$ = 20 min), ^{18}F ($T_{\frac{1}{2}}$ = 110 min) and ^{75}Br ($T_{\frac{1}{2}}$ = 98 min) or the single photon emitter ^{123}I ($T_{\frac{1}{2}}$ = 13.3 h) can be introduced into most of the compounds important for the characteristic metabolism or function of the brain with acceptable alterations in their physico-chemical behaviour (2). They also lend themselves to 3-dimensional imaging, the positron emitters to positron-emission computed tomography (PECT) and the single photon emitters to single photon emission computed tomography (SPECT).

Using these radionuclides in conjunction with emission tomography for regional functional imaging of the brain, a biochemical approach will lead to the following classes of radiopharmaceutical:

- Metabolites and analogs
  D-glucose and analogs
  oxygen
  amino acids
- Receptor-specific radiopharmaceuticals
  neurotransmitters (dopamine, serotonin, etc)
  neurotransmitters antagonists (centrally acting drugs)
- Perfusion agents
  noble gases
  water, ammonia
  iodoantipyrine
  iodoamphetamine

This approach has also been named "in-vivo autoradiography"
and relies heavily on the results of classical in-vitro autoradiographic studies performed with ^{3}H and ^{14}C-labelled compounds. For the purpose of this review we shall restrict ourselves to D-glucose and its analogs and receptor-specific
radiopharmaceuticals.

D-GLUCOSE AND ITS ANALOGS

In contrast to all other organs, the brain meets its energy
needs exclusively by oxidative degradation of a single substrate
namely D-glucose. Thus, labelled derivatives of D-glucose (and
oxygen) are the only radiopharmaceuticals that allow the study
of brain energy metabolism. Consequently, a large number of
D-glucose analogs have been investigated as potential D-glucose
tracers, apart from D-glucose itself.

D-glucose is a hydrophilic molecule that cannot freely
enter the brain due to the restrictions of the BBB. There is,
however, a specialized carrier system for D-glucose, namely
the hexose carrier, that allows adequate glucose flux across
the BBB to maintain brain energy metabolism at a high level
(3). The hexose carrier imposes strict sterochemical requirements on D-glucose analogs that are transported across the
BBB: their electronegative substituents must be in the same
configuration as D-glucose itself, that is all-trans as well
as all-equatorial. In some positions, -OH-groups may be replaced by - H (giving the respective deoxy sugar) whereas

Table 1: D-Glucose analogs used or suggested as tracers for glucose metabolism or transport in-vivo

Compound	Synthesis (Ref.)	Model (Ref.)	Remarks
U-[^{11}C]-D-glucose	[4],[5],[9]	[6],[7]	quantitation difficult; tracer for overall glucose metabolism
2-[^{18}F]-2-deoxy-2-fluoro-D-glucose (2-FDG)	[15],[19],[20], [24],[26]	[17],[18]	well established tracer for transport and hexokinase (glucose utilization)
1-[^{11}C]-2-deoxy-D-glucose (2-FDG)	[36]	[13],[38]	shorter-lived alternative to 2-FDG
3-[^{11}C]-O-methyl-D-glucose (MG)	[39]	[41]	tracer for glucose transport only
2-[*Br]-2-deoxy-2-bromo-D-glucose (2-BDG)	[54]	-	low brain uptake, unknown mechanism
3-[^{18}F]-3-deoxy-3-fluoro-D-glucose (3-FDG)	[47]	-	low affinity substrate for hexo-kinase; difficult to treat quantitatively
3-[^{75}Br]-3-deoxy-3-bromo-D-glucose (3-BDG)	[53]	-	low brain uptake; unknown mechanism
2-[^{75}Br] methyl 3,4,6-tri-O-acetyl-2-deoxy-2-bromo-ß-D-glucopyranoside (MTBG)	[53]	-	possible longer-lived alternatives for MG as glucose transport tracer; carrier mediated uptake not yet demonstrated
2-[^{18}F]-2-deoxy-2-fluoro-3-O-methyl-D-glucose	[57]	-	

others are essential (3). Thus, all analogs studied so far
(table 1) have that particular configuration.

D-Glucose. Historically, the first compounds used as an
in-vivo tracer for glucose metabolism was U-(^{11}C)-D-glucose.
It was first prepared in 1971 by the St. Louis group (4,5)
using a photosynthetic procedure. They also used this compound
in conjunction with PECT to obtain tomographic images of
primate brains and also presented a mathematical model that
allowed computation of metabolic rates of glucose consumption
(6,7).

(^{11}C)-D-glucose has the advantage of identity with the
substrate to be traced. Thus, no corrections for different
affinities to carriers or enzymes have to be made. This greatly facilitates the data analysis. On the other hand, (^{11}C)-D-
glucose has a serious disadvantage: it is extensively metabolized via the glycolytic pathway yielding $^{11}CO_2$ and a number of
labelled compound that have been shown to be amino acids (8).
By this reutilization into amino acids the (^{11}C)-label remains
in the brain where it is indistinguishable from (^{11}C)-D-glucose
for the PECT. Thus assumptions have to made as to the extent
of this reutilization or data have to be taken at very short
intervals after administration which makes the interpretation
of the biodistribution data rather difficult.

Nevertheless, there is renewed interest in (^{11}C)-D-glucose
recently. An improved synthesis was presented (9,10), and
application of (^{11}C)-D-glucose in patient studies was also
reported (10,11). However, no solution to the inherent problems
of (^{11}C)-D-glucose metabolism has been put forward.
On the basis of animal experiments with (^{14}C)-D-glucose, an
elaborate sequence of injections of specifically labelled
(^{11}C)-D-glucoses ((3,4-^{11}C), (2,5-^{11}C), and 1-^{11}C) respectively) has been proposed in order to get meaningful information
on glucose metabolism (12). This sequence, however, seems very
difficult to implement with a short-lived radionuclide like
^{11}C.

2-Fluoro-2-deoxy-D-glucose. In order to avoid the problems
stemming from the extensive metabolism of D-glucose, a differ-

ent approach was proposed to develop a tracer that is involved
in only a few steps of the metabolic sequence. This approach
was first implemented by the NIMH group using (^{14}C)-2-deoxy-
D-glucose (2-DG) as a tracer for glucose metabolism in conjunction with rat brain autoradiography (13,14). The application of 2-DG is based on the fact that this analog is a competitive substrate of D-glucose on the hexose carrier at the
BBB while it is only metabolized in the first step of the
glycolytic pathway, namely the phosphorylation at C-6 by
hexokinase, thus forming an ionic compound that cannot leave
the brain. An extensive model was developed on this basis and
tested. It allows to calculate regional metabolic rates for
glucose directly from the isotope densities of the autoradiographs taken 45 min after (^{14}C)-2-DG application and the
arterial blood activity integrated over that time (13).

Adaptation of this technique to "in vivo autoradiography"
in patients for noninvasive measurement of glucose metabolic
rates made it necessary to introduce a version of 2-DG labelled
with a radionuclide that can be measured tomographically from
outside. The first such compound was 2-(^{18}F)-2-fluoro-2-deoxy-
D-glucose (2-FDG) which was introduced by the Brookhaven-group
in 1978 (15). Like 2-DG, 2-FDG is a substrate for the hexose
carrier at the BBB and a substrate for hexokinase. 2-FDG-6-
phosphate formed by the hexokinase reaction is a substrate for
neither phosphoglucose-isomerase nor glucose-6-phosphate
dehydrogenase; thus, it is effectively trapped in tissues low
in glucose-6-phosphates like brain and heart (16). Owing to
these attributes it can be used noninvasively in the same way
as 2-DG was used in autoradiographs. The same theory for
quantitation of regional cerebral glucose metabolism as for
2-DG can be applied for 2-FDG, provided some of the constants
specific for 2-DG are redetermined for 2-FDG. This theory has
been presented and was tested by two groups independently
(17,18).

The success of 2-FDG in neurological research that rapidly
followed its introduction increased the pressure on chemists
to devise syntheses that have higher yields than the 8-10%

observed for the original synthesis (15) by addition of $^{18}F_2$ (carrier added) to tri-O-acetyl-D-glucal, followed by isomer separation and hydrolysis of the protecting acetyl groups. A number of synthetic procedures has been tested towards this end (table 1). Two groups (19,20) independently used ^{18}F-labelled acetyl hypofluorite (prepared from ^{18}F-F_2 and acetate in acetic anhydride) as a tamed form of elemental fluorine. Acetyl hypofluorite adds to tri-O-acetyl-D-glucal and exclusively furnishes 1,3,4,6-tetra-C-acetyl-2-deoxy-2-(^{18}F)-fluoro-D-glucose without any of the manno-isomer. After hydrolysis of the acetyl-groups, 2-FDG is obtained in 20-25% yields (19, 20). Another form of tamed elemental fluorine, namely (^{18}F-XeF$_2$, has been used by two groups (21,22) to add fluorine across the double bond of tri-O-acetyl-D-glucal. Radiochemical yields for 2-FDG from (^{18}F)-XeF$_2$ were 15-20%; however, to make this a viable alternative to the acetyl hypofluorite method, a high yield method for preparation of large amounts of (^{18}F)-XeF$_2$ is mandatory.

Two other synthetic methods starting from (^{18}F)-fluoride ion have recently been reported (23-26). The use of fluoride ion as starting material has inherent advantages: maximum radiochemical yields of 100% are possible in contrast to methods starting from F_2, where only a 50% radiochemical yield is possible. Second, it can be used in a larger number of laboratories, since this is the only species obtainable from a low-energy one-particle cyclotron or a reactor. Most important, these methods have the principal advantage that high specific activity products can be obtained, although specific activity is generally not a physiological problem with 2-FDG. Both procedures use D-mannose derivatives protected with groups stable against nucleophilic substitution by fluoride ion on all hydroxyls except that on carbon 2. The first one (23,24) uses triflate on C-2 as a leaving group; however, one of the protecting groups, a methyl ether on C-3, is rather resistant against hydrolytic cleavage. Thus, harsh reaction conditions have to be used for hydrolysis and the overall radiochemical yield is rather low at 10%. The second one (25,26) uses a cyclic sulfate ester of C-2 and C-3 which selectively forms the 2-fluoro-3-sulfate by nucleophilic substitution. After hydrolysis of the protecting groups and chromatographic purification, 2-FDG was isolated in 70% radiochemical yield at a purity of 85% or 40% yield at a purity of >98% The purification, however, seems to be the most difficult part of this synthesis.

Routine production of large amounts of 2-FDG can only be carried out in lead cells using remotely controlled synthesis apparatures. Two such systems, based on the original 2-FDG synthesis (15), have been described (27,28). For large-scale synthesis, the acetyl hypofluorite method (19,20) or the method using nucleophilic substitution of the cyclic sulfate (25,26) seem to be the most promising due to the high yields obtained by these two methods.

The advent of 2-FDG as the first metabolic tracer for D-glucose that can be used noninvasively to obtain regionally quantitative metabolic rates for glucose in conjunction with PECT had a great impact on neurological research. Consequently, a large number of groups are engaged in extensive studies evaluating the clinical usefulness of 2-FDG in various states in normal controls and patients. It is beyond the scope of this review to provide even a list of the various investigations that have been performed; however, a number of recent reviews (29-32) may serve the interested reader to find his way into the original papers.

A point of continuing controversy in the quantification of 2-FDG tomography seems to be the value of the so-called lumped constant and/or the various rate constants in severe disease states. At present, these constants cannot all be calculated simultaneously from the data obtained in the patient study; thus, some have to be taken from investigations in normals. It is still open to question whether this is permissible and how accurate quantitative data are in severely diseased patients. This problem is addressed in experimental investigations (for example 33) in various laboratories.

Occasionally, basic assumptions of the 2-DG model have

been questioned in the literature (34,35). Alterations of the
model (18) have taken into account some of these objections
(34). Nevertheless, quantitative values obtained by the 2-DG
and 2-FDG method correlate well with global metabolic data
obtained by classical physiological techniques.

   2-Deoxy-D-glucose. The relatively long physical half-life
of ^{18}F (110 min) allows shipment of 2-FDG to distant laboratories for use at a site not having a cyclotron. On the other
hand, this long half-life in combination with the long biological half-time of 2-FDG-6-phosphate in the brain severely
restricted repeat studies in humans; they could at best be
performed on consecutive days. The use of ^{11}C-labelled 2-deoxy-
D-glucose (2-DG), however, makes these repeat studies possible
after a 2 hour interval due to the short half-life of ^{11}C
(20 min). Thus, (1-^{11}C)-2-DG has been synthetized from H^{11}CN
and a suitably protected arabinitol derivative (36), followed
by a reduction of the nitrile to the corresponding alcohol.
Radiochemical yields of 30-40% have been obtained with a
synthesis time of 45 min. The quality control of 2-DG was
studied in detail (37).

   Studies in humans showed that the coefficient of variation
for repeated measurements of regional glucose metabolism with
2-DG was 5.5 - 8.7% for various gray matter structures and
9.7 - 14.0% for white matter structures (38). The authors
conclude that the pattern of cerebral metabolic rates is
relatively constant in a given individual when the conditions
of the study are unchanged.

   Thus, 2-DG seems to be preferable to 2-FDG for institutions
having an on-site cyclotron since a) the patient can be used
as his own control in repeat measurements and b) radiation
dose to the patient is lower for 2-DG.

   3-0-Methyl-D-glucose. Studies using 2-FDG and 2-DG for the
determination of regional cerebral metabolic rates for glucose
give an average metabolic rate over the time needed for the
study (around 45-60 min). Rapid changes during this interval
will be averaged out. Using a glucose analog that will not be
metabolically trapped inside the cell one should principally

be able to monitor such rapid changes. Such a glucose analog
is 3-0-methyl-D-glucose (MG). MG is a substrate for the hexose
carrier at the BBB (3), but does not enter any of the metabolic
reactions of the glycolytic pathway. MG is eliminated unchanged
from the body.

Based on these facts, we at Jülich chose $(3-^{11}C)$-MG as a
glucose analog to trace transport only (39). MG was synthesized
from (^{11}C)-CH_3I and the potassium salt of 1,2:5,6-diisopropyl-
idene-D-glucose, a glucose derivative fully protected on all
hydroxyls except that on C-3. After hydrolysis of the ketal
groups and chromatographic purification, MG was obtained in
35% radiochemical yield with a synthesis time of 30 min (39).
A remotely controlled highly shielded apparatus for large-
scale synthesis was also described (40).

Investigations in normals and patients showed that MG is
distributed in a manner expected for a glucose transport
tracer, having a constant cortex-to-blood concentration ratio
of about 0.8 later than 6 min following administration (41).
Similar to 2-FDG, functional defects not visible in the CT-
scan were demonstrated (42).

A compartmental model for quantitation of regional cerebral
glucose transport rate analogous to the 2-DG model (13) was
developed and tested in patients (41,43,44). Although the
model contains assumptions that were extrapolated from
studies in small mammals or were introduced to simplify the
numerical treatment, which still have to be proven by independent measurements, glucose transport seems to correlate satisfactorily with data obtained by classical physiological measurements.

Apart from giving data for the regional undirectional
glucose transport rate constants at the BBB, MG may also be
used to obtain in vivo values of regional glucose content of
the brain, as suggested by data determined autoradiographically
in rat brain (45). These data may also be important for the
2-FDG and 2-DG model, since they can be used to get a better
estimate of the value of the lumped constant and the amount of
non-phosphorylated 2-FDG or 2-DG in the tissue (46). Studies

along these lines are in progress in humans.

3-Fluoro-3-deoxy-D-glucose. Another potential glucose
analog whose properties are intermediate between 2-FDG or 2-DG
and MG is 3-fluoro-3-deoxy-D-glucose (3-FDG). Again, 3-FDG is
a substrate for the hexose carrier at the BBB; it is, however,
only a poor substrate for hexokinase. Thus, it was claimed to
be an alternative glucose transport tracer.

(^{18}F)-3-FDG was synthetized by nucleophilic substitution
of 3-0-trifluoromethansulphonyl-1,2:5,6-diisopropylidene-D-
allose with (^{18}F)-fluoride ion. A radiochemical yield of 15%
was obtained after hydrolysis of the protecting groups and
chromatography. Synthesis and biodistribution data were first
published by the St. Louis group (47) and later republished by
others (49,50).

Biodistribution data show a rather prolonged retention of
the tracer 3-FDG in the brain (47,48) indicating significant
phosphorylation by hexokinase resulting in trapped 3-FDG-6-
phosphate. Compared to 2-FDG, however, the phosphorylation
rate was rather low (51).

Thus, 3-FDG does not seem to be a viable alternative either
for 2-FDG as a metabolic tracer since phosphorylation rate
was too low for this purpose or for MG as a glucose transport
tracer since the phosphorylation rate was too high for that
purpose (51).

Brominated and iodinated D-glucose analogs. Several attempts
have been made to synthesized Br- and I-labelled analogs of
D-glucose. All attempts to prepare an injectable solution of
2-iodo-2-deoxy-D-glucose (labelled with either ^{123}I or ^{131}I)
failed completely (52,53). 2-Bromo-2-deoxy-D-glucose was prepared labelled with ^{82}Br, but the biodistribution data were
inferior to those of 2-FDG (54).

3-Bromo-3-deoxy-D-glucose and 3-iodo-3-deoxy-D-glucose
were prepared (53) labelled with ^{77}Br or ^{123}I, but again biodistribution data were disappointing (55). The methyl glucosides
of both 2-bromo-2-deoxy-D-glucose and 2-iodo-2-deoxy-D-glucose
were also prepared (53), but again biodistribution data, though
better than for the 3-deoxy sugars, were not encouraging (55).

2-Bromo-2-deoxy-D-glucosyl bromide, synthesized by Br_2 addition (^{82}Br) to D-glucal, was claimed to accumulate in brain; however, nothing is known about in vivo stability of the label (56).

Finally, two compounds obtained as intermediates in syntheses aimed at other D-glucose analogs, namely methyl 3,4,6-trio-0-acetyl-2-bromo-2-deoxyde-D-glucoside (53,55) and 2-deoxy-2-fluoro-3-0-methyl-D-glucose (57) may be potential longer-lived alternatives as D-glucose transport tracers to MG. Both can be radiolabelled in good yields and have biodistribution data similar to MG. However, more basic biochemical work is mandatory for both to prove that they are substrates for the hexose carrier at the BBB, a feature necessary for a D-glucose transport tracer.

D-glucose analogs: summing up. 2-FDG is the most widely used and the most thouroughly evaluated sugar among the many D-glucose analogs investigated. Actually, it is the workhorse for in vivo determination of glucose metabolic rates in the brain. 2-DG will most probably be the preferable tracer for all institutions having an in-house cyclotron. Both compounds yield the same biological information.

Other compounds that have already been tested clinically and seem promising tracers are MG and D-glucose itself. Both these compounds trace biochemical mechanisms that are clearly different from each other and 2-FDG or 2-DG. MG isolates the transport step at the BBB, 2-FDG and 2-DG record the effects of transport and the hexokinase reaction, while D-glucose yields an overall picture of the glycolytic pathway including reutilization of CO_2. Thus these tracers seem to be complimentary rather than competitive in the long run. In disease states it may be necessary to study alterations at different steps of glucose metabolism with different radioactive tracers, including a perfusion tracer, to obtain an in-depth understanding of the underlying pathology. Nevertheless, 2-FDG or 2-DG will probably remain the D-glucose tracer most widely used.

RECEPTOR-SPECIFIC RADIOPHARMACEUTICALS

Nerve conduction in the mammalian CNS is a process of both electrical and chemical transmission. While the impulse is transmitted electrically along the nerve cell body, it has to be altered into a chemical signal to bridge the synaptic cleft between two neurons. Different chemical substances called neuro-transmitters are used in different areas of the brain and for excitatory as well as inhibitory neurons. After being released into the synaptic cleft the neurotransmitters (i.e. dopamine), serotonin or GABA) bind to specific receptors at the postsynaptic membrane to again effect an electrical nerve impulse. Altered binding of neurotransmitters to their respective receptors or altered response of the receptors to their neurotransmitters have been involved in a large number of neurological diseases. Thus, in vivo studies of regional receptor densities and/or their binding characteristics is an important field in experimental neurology.

Receptors respond very specifically to chemical structures and bind very selectively certain molecules while rejecting others. Their specificity can be compared to that of enzymes. But a number of chemically different substances, so-called receptor antagonists, are known to also specifically bind to the receptor without effecting signal transmission. These antagonists only inhibit the binding of agonists (neurotrans-mitters).

Most of the drugs used in the treatment of neurological disorders are antagonists for one or more neurotransmitter receptors. All of them have a structure totally different from the corresponding receptor agonists. They are rather lipophilic molecules that can cross the BBB by passive diffusion due to their lipophilicity (58-60). An octanol: water partition coeeficient (P) of 0.5 or more is the minimal requirement for efficient penetration into the brain (59), while a P of about 100 yields optimum brain concentrations (58,60) for a number of structurally different drugs.

Apart from lipophilicity a number of other important criteria have to be fulfilled for a successful receptor-specific radiopharmaceutical (for a recent review see 61): (a) they should have high specific binding to a single receptor while having far lower specific binding to all other receptors; (b) they should have a high specific (receptor) to nonspecific (membrane solubility, protein binding) binding ratio; (c) as specific binding is saturable while nonspecific binding is not, high specific activities for radiolabelled receptor-specific tracers are mandatory (62). Specific activities of larger than 500 Ci/mmol seem to be desirable.

It is very difficult to obtain such high specific activities with either ^{11}C or electrophilic ^{18}F for various reasons. The use of either nca (^{18}F)-fluoride in nucleophilic reactions or nca ^{75}Br (63) will yield high specific activity products. Chemically, the use of ^{75}Br is advantageous in large molecules usually containing aromatic rings like most receptor antagonists.

For preparation of these high specific activity radiopharmaceuticals labelled regiospecifically in positions that do not interfere with receptor binding, radiohalogenation methods are mandatory that allow labelling in specified positions at extremely high specific activities. Radiochemical procedures towards this end have recently been reviewed for the heavy halogens ^{75,77}Br and ^{123}I (64).

The collection of receptor-specific radiopharmaceuticals treated in more detail below (table 2) is by no means complete. We present here a selection of compounds which we feel show the greatest promise for in vivo mapping of receptors in conjunction with PECT.

Dopamine receptor. Dopamine receptor involvement has been invoked in a number of neurological diseases like schizophrenia, Parkinson's disease, Huntington's chorea or tardive diskinesia. Thus, this receptor has attracted much interest recently in investigations aimed at monitoring its density in various brain regions in vivo.

Dopamine receptors in the mammalian brain have the highest density in the corpus striatum and low density in most other regions, especially the cerebellum. A promising radiopharmaceutical for in vivo mapping of the dopamine receptor, thus, le 2: Selected compounds investigated as receptor-specific radiopharmaceuticals or neurotransmitter analog tracers.

Dopamine receptor:

	synthesis (ref.)	spec. activity (Ci/mmol)	biodistribution (ref.)	remarks
F]-Haloperidol	[67]	$\sim 10^5$	[70]	constant striatum: cerebellum ratio; no receptor-specific binding
C]-Spiroperidol	[71],[72]	650	[72]	binding receptor-specific and displaceable; monkey data
F]-Spiroperidol	[73],[70]	nca	[70]	
C]-N-Methyl-spiroperidol	[75]	10-263	[75]	binding receptor-specific and displaceable; monkey and human data
Br]-p-Bromo-spiro-idol	[78],[79]	80-140	[76],[77],[79],[80]	binding receptor-specific and displaceable; human data; isotope not optimal
Br]-Bromobenperidol	[82],[82]	> 8000	[81],[82]	binding receptor-specific and displaceable; preliminary monkey data
C]-Pimozide	[83]	20-295	-84]	binding receptor-specific and displaceable; human patient data (dynamic)

2: continued

__amine analog tracers:__

	synthesis (ref.)	spec. activity (Ci/mmol)	biodistribution (ref.)	remarks
-DL-DOPA	[85],[86]	not relevant	[87]	cold-spot agent; not very suitable for PECT due to partial volume effect
-6-Fluoro-DOPA	[88]	not relevant	[89],[90]	monkey and human data
__rotonin receptor:__				
-Ketanserin	[91]	25o	[91]	only mouse data available
-Mesulergin	[92]	1o	-	only preliminary biodistribution data available
__nzodiazepine receptor:__				
-Flunitrazepam	[93]	3oo-9oo	[93],[94]	binding receptor-specific and displaceable; monkey data
l-Ro 15-1788	[94]			
e]-7-Bromobenzo- epine (BFB/see text)	[95]	> 2o.ooo	[95]	binding not displaceable by Ro 15-1788 in monkeys

able 2: continued

) Acetylcholine receptor:

	synthesis (ref.)	spec. activity (Ci/mmol)	biodistribution (ref.)	remarks
123I] 4-Iodo-uinuclidinyl-enzilate	[99]	9oo-12oo	[98]	species differences in receptor specificity; human data available (SPECT)
123I] 3-Iodo-4-ydroxi-quinuclidinyl enzilate	[97]	71-17o	[97]	calf brain data; binding displaceable; agent not ideal

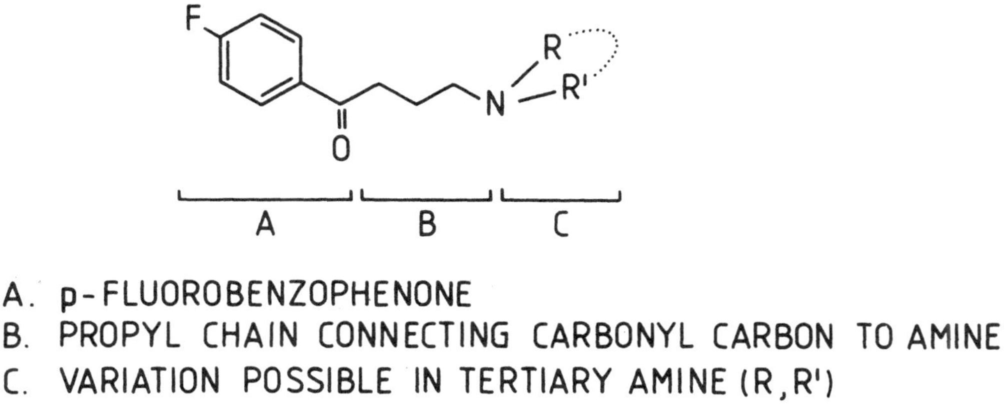

A. p-FLUOROBENZOPHENONE
B. PROPYL CHAIN CONNECTING CARBONYL CARBON TO AMINE
C. VARIATION POSSIBLE IN TERTIARY AMINE (R,R')

Fig. 1. General structure of butyrophenone neuroleptics. A,B: parts essential for receptor recognition. C: part not essential for receptor recognition.

should be highly concentrated in the striatum and have a high striatum: cerebellum concentration ratio. Furthermore, the specific binding to the receptor should be long-lasting and largely independent of blood concentrations, while non-specific binding should be of shorter duration and coupled to blood concentrations of the radiopharmaceutical. Thus, target-to-nontarget ratios are expected to be higher at later time intervals.

   Among the neuroleptic drugs used in the treatment of disease states ascribed to dopamine receptor interactions, the butyrophenone class has found the greatest interest as potential radiopharmaceuticals for the dopamine receptor. Only part of their structure is essential for receptor binding while considerable variation is possible in the nonessential part of the molecule (fig 1). Many of the butyrophenone neuroleptics show high specificity for the dopamine-D_2-receptor with affinities to the serotonin-S_2-receptor being next while they do not bind to most of the other neurotransmitter receptors. The higher the specificity for one receptor over all the others, the

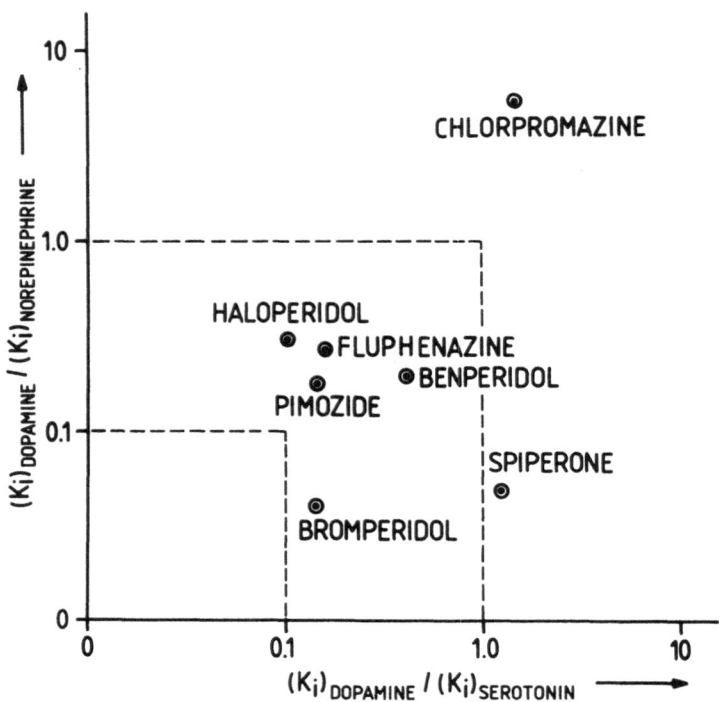

Fig. 2. Relative affinity constants of neuroleptics for the dopamine and competitive receptors (in vitro data for rat brain homogenate, ref. 102).

higher is the expected chance for that compound as a receptor-specific radiopharmaceutical (fig 2).

Haloperidol (HP), labelled with ^{18}F (^{18}F-for-^{19}F) in the part of the molecule that is essential for receptor binding, has first been prepared in 1975 by decomposition of a diazonium salt in the presence of (^{18}F)-fluoride ion (65). The specific activity of this preparation was very low ($\sim$ 2Mci/mmol). It was also used in biodistribution studies; however, only organ radioactivity contents were reported which give no information on possible receptor-specific binding (66). The first synthesis of (^{18}F)-HP using nca (^{18}F)-fluoride was performed in 1980 by triazene decomposition (67). Specific activity was high ($\sim 10^5$ Ci/mmol) although the yields seemed rather low. In bio-distribution studies using a single collimated detector, different uptake and elimination patterns in the brain were noted before and after a therapeutic dose of haloperidol (67). This was attributed to a significant fraction of (^{18}F)-HP bound to specific receptors in the brain. However, no detailed regional distribution data were available. Another study using (^{18}F)-HP at low specific activity (40 mCi/mmol) prepared by the Balz-Schiemann reaction reported extremely high brain uptake in mouse brain (69). Examination of the original data (68), however, raised serious doubts whether the methods used for determination of this extraordinarily high brain uptake are adequate for the problem investigated. As they contradict all data obtained by more suitable methods they should only be used with extreme criticism. Finally, (^{18}F)-HP was prepared by nucleophilic (^{18}F)-fluoride for -NO$_2$ exchange at high specific activities and compared to (^{18}F)-spiroperidol (SP) in rat studies (70). These authors conclude that no receptor-specific binding is observable for HP (constant striatum: cerebellum ratio) while specific binding is observed for SP.

Spiroperidol (SP) was labelled with (^{11}C) (71,72) or (^{18}F) (73) in the part essential for receptor binding by a sequence of radioactive synthetic steps similar to total synthesis of SP. Yields for nca (^{18}F)-SP from (^{18}F)-fluoride were 8-10% (73), while those for (^{11}C)-SP from (^{11}C)-CN were 20-30% at a specific activity of 650 Ci/mmol at the end of synthesis (71). In biodistribution studies in rats, specific binding was demonstrated (a) by the high striatum: cerebellum ratio of 4 after 60 min (72) or 10.6 after 120 min (70) and (b) by the displacement of SP from specific binding sites by excess (+)-butaclamol which is a dopamine receptor antagonist, but not by excess (-)-butaclamol which is not an antagonist (72). In a monkey study in conjunction with PECT the striatum was clearly visualized by SP labelled with either (^{18}F) (70,74) or (^{11}C) (74); furthermore the activity in the striatum could be displaced by injection of excess (+)-butaclamol (74).

HP and SP were the only butyrophenone neuroleptics labelled isotopically in the part essential for molecular recognition by the receptor. A number of other compounds was reported for the same purpose where the label was in the part nonessential

108

for binding. Some of these molecules are different from the
neuroleptics used therapeutically.

3-N-methyl-spiroperidol (NMSP) was prepared by methylation
with (^{11}C)-methyl iodide of spiroperidol. No yields were given
but specific activities ranged from 263 Ci/mmol to 10 Ci/mmol
(75). Biodistribution studies in monkeys using PECT clearly
visualized the striatum 40-60 min after NMSP administration.
Coinjection of a therapeutic dose of SP along with (^{11}C)-
NMSP displaced the activity from the striatum. In a human, the
striatum was clearly visible 40-60 and 70-130 min after NMSP
administration. Striatum: cerebellum ratios observed were
2.03 at 60 min for the monkey and 4.4 at 130 min in the human
(75).

p-Bromospiroperidol (BSP) has been labelled with ^{77}Br by
electrophilic bromination of SP with nca ^{77}Br (78,79). Radiochemical yields of 80 to 90% were obtained. Specific activities
reported were 80-140 Ci/mmol (78). BSP reached rather high
concentrations in rat striata with striatum: cerebellum ratios
peaking at 6.3 8 hours after BSP administration (76). For
the rat brain, striatum: cerebellum ratios of 3.8 were observed
5 hours after BSP administration (77). The radioactivity was
displaceable from the specific binding sites by either SP (76)
or α-flupenthixol (79) indicating receptor-specific binding.
In a human, selective BSP uptake in the striatum was demonstrated using ^{77}Br and SPECT (80). However, ^{77}Br is an isotope
difficult to detect in good spatial resolution in SPECT since
it has an abundant high-energy γ-line. Furthermore, the use of
^{77}Br results in rather high radiation doses due to the long
half-life (56 hours) of the isotope. ^{75}Br in conjunction with
PECT is a better choice for in vivo imaging.

At Jülich, we are investigating the suitability of a ^{75}Br-
labelled butyrophenone neuroleptic, namely (^{75}Br)-bromben-
peridol (BBP), as a dopamine receptor-specific radiopharmaceutical (81,82). BBP is a derivative of benperidol which is more
selective for the dopamine receptor than SP. BBP was synthetized
by electrophilic bromination of benperidol using (^{75}Br)-
bromide and dichloramine T; bromination takes place in the
aromatic ring at the site nonessential for receptor binding.

Yields of 40% were obtained using nca (^{75}Br)- or (^{77}Br)-bromide
(81,82). The specific activity observed was larger than 8000
Ci/mmol (82). In biodistribution studies in rats BBP reached
higher brain radioactivity concentrations than HP or SP.
Binding in the striatum was displaceable by an excess of unlabelled benperidol indicating receptor-specific binding. The
striatum: cerebellum ratio rose to 3 at 120 min and 4 at 240
min after BBP administration (82). Preliminary investigations
using BBP in vivo in monkeys in conjunction with PECT are
encouraging.

Although not strictly a butyrophenone neuroleptic, pimozide
bears great structural similarity to this class of compounds.
Again, it is more selective for the dopamine receptor than SP.
Pimozide was labelled with ^{11}C via (^{11}C)-$COCl_2$ by phosgenation
of a suitable precursor. Radiochemical yields of 20% from
(^{11}C)-CO_2 were obtained. Specific activities reported were
20-295 Ci/mmol, which is rather high for (^{11}C)-compounds (83).
Studies in patients in conjunction with PECT (84) demonstrated
that pimozide is taken up in the brain. The regional kinetics
in the striatum and cerebellum were different during 60 min
after administration. Although this difference was small the
authors found it to be significant. Coadministration of a
therapeutic dose of cold HP abolished this different behaviour.
Striatum: cerebellum concentration ratios, however, were not
significantly different from 1 in untreated patients, casting
some doubt on the claim that binding is receptor-specific. A
relatively large amount of nonspecific binding may be the
reason for this fact (84). Nevertheless, to our knowledge this
is the only study presenting dynamic data in patients for a
receptor-specific radiopharmaceutical.

Two potential radiopharmaceuticals also have to be mentioned
at this point, altough they are not directly dopamine receptor-
specific compounds. However, they may be useful compounds for
tracing specific components of the dopaminergic system. These
two compounds are $(1-^{11}C)$-DOPA and (^{18}F)-6-fluoro-DOPA, respectively. For this purpose, high specific activity compounds
are not necessary since DOPA is present in relatively large

quantities in blood.

DOPA was prepared by carboxylation with (^{11}C)-CO_2 of a suitably protected isonitrile precursor via the Li-salt. After hydrolysis of the protecting groups and purification, yields of 25-30% were obtained for DL-DOPA (85,86). A method for preparation of the isometric D- or L-DOPA was described recently; yields of up to 3-5% were obtained for the different isomers (not corrected for decay) (86). DOPA is a prodrug for dopamine and is used therapeutically in Parkinson's disease. To prevent decarboxylation of DOPA at the BBB a peripheral DOPA-decarboxylase inhibitor has to be coinjected. Studies using the same protocol in rats showed that less radioactivity was found in the striatum due to loss of (^{11}C)-CO_2 from the C-1 position by action of striatal DOPA-decarboxylase (87). This approach, a cold-spot technique, however, was not implemented further since a cold-spot technique for a small brain structure (striatum) is not particularly favorable in conjunction with PECT due to partial volume effects.

For these reasons, 6-fluoro-DOPA is expected to be a superior prodrug for dopamine and, consequently, a tracer for regional cerebral dopamine content since on decarboxylation the label will be retained in the dopamine analog formed, namely 6-fluoro-dopamine. After they had previously investigated 5-fluoro-DOPA the Hamilton group recently changed their interest towards 6-fluoro-DOPA as the superior compound. L-6-(^{18}F)-fluoro-DOPA was synthesized by (^{18}F)-fluorination with (^{18}F)-XeF_2 of L-3-methoxy-4-hydroxy-phenylalanine methylester. Subsequent removal of the protecting groups yielded L-6-fluoro-DOPA (88). No radiochemical yields were reported. In a monkey study in conjunction with PECT, the striatum was clearly visualized as a site of dopamine storage; the 6-fluoro-dopamine formed on decarboxylation probably acts as a false neurotransmitter. After administration of Ro 4-4046 a DOPA-decarboxylase inhibitor, twice the amount of radioactivity was accumulated in the striata, while after administration of reserpine, which discharges dopamine from its neuronal storage sites, the concentration of radioactivity in the striatum was reduced by

50% (90). This seems to be sufficient evidence that 6-fluoro-
dopamine, formed from the prodrug 6-fluoro-DOPA, is a suitable
tracer for dopamine. In a human, the striatum was clearly
delineated 3 hours after 6-fluoro-DOPA administration substant-
iating the monkey data obtained previously (89).

Other cerebral receptors. Effects of serotonin have been
hypothesized in a number of neurological diseases like sleep
disorders, affective disorders and migraine. Thus, ligands
for in vivo mapping of the serotonin receptor seem desirable.
Many dopamine receptor antagonists have high affinity towards
the serotonin receptor as well. Thus, selective serotonin
receptor-specific radiopharmaceuticals can be expected to
also be useful agents for differentiation in dopamine receptor
studies.

Ketanserin is a new investigational drug that is rather
selective to serotonin-S_2-receptor sites in vitro. The synthesis of (^{11}C)-ketanserin by phosgenation using (^{11}C)-$COCl_2$
of a suitably substituted diamino-compound was recently described (91). Radiochemical yields of 25-50% from (^{11}C)-CO_2
were obtained. Specific activities of up to 250 Ci/mmol were
observed. The biodistribution in mice showed brain uptake and
cerebellum: cerebrum ratios similar to (^{3}H)-ketanserin (91).
No data from larger mammals are available yet.

Mesulergin is another new investigational drug that is
rather selective for the serotonin-S_2-receptor in vitro. We
labelled mesulergin, an ergoline derivative, on N-6 with ^{11}C
via (^{11}C)-CH_3I by methylation of the N_6-desmethyl compound.
Radiochemical yields obtained were 40-50% at a specific activity of about 10 Ci/mmol. Preliminary in vivo investigations
in monkeys, based on the data obtained in (^{3}H)-mesulergin
(100) studies in animals, showed encouraging results (92).

Benzodiazepines are a class of widely used centrally acting
tranquilizers. They are hypothesized to act at central benzo-
diapine receptors coupled to the inhibitory GABA neuronal
pathways. Thus, labelled benzodiazepines are potential tools
for studying receptor changes in anxiety and other states.

Flunitrazepam (FN) is an agonistic ligand with high

affinity to the benzodiazepine receptor. Like all other benzodiazepines, it is highly selective towards the benzodiazepine
receptor and almost exclusively binds to this receptor. FN was
labelled with ^{11}C at the N-1 position via (^{11}C)-CH$_3$I alkyla-
tion of the corresponding nor-compound. Specific activities of
300-900 Ci/mmol were obtained (93). Good brain uptake of FN
was observed in biodistribution studies in baboons using PECT,
with a rather homogeneous distribution through the brain
corresponding to the similar concentrations of benzodiazepine
receptors in many brain structures. Displacement studies using
lorazepam as displacer showed a relatively slight displacement
(93,94). Using Ro-15-1788, a benzodiazepine antagonist, also
labelled with ^{11}C, in a monkey, brain radioactivity was dramatic·
ally displaced using unlabelled Ro-15-1788 as displacer (94).
Thus, the antagonist clearly has advantages over the agonist.

As very high specific activity compounds can only be
prepared using appropriate halogen radionuclides like ^{75}Br, we
have investigated 7-(^{75}Br)-bromo-5-(2-fluorophenyl)-1-methyl-1,
3-dihydro-2H-1,4-benzodiazepin-2-one (BFB) as a benzodiazepine
agonist. BFB was labelled with ^{75}Br from (^{75}Br)-bromide and a
piperidyl triazene prepared from the corresponding 7-amino-
benzodiazepine. Radiochemical yields in this Wallach reaction
were 25% with a specific activity of > 20,000 Ci/mmol (95).
Biodistribution in mice showed rapid BFB uptake into brain
and retention in the brain at useful concentrations for a
significant period of time (95). In a monkey study using PECT,
BFB taken up into brain was not displaceable by unlabelled
Ro-15-1788, although in vitro studies had shown high affinity
to the benzodiazepine receptor (unpublished results, see 95).
Thus, the reasons for BFB brain uptake seem different from
receptor-specific binding.

Finally, attempts have been made to visualize specific
binding to the muscarinic acetylcholine receptor with compounds
labelled with ^{123}I and SPECT (96-99). The compound used was
4-iodo-quinuclidinyl benzilate (4-IQNB) which shows higher
binding to the receptor than the non-iodinated QNB (96) or
its 3-iodo-4-OH derivative (97). 4-IQNB was synthetized by

triazene decomposition in the presence of (^{123}I)- or (^{125}I)-
iodide; the yield in this Wallach reaction was 20%. Specific
activities stated were 900-1200 Ci/mmol for ^{125}I (99). Biodistribution data in calf brain with 3-I-4-OH-QNB (97) or
humans with 4-IQNB (98) using SPECT show a distinct regional
distribution that seems to be related to regional receptor
concentration. In the rat, however, 4-IQNB does not provide
localization in striatum and cerebellum that is consistent
with the concentration of receptor in these areas (99). The
reason for these obvious species differences is still unclear.

Receptor-specific radiopharmaceuticals: summing up.
In contrast to the situation for the D-glucose analogs, the
field of receptor-specific radiopharmaceuticals is still in
its infancy. Many compounds still bear promise as suitable
receptor-specific tracers, and no quantitative model has yet
been presented for any of these tracers investigated. Actually,
only very few studies have been performed in a dynamic mode
yielding time-dependent data on regional concentrations of
these radiopharmaceuticals. Most of the studies reported in
the literature have accumulated data for very long time intervals in order to obtain a static image of receptor areas with
the greatest possible contrast. Again, most of the studies
presented static images of normal healthy volunteers; only
very few data on patients were reported. Agents used pharma-
cologically for the treatment of neurological diseases are not
specific for a single receptor; on the contrary, some of them,
like SP, have nearly equal binding constants for two different
receptors. So, further progress in pharmacology to demonstrate
receptor-specific pharmaceuticals will certainly fertilize
the development of receptor-specific radiopharmaceuticals.
Even if a compound that is specific for a single receptor is
not a suitable pharmaceutical owing to possible side-reactions,
it will be a desirable development to implement in the area of
radiopharmaceuticals, since these are used in small doses and
only intermittently.

The results obtained so far with non-ideal receptor-specific
radiopharmaceuticals are highly encouraging. Undoubtedly, they

will enhance our knowledge of receptor involvement in neurological diseases. Apart from the development of more specific
radiopharmaceuticals, a theory to interpret dynamic changes in
the pharmacokinetics of receptor-specific radiopharmaceuticals
has to be developed most urgently to obtain quantitative data
that can be compared among different groups in the field.
Furthermore, more research is needed to obtain higher specific
activity compounds for these investigations, particularly in
the case of carbon-11 and fluorine-18. In the latter case
improved nca aromatic radiofluorination methods are also
needed. Ultra-high-specific activity compounds, however, may
not be needed for in vivo receptor studies, since there are
indications that optimum target-to-nontarget ratios should be
obtained at intermediate specific activities (99,101).

ACKNOWLEDGEMENT

We thank Dr S.M. Moerlein for valuable discussions on
receptor-specific radiopharmaceuticals and for the design of
figures 1 and 2.

REFERENCES

1. Oldendorf WH, Nuclear medicine in clinical neurology: an update. Ann. Neurol. 10:207, 1981.

2. Stöcklin G, Kloster G, Metabolic analogue tracers. In: Computed emission tomography. Ell PJ, Holman BL (eds), Oxford, Oxford University Press, pp 299-338, 1982.

3. Pardridge WM, Oldendorf WH, Kinetics of blood-brain barrier transport of hexoses. Biochim. biophys. Acta 382:377, 1975.

4. Lifton JF, Welch MJ, Preparation of glucose labeled with 20-minute half-lived carbon-11. Radiat. Res. 45:35, 1971.

5. Straatmann M, Welch MJ, The liquid chromatographic purification of carbon-11 labeled glucose. Int. J. appl. Radiat. Isot. 24:234, 1973.

6. Raichle ME, Larson KB, Phelps ME, Grubb RL, Welch MJ, Ter-Pogossian MM, In vivo measurement of brain glucose transport and metabolism employing glucose-[11]C. Amer. J. Physiol. 228:1936, 1975.

7. Raichle ME, Welch MJ, Grubb RL, Higgins CS, Ter-Pogossian MM, Larson KB, Measurement of regional substrate utilization rates by emission tomography. Science 199:986, 1978.

8. Jones SC, Ackerman RH, Hoop B, Baron JC, Brownell GL, Taveras JM, Brain uptake and organ distribution of ^{11}C from ^{11}C-labeled glucose. Int. J. Nucl. Med. Biol. 10:173, 1983.

9. Ehrin E, Westman E, Nilsson SO, Nilsson JLG, Widen L, Greitz T, Larson CM, Tillberg JE, Malmborg P, A convenient method for production of ^{11}C-labelled glucose. J. Lab. Comp. Radiopharm. 17:453, 1980.

10. Ehrin E, Stone-Elander S, Nilsson JLG, Bergström M, Blomqvist G, Brisman T, Eriksson L, Greitz T, Jansson PE, Litton JE, Malmborg P, af Ugglas M, Widen L, C-11-labeled glucose and its utilization in positron-emission tomography. J. nucl. Med. 24:326, 1983.

11. Bergström M, Collins VP, Ehrin E, Ericson K, Eriksson L, Greitz T, Halldin C, Von Holst H, Langström B, Lilja A, Lundqvist H, Nagren K, Discrepancies in brain tumor extent as shown by computed tomography and positron emission tomography using (^{68}Ga) EDTA, (^{11}C) glucose and (^{11}C) methionine. J. Comput. Assist. Tomogr. 7:1062, 1983.

12. Sacks W, Sacks S, Badalamenti A, Fleischer A, A proposed method for the determination of cerebral regional intermediary glucose metabolism in humans in vivo using specifically labeled ^{11}C-glucose and positron emission transverse tomography (PETT). I. An animal model with ^{14}C-glucose and rat brain autoradiography. J. Neurosci. Res. 7:57, 1982.

13. Sokoloff L, Reivich M, Kennedy C, DesRosiers MH, Patlak CS, Pettigrew KD, Sakurada O, Shinohara M, The (^{14}C) deoxyglucose method for the measurement of local cerebral glucose utilization: theory, procedure and normal values in the conscious and anesthetized albino rat. J. Neurochem. 28:897, 1977.

14. Sokoloff L, Localization of functional activity in the central nervous system by measurement of glucose utilization with radioactive deoxy-glucose. J. Cereb. Blood Flow Metabol. 1:7, 1981.

15. Ido T, Wan CN, Casella V, Fowler JS, Wolf AP, Reivich M, Kuhl DE, Labeled 2-deoxy-D-glucose analogs. ^{18}F-labeled 2-deoxy-2-fluoro-D-

16. Gallagher BM, Fowler JS, Gutterson NI, MacGregor RR, Wan CN, Wolf AP, Metabolic trapping as a principle of radiopharmaceutical design: Some factors responsible for the biodistribution of (^{18}F) 2-deoxy-2-fluoro-D-glucose. J. nucl. Med. 19:1154, 1978.

17. Reivich M, Kuhl D, Wolf A, Greenberg J, Phelps M, Ido T, Casella V, Fowler J, Hoffman E, Alavi A, Som P, Sokoloff L, The (^{18}F) fluoro-deoxyglucose method for the measurement of local cerebral glucose utilization in man. Circulat. Res. 44:127, 1979.

18. Phelps ME, Huang SC, Hoffman EJ, Selin C, Sokoloff L, Kuhl DE, Tomographic measurement of local cerebral glucose metabolic rate in humans with (F-18) 2-fluoro-2-deoxy-D-glucose: Validation of method. Ann. Neurol. 6:371, 1979.

19. Shiue CY, Salvadori PA, Wolf AP, Fowler JS, MacGregor RR, A new improved synthesis of 2-deoxy-2(^{18}F)fluoro-D-glucose from ^{18}F-labeled acetyl hypofluorite. J. nucl. Med. 23:899, 1982.

20. Diksic M, Jolly D, New high-yield synthesis of ^{18}F-labelled 2-deoxy-2-fluoro-D-glucose. Int. J. appl. Radiat. Isot. 34:893, 1983.

21. Shiue CY, To KC, Wolf AP, A rapid synthesis of 2-deoxy-2-fluoro-D-glucose from xenon difluoride suitable for labelling with [18]F. J. lab. Comp. Radiopharm. 20:157, 1983.

22. Sood S, Firnau G, Garnett ES, Radiofluorination with xenon difluoride: A new high yield synthesis of (^{18}F)2-fluoro-2-deoxy-D-glucose. Int. J. appl. Radiat. Isot. 34:743, 1983.

23. Levy S, Livni E, Elmaleh D, Curatolo W, Direct displacement with anhydrous fluoride of the C-2 trifluoromethylsulphonate of methyl 4,6-0-benzylidene-3-0-methyl-2-0-trifluoromethyl-sulphonyl-β-D-mannopyranoside. J. chem. Soc. Chem. Comm. pp 972-973, 1982.

24. Levy S, Elmaleh DR, Livni E, A new method using anhydrous (^{18}F) fluoride to radiolabel 2-(^{18}F)fluoro-2-deoxy-D-glucose. J. nucl. Med. 23:918, 1982.

25. Tewson TJ, Cyclic sulfur esters as substrates for nucleophilic substitution. A new synthesis of 2-deoxy-2-fluoro-D-glucose. J. Org. Chem. 48-3507, 1983.

26. Tewson TJ, Synthesis of no-carrier-added fluorine-18 2-fluoro-2-deoxy-D-glucose. J. nucl. Med. 24:718, 1983.

27. Barrio JR, MacDonald NS, Robinson GD, Najafi A, Cook JS, Kuhl DE, Remote, semiautomated production of F-18 labeled 2-deoxy-2-fluoro-D-glucose. J. nucl. Med. 22:372, 1981.

28. Fowler JS, MacGregor RR, Wolf AP, Farrell AA, Karlstrom KI, Ruth TJ, A shielded synthesis system for production of 2-deoxy-2-(^{18}F) fluoro-D-glucose. J. nucl. Med. 22:376, 1981.

29. Reivich M, Alavi A, Greenberg J, Farkas T, Wolf A, ^{18}F-fluorodeoxy-glucose method for measuring local cerebral glucose metabolism in man: Technique and results. Progr. Nucl. Med. 7:138, 1981.

30. Alavi A, Reivich M, Greenberg JH, Wolf AF, Positron emission tomography of the brain. In: Computed emission tomography. Ell PJ, Holman BL (eds) Oxford University Press, Oxford, pp 134-187, 1982.

31. Phelps ME, Mazziotta JC, Huang SC, Study of cerebral function with positron computed tomography. J. Cereb. Blood Flow Metabol. 2:113, 1982.

32. Heiss WD, Phelps ME, (eds), Positron emission tomography of the brain. Berlin, Springer Verlag, 1983.

33. Hawkins RA, Phelps ME, Huang SC, Kühl DE, Effect of ischemia on quantification of local cerebral glucose metabolic rate in man. J. Cereb. Blood Flow Metabol. 1:37, 1981.

34. Hawkins RA, Miller AL, Loss of radioactive 2-deoxy-D-glucose-6-phosphate from brains of conscious rats: Implications for quantitative autoradiographic determination of regional glucose utilization. Neurosci. 3:251, 1978.

35. Sacks W, Sacks S, Fleischer A, A comparison of the cerebral uptake and metabolism of labeled glucose and deoxygluxose in vivo in rats. Neurochem. Res. 8:661, 1983.

36. MacGregor RR, Fowler JS, Wolf AP, Shiue CY, Lade RE, Wan CN, A synthesis of 2-deoxy-D-(1-^{11}C)glucose for regional metabolic studies: Concise communication. J. nucl. Med. 22:800, 1981.

37. Vora MM, Boothe TE, Finn RD, Smith PM, Gilson AJ, Quality control procedures in the preparation of 2-deoxy-D-(1-^{11}C) glucose radio-pharmaceutical. J. Lab. Com. Radiopharm. 20:147, 1983.

38. Reivich M, Alavi A, Wolf A, Greenberg JH, Fowler J, Christman D, MacGregor R, Jones SC, London J, Shiue C, Yonekura Y, Use of 2-deoxy-D-(1-^{11}C)glucose for the determination of local cerebral glucose metabolism in humans: Variation within and between subjects. J. Cereb. Blood Flow Metabol. 2:307, 1982.

39. Kloster G, Müller-Platz C, Laufer P, 3-(^{11}C)-methyl-D-glucose, A potential agent for regional cerebral glucose utilization studies: synthesis, chromatography and tissue distribution in mice. J. Lab. Comp. Radiopharm. 18:855, 1981.

40. Laufer P, Kloster G, Remote control synthesis of 3-(^{11}C)-methyl-D-glucose. Int. J. appl. Radiat. Isot. 33:775, 1982.

41. Vyska K, Freundlieb C, Höck A, Becker V, Schmid A, Feinendegen LE, Kloster G, Stöcklin G, Heiss WD, Analysis of local perfusion rate and local glucose transport rate in brain and heart in man by means of C-11-methyl-D-glucose and dynamic positron emission tomography. Radioakt. Isot. Klin. Forsch. 15:129, 1982.

42. Heiss WD, Vyska K, Kloster G, Traupe H, Freundlieb C, Höck A, Feinendegen LE, Stöcklin G, Demonstration of decreased functional activity of visual cortex by (^{11}C) methylglucose and positron emission tomography. Neuroradiol. 23:45, 1982.

43. Kloster G, Stöcklin G, Vyska K, Freundlieb C, Höck A, Feinendegen LE, Traupe H, Heiss WD, 3-(^{11}C)-methyl-D-glucose, an agent for the assessment of regional glucose transport across the blood-brain barrier. In: Progress in Radiopharmacology, Vol. 3, Cox PH (ed), Martinus Nijhoff, Den Haag, pp 199-211, 1982.

44. Vyska K, Kloster G, Feinendegen LE, Heiss WD, Stöcklin G, Höck A, Freundlieb C, Aulich A, Schuier F, Thal HU, Becker V, Schmid A, Regional perfusion and glucose uptake determination with 11C-methyl-glucose and dynamic positron emission tomography. In: Positron

118

emission tomography of the brain. Heiss WD, Phelps ME, (eds), Berlin, Springer Verlag, pp 169-180, 1983.

45. Gjedde A, Diemer NH, Autoradiographic determination of regional brain glucose content. J. Cereb. Blood Flow Metabol. 3:303, 1983.

46. Gjedde A, Calculation of cerebral glucose phosphorylation from brain uptake of glucose analogs in vivo: A reexamination. Brain Res. 4:237, 1982.

47. Tewson TJ, Welch MJ, Raichle ME, (^{18}F)-labeled 3-deoxy-3-fluoro-D-glucose: Synthesis and preliminary biodistribution data. J. nucl. Med. 19:1339, 1978.

48. Goodman MM, Elmaleh DR, Kearfott KJ, Ackerman RH, Hoop B, Brownell GL, Alpert NM, Strauss HW, F-18-labeled 3-deoxy-3-fluoro-D-glucose for the study of regional metabolism in the brain and heart. J. nucl. Med. 22:138, 1981.

49. Knust EJ, Machulla HJ, Dutschka K, ^{18}F-labelling with water target produced [18]F. Synthesis and quality control of ^{18}F-3-deoxy-3-fluoro-D-glucose. Radiochem. Radioanal. Lett. 55:21, 1982.

50. Knust EJ, Machulla HJ, Dutschka K, Molls M, Kafka C, Graebe KJ, ^{18}F-3-Desoxy-3-fluor-D-glukose als potentieller Tracer für die Hirn- und Herzdiagnostik Synthese und tierexperimentelle Untersuchungen. NucCompact 14:40, 1983.

51. Holder JE, Gatley SJ, Koeppe RA, Halama JR, Polcyn RA, Tomographic measurement of unidirectional transport rate of glucose across the blood-brain barrier. J.Cereb. Blood Flow Metabol. 3 (suppl. 1) pp S476-S477, 1983.

52. Fowler JS, Lade RE, MacGregor RR, Shiue C, Wan CN, Wolf AP, Agents for the armamentarium of regional metabolic measurement in vivo via metabolic trapping: ^{11}C-2-deoxy-D-glucose and halogenated deoxy-glucose derivatives. J. Lab. Comp. Radiopharm. 16:7, 1979 (abstract).

53. Kloster G, Laufer P, Stöcklin G, D-glucose derivatives labelled with [75,77] Br and [123]I. J. Lab. Comp. Radiopharm. 20:391, 1983.

54. Zhou YG, Shiue CY, Wolf AP, Arnett CD, Syntheses and biodistribution of (Br-82)-2-deoxy-2-bromo-D-glucose and (Br-82)-2-deoxy-2-bromo-D-mannose. J. nucl. Med. 23:105, 1982 (abstract).

55. Kloster G, Laufer P, Wutz W, Stöcklin G, [75,77]Br- and ^{123}I-analogues of D-glucose as potential tracers for glucose utilisation in heart and brain. Eur. J. Nucl. Med. 8:237, 1983.

56. Homma Y, Murase Y, Ishii M, Brain uptake of halogenated products of D-glucal. J. Radioanal. Chem. 76:283, 1983.

57. Levy S, Livni E, Elmaleh DR, Varnum DA, Brownell GL, 2-Deoxy-2-(^{18}F) fluoro-3-0-methyl-D-glucose. Synthesis and animal biodistribution studies. Int. J. appl. Radiat. Isot. 34:1560, 1983.

58. Hansch C, Stewart AR, Anderson SM, Bentley D, The parabolic dependence of drug action upon lipophilic character as revealed by the study of hypnotics. J. Med. Chem. 11:1, 1968.

59. Oldendorf WH, Lipid solubility and drug penetration of the blood brain barrier. Proc. Soc. exp. Biol. Med. 147:813, 1974.

60. Dischino DD, Welch MJ, Kilbourn MR, Raichle ME, Relationship between lipophilicity and brain extraction of C-11-labeled radiopharmaceuticals. J. nucl. Med. 24:1030, 1983.

61. Eckelman WC, Receptor-specific radiopharmaceuticals. In: Computed emission tomography. Ell PJ, Holman BL, (eds), Oxford University Press, Oxford, pp 263-284, 1982.

62. Eckelman WC, Reba RC, Gibson RE, Rzeszotarski WJ, Vieras F, Mazaitis JK, Francis B, Receptor-binding radiotracers: A class of potential radiopharmaceuticals. J. nucl. Med. 20:350, 1979.

63. Blessing G, Weinreich R, Qaim SM, Stöcklin G, Production of ^{75}Br and ^{77}Br via the ^{75}As (^{3}He,3n) ^{75}Br and ^{75}As(α,2n) ^{77}Br reactions using Cu3As-allow as a high-current target material. Int. J. appl. Radiat. 33:333, 1982.

64. Coenen HH, Moerlein SM, Stöcklin G, No-carrier added radiohalogenation methods with heavy halogens. Radiochim. Acta (in press).

65. Kook CS, Reed MF, Digenis GA, Preparation of (^{18}F) haloperidol. J. Med. Chem. 18:533, 1975.

66. Digenis GA, Vincent SH, Kook CS, Reiman RE, Russ GA, Tilbury RS, Tissue distribution studies of (^{18}F) haloperidol, (^{18}F)-β-(4-fluorobenzoyl)propionic acid, and (^{82}Br)bromperidol by external scintigraphy. J. pharm. Sci. 70:985, 1981.

67. Tewson TJ, Raichle ME, Welch MJ, Preliminary studies with (^{18}F) haloperidol: A radioligand for in vivo studies of the dopamine receptors. Brain Res. 192:291, 1980.

68. Zanzonico PB, The development of (carbon-11)-alpha-amino-isobutyric acid and (fluorine-18)-haloperidol as substrate-specific radiotracers. Ph.D. Thesis, Cornell Univ. Medical College, 1982.

69. Zanconico PB, Bigler RE, Small B, Neuroleptic binding sites: Specific labeling in mice with (^{18}F)haloperidol, A potential tracer for positron emission tomography. J. nucl. Med. 24:408, 1983.

70. Welch MJ, Kilbourn MR, Mathias CJ, Mintun MA, Raichle ME, Comparison in animal models of ^{18}F-spiroperidol and ^{18}F-haloperidol: Potential agents for imaging the dopamine receptor. Life Sci. 33:1687, 1983.

71. Fowler JS, Arnett CD, Wolf AP, MacGregor RR, Norton EF, Findley AM, (^{11}C) Spiroperidol: Synthesis, specific activity determination, and biodistribution in mice. J. nucl. Med. 23:437, 1982.

72. Arnett CD, Fowler JS, Wolf AP, MacGregor RR, Specific binding of (^{11}C) spiroperidol in rat brain in vivo. J. Neurochem. 40:455, 1983.

73. Wolf AP, Watanabe M, Shiue CY, Salvadori P, Fowler JS, No-carrieradded (nca) ^{18}F-spiroperidol. J. nucl. Med. 24:52, 1983 (abstract).

74. Arnett CD, Shiue CY, Wolf AP, Fowler JS, Logan J, Comparative evaluation by positron emission tomography of three ^{18}F-labeled butyrophenone neuroleptic drugs in the baboon. J. Neurochem. (submitted for publication).

75. Wagner HN, Burns HD, Dannals RF, Wong DF, Langstrom B, Duelfer T, Frost JJ, Ravert HT, Links JM, Rosenbloom SB, Lukas SE, Kramer AV, Kuhar MJ, Imaging dopamine receptors in the human brain by positron tomography. Science 221:1264, 1983.

120

76. Kulmala HK, Huang CC, Dinerstein RJ, Friedman AM, Specific in vivo binding of [77]Br-p-bromospiroperidol in rat brain: A potential tool for gamma ray imaging. Life Sci. 28:1911, 1981.

77. Friedman AM, Huang CC, Kulmala HK, Dinerstein R, Navone J, Brunsden B, Gawlas D, Cooper M, The use of radiobrominated p-bromospiroperidol for γ-ray imaging of dopamine receptors. Int. J. Nucl. Med. Biol. 9:57, 1982.

78. DeJesus OT, Friedman AM, Prasad A, Revenaugh JR, Preparation and purification of [77]Br-labelled p-bromo-spiroperidol suitable for in vivo dopamine receptor studies. J. Lab. Comp. Radiopharm. 20:745, 1983.

79. Owen F, Poulter M, Mashal RD, Crow TJ, Veall N, Zanelli GD, [77]Br-p-bromospiperone: A ligand for in vivo labelling of dopamine receptors. Life Sci. 33:765, 1983.

80. Crawley JCW, Smith T, Veall N, Zanelli GD, Crow TJ, Owen F, Dopamine receptors displayed in living human brain with [77]Br-p-bromospiperone. Lancet 975, 1983.

81. Moerlein SM, Stöcklin G, Synthesis of no-carrier-added [75,77]Br-benperidol: A potential radiopharmaceutical for quantitating cerebral dopamine receptors. J. nucl. Med. 24:42, 1983 (abstract).

82. Moerlein SM, Stöcklin G, Specific in vivo binding of [77]Br-brombenperidol in rat brain. Life Sci. (submitted for publication).

83. Crouzel C, Mestelan G, Kraus E, Lecomte JM, Comar D, Synthesis of a ^{11}C-labelled neuroleptic drug: pimozide. Int. J. appl. Radiat. Isot. 31:545, 1980.

84. Baron JC, Comar D, Zarifian E, Crouzel C, Mestelan G, Loo H, Agid Y, An in vivo study of the dopaminergic receptors in the brain of man using ^{11}C-pimozide and positron emission tomography. In: Functional radionuclide imaging of the brain. Magistretti PL (ed), Raven Press, New York, pp 337-345, 1983.

85. Reiffers S, Berling-Van der Molen HD, Vaalburg W, Ten Hoeve W, Paans AMJ, Korf J, Woldring MG, Wynberg H, Rapid synthesis and purification of carbon-11 labelled DOPA: A potential agent for brain studies. Int. J. appl. Radiat. Isot. 28:955, 1977.

86. Bolster JM, Vaalburg W, Van Veen W, Van Dijk T, Van der Molen HD, Wynberg H, Woldring MG, Synthesis of no-carrier-added L- and D-(1-^{11}C)-DOPA. Int. J. appl. Radiat. Isot. 34:1650, 1983.

87. Korf J, Reiffers S, Beerling-Van der Molen HD, Lakke JPWF, Paans AMJ, Vaalburg W, Woldring MG, Rapid decarboxylation of carbon-11 labelled DL-DOPA in the brain: A potential approach for external detection of nervous structures. Brain Res. 145:59, 1978.

88. Firnau G, Chirakal R, Sood S, Garnett S, Aromatic fluorination with xenon difluoride: L-3,4-dihydroxy-6-fluoro-phenylalanine. Canad. J. Chem. 58:1449, 1980.

89. Garnett ES, Firnau G, Nahmias C, Dopamine visualized in the basal ganglia of living man. Nature 305:137, 1983.

90. Garnett S, Firnau G, Nahmias C, Chirakal R, Striatal dopamine metabolism in living monkeys examined by positron emission tomography. Brain Res. 280:169, 1983.

91. Berridge M, Comar D, Crouzel C, Baron JC, ^{11}C-labelled ketanserin: A selective serotonin S_2 antagonist. J. Lab. Comp. Radiopharm. 20:73, 1983.

92. Kloster G, Hanus J, Voges R, Stöcklin G, ^{11}C-Mesulergin, a potential agent for mapping the serotonin receptor: synthesis and animal experiments. J. Lab. Comp. Radiopharm. (in press, abstract).

93. Comar D, Maziere M, Godot JM, Berger G, Soussaline F, Menini C, Arfel G, Naquet R, Visualization of ^{11}C-flunitrazepam displacement in the brain of the live baboon. Nature 280:329, 1979.

94. Maziere M, Prenant C, Sastre J, Crouzel M, Comar D, Hantraye P, Kaisima M, Guibert B, Naquet R, ^{11}C-Ro 15-1788 et ^{11}C-flunitrazepam, deux coordinats pour l'étude par tomographie par positrons des sites de liason des benzodiazépines. C.R. Acad. Sci. Paris 296:871 1983.

95. Scholl H, Kloster G, Stöcklin G, Bromine-75-labeled 1,4-benzodiazepines: potential agents for the mapping of benzodiazepine receptors in vivo: concise communication. J. nucl. Med. 24:417, 1983.

96. Rzeszotarski WJ, Gibson RE, Eckelman WC, Simms DA, Jagoda EM, Ferreira NL, Reba RC, Analogues of 3-quinuclidinyl benzilate. J. Med. Chem. 25:1103, 1982.

97. Drayer B, Jaszczak R, Coleman E, Storni A, Greer K, Petry N, Lischko M, Flanagan S, Muscarinic cholinergic receptor binding: In vivo depiction using single photon emission computed tomography and radio-iodinated quinuclidinyl benzilate. J. Comput. Assist. Tomogr. 6:536, 1982.

98. Eckelman WC, Reba RC, Rzeszotarski WJ, Gibson RE, Hill T, Holman BL, Budinger T, Conklin JJ, Eng R, Grissom MP, External imaging of cerebral muscarinic acetylcholine receptors. Science 223:291, 1984.

99. Gibson RE, Weckstein DJ, Jagoda EM, Rzeszotarski WJ, Reba RC, Eckelman WC, The characteristics of I-125 4-IQNB and H-3 QNB in vivo and in vitro. J. nucl. Med. 25:214, 1984.

100. Closse A, (^{3}H) Mesulergine, a selective ligand for serotonin-2-receptors. Life Sci. 32:2485, 1983.

101. Selikson M, Gibson RE, Eckelman WC, Reba RC, Calculation of binding isotherms when ligand and receptor are in different volumes of distribution. Ann. Biochem. 108:64, 1980.

CEREBRAL UPTAKE OF RADIOIODINATED AMPHETAMINES -
BASIC RESEARCH AND CLINICAL RESULTS

H.J. BIERSACK, H. KLÜNENBERG, G. FRIEDRICH, R. KNOPP, R. LEDDA,
E. DOPPELFELD, C. WINKLER

INTRODUCTION

In 1975, Sargent et al (1) were the first to point out the
potentialities of scintigraphic brain imaging with radioactive
amphetamines using Br^{77} labelled dimethoxy phenyl isopropyl
amphetamine as a tracer. Five years later Winchell et al (2,3)
published their pioneer work on cerebral uptake and organ
kinetics of amphetamine derivatives which led to the clinical
use of N-isopropyl amphetamine (IMP). At present IMP and HIPDM
SPECT has become a routine tool for nuclear brain imaging
(4-12).Since 1983 we had the opportunity to perform brain
SPECT with I^{123}-IMP provided by Amersham Buchler for research
purposes (4). However,due to the fact that there is only 5 to
10% cerebral uptake (13) relatively high amounts of the I^{123}
labelled tracer have to be administered resulting in high
costs. Above that, its extensive pulmonary retention leads to
a high radiation burden to this organ. These reasons prompted
us to evaluate other tracers with superior properties for
brain imaging.

EXPERIMENTAL STUDIES

Five amphetamine derivatives namely N-isopropyl amphetamine
(IMP), fenetylline, pentyl amphetamine, benzyl amphetamine,
and N-sec. butyl amphetamine (BMP) were tested. The dog was
the first animal used for general evaluation of the organ
kinetics of all of the respective tracers (with exception of
benzyl amphetamine). Sequential camera scintigraphy following
i.v. injection of 500 µCi I^{131} labelled compounds revealed
cerebral uptake of the afore mentioned amphetamines (14,15).
The second experimental series consisted of wistar rats

Table 1. Brain uptake of amphetamines

Derivatives	(% dose/g tissue)		
	15'	30'	60'
IMP	1.7	0.9	1.7
BMP	1.2	1.9	0.7
Fenetylline	0.4	0.2	0.5
Benzyl amphetamine	1.1	0.9	1.0
Pentyl amphetamine	0.9	1.0	1.1

Table 2. Lung and liver kinetic of BMP and IMP

	(% dose/g tissue)									
	10'		15'		30'		60'		120'	
	IMP	BMP	IMP	BMP	IMP	BMP	IMP	BMP	IMP	BMP
Lung	31.8	14.0	14.1	7.6	5.3	18.1	10.5	3.4	11.7	6.4
Liver	2.5	1.1	2.9	1.6	1.5	3.5	1.7	1.6	3.5	0.7

weighing 180 - 200 g; 5 to 10 µCi I^{125} or I^{131} labelled IMP, fenetylline, pentyl amphetamine, benzyl amphetamine, or BMP were administered intravenously. The animals were sacrificed 10,15,30,60, and 120 min p.i. and the radioactivity content of tissue specimens (brain, cerebellum, liver, lung, spleen, kidney, myocardium, muscle) as well as that in urine and blood samples were measured in a well counter (%dose/g tissue). The most important data of this series are summarized in table 1. BMP showed the highest brain uptake (1.9 %/g) after 30 min, followed by IMP (1,7 %/g) at 60 min. Fenetylline reached its maximum brain uptake (1,3 %/g) at 10 min followed by a fast

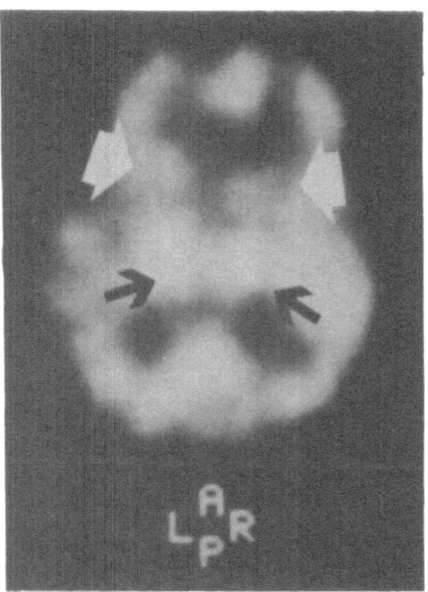

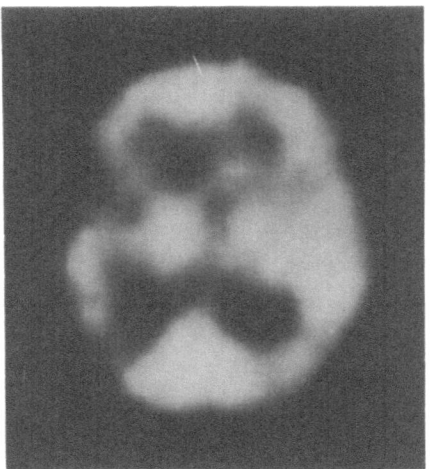

Fig. 1.IMP SPECT (I^{123}), basal
transverse section, with regular
activity accumulation; the arrows
are marking nucleus caudatus
and thalamus.

Fig. 2. BMP SPECT (I^{123}) of a
patient with brain infarction
in the anterior part of the
left temporal lobe and hypoperfusion of the entire left
hemisphere.

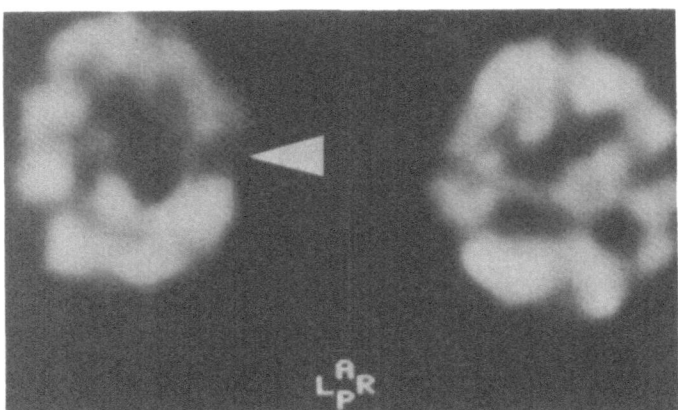

Fig. 3. Fenetylline SPECT (I^{123}) of a patient with epilepsy (EEG focus
temporal right during ictus) and hypoperfusion of the temporal lobe
(arrow).

Table 3. Comparison of CT and IMP SPECT results in 59 patients

	Epilepsy (n=24)	Cerebrovascular disease (n=30)	Migraine (n=3)	Tumour (n=2)
CT and SPECT normal	5	1	0	0
CT and SPECT abnormal	12	25	0	2
CT normal SPECT abnormal	6	4	3	0
CT abnormal SPECT normal	1	0	0	0

decrease, thus appearing to be suitable for a perfusion marker. Benzyl amphetamine and pentyl amphetamine did not show any significant cerebral accumulation.

A comparison of lung and liver kinetics of IMP and BMP (table 2) reveals BMP to have a pulmonary retention much less than that of IMP and a peak liver uptake (3,5 %/g) after 30 min, followed by a fast decrease to 1,2 %/g (liver) at 2 hours; IMP having 3,5 %/g at 2 hours. With respect to extra-cerebral radiation burden BMP seems to be superior to IMP (15). In the third series of experiments I^{123} labelled BMP was injected in a baboon, SPECT using a rotating camera system allowed excellent cross-sectional visualization of the brain (15).

CLINICAL RESULTS

SPECT of the brain was performed 60 min after injection of 6,5 mCi I^{123} labelled IMP (n=51, fig. 1), BMP (n=5, fig 2), and fenetylline (n=3, fig 3) provided by Amersham Buchler. The I^{124} content was less than 2% as the investigations were performed only about 12 hours after cyclotron production of the I^{123}.

For SPECT, a rotating gamma camera system (Gammatome

T9000/CGR) equiped with a high resolution low energy collimator
was used. During one 360 rotation 64 frames with 4K matrix were
acquired within 20 min. Transversal, sagittal, and coronal slice
were reconstructed within short time using an array processor.
The study included patients who suffered from cerebrovascular
disease (n=30), epilepsy (n=24), migraine (n=3), and tumour
(n=2). In 5 patients follow-up brain imaging was performed
one week after the first investigation. In all patients X-ray
CT was performed. EEG was additionally done in patients with
epilepsy and migraine.

Our clinical results are summarized in table 3. From the
24 patients with epilepsy 5 had concordant negative CT and
SPECT findings and 12 concordant positive CT and SPECT results.
One patient with cerebral atrophy had positive CT but negative
SPECT. However, in 6 patients with normal CT, SPECT revealed
lesions consistent with the EEG abnormalities. A comparison
of CT and SPECT with respect to the extent of lesions showed
SPECT lesions to be larger than that of CT in 5 patients.
Concordant extent of the lesions as estimated with both imaging
procedures was demonstrated in 6 patients. There was one
patient whose CT lesions appeared to be larger than that on
the SPECT image.

From the 30 patients with cerebrovascular disease one
presented with similar negative CT and SPECT findings; 25 with
concordant positive CT and SPECT results. There was no patient
with positive CT and negative SPECT, but 4 patients revealed
SPECT lesions despite normal CT. As to the extent of the
lesions, the respective SPECT defects were found to be larger
than those on the CT image in 13 out of 25 cases. 12 patients
had concordant extent of the lesions as estimated with both
imaging procedures. In 12 out of 30 patients with cerebrovascular disease crossed cerebellar diaschisis (hypoperfusion of
the contralateral cerebellar hemisphere in patients with uni-
lateral cerebral lesions) was observed. Two of the 3 patients
who suffered from migraine had focal hyperperfusion; one had
regional diminished perfusion consistent with an EEG focus.
CT was negative in all 3 patients. Two patients with brain
tumours (glioblastoma, metastases) revealed SPECT defects

128

in accordance with the CT findings.

CONCLUSIONS

From our experimental studies BMP appears to be the tracer of choice for functional brain imaging based on the following reasons. First, its brain uptake is slightly higher than that of IMP and second, its radiation burden to the lung is considerably lower than that of IMP. Our clinical results show that 13 out of 57 (23%) patients with epilepsy, cerebrovascular disease, and migraine had positive amphetamine SPECT despite negative CT findings. Here, SPECT was the only imaging procedure which demonstrated the lesions underlying the respective diseases. Moreover, the exact functional extent of CT-proven lesions was better evaluated by SPECT in 18 out of 37 cases (50%).

In conclusion, amphetamine SPECT has 2 main advantages over CT:

1. In patients with cerebrovascular disease regional hypo-perfusion can be detected even in the absence of morphological (structural) changes.
2. Functional epileptic foci can be delineated in patients with partial epilepsy which is of great importance when surgery (temporal lobectomy) is being considered.

The diagnostic value of amphetamine SPECT in migraine and brain tumours warrant further investigation. It, however, seems possible to evaluate the grade of malignancy of brain tumours by amphetamine imaging (16,17).

REFERENCES

1. Sargent T, Kalbhen A, Shulgin AT, Stauffer H, Kusubor N, A potential new brain-scanning agent: 4-[77]Br-2,5-Dimethoxy-phenylisopropyl-amphetamine (4-Br-DPIA). J. nucl. Med. 16:243, 1975.

2. Winchell HS, Baldwin RM, Lin TH, Development of I-123 labeled amines for brain studies: Localization of I-123 iodophenylalkyl amines in rat brain. J. nucl. Med. 21:940, 1980.

3. Winchell HS, Horst WD, Braun L, Oldendorf WH, Hattner R, Parker M, N-Isopropyl-(^{123}I)-p-Iodoamphetamine: Single pass brain uptake and washout; binding to brain synaptosomes; and localization in dog and monkey brain. J. nucl. Med. 21:947, 1980.

4. Biersack HJ, Fröscher W, Klünenberg H, Reske SN, Rasche A, Reichmann K, Winkler C, SPECT des Hirns mit [123]J-Isopropylamphetamin bei Epilepsie. NucCompact 14:62, 1983.

5. Biersack HJ, Hartmann A, Fröscher W, Reske SN, Reichmann K, Knopp R, Winkler C, Cerebrale Emissions-Computertomographie mit einer rotieren-den Gammakamera - klinische Ergebnisse mit [123]J-Isopropylamphetamin und erste Erfahrungen mit [123]J-Fenetyllin. In: Radioaktive Isotope in Klinik und Forschung. Höfer R, Bergmann H (eds), Verlag Egermann, Wien 16, S 11, 1984.

6. Ell PJ, Cullum I, Donaghy M, Lui D, Jarritt PH, Harrison MJG, Cerebral blood flow studies with [123]Iodine-labeled amines. Lancet, 1348, June 1984.

7. Hill TC, Holman BL, Lovett R, O'Leary DH, Front D, Magistretti P, Zimmermann RE, Moore S, Clouse ME, Wu JL, Lin TH, Baldwin RM, Initial experience with SPECT (Single-photon computerized tomography) of the brain using N-isopropyl I-123 p-iodoamphetamine: Concise comminucation. J. nucl. Med. 23:191, 1982.

8. Holman BL, Hill TC, Magistretti PL, Brain imaging with emission computed tomography and radiolabeled amines. Invest. Radiol. 17:206, 1982.

9. Kuhl DE, Barrio JR, Huang SC, Tomographic mapping of local cerebral blood flow using N-isopropyl-p (^{123}I)-iodoamphetamine (IMP). In: Proc. III World Congr. Nucl. Med. and Biol. Raynaud C, (ed), Pergamon Press, p 1731, 1982.

10. Kung HF, Tramposch KM, Blau M, A new brain perfusion imaging agent (I-123) HIPDM:N,N.N'-Trimethyl-N'-(2-Hydrox-3-Methyl-S-Iodobenzyl)-1,3 Propanediamine. J. nucl. Med. 24:66, 1983.

11. Magistretti P, Uren R, Shomer D, Blume H, Holman BL, Hill T, Emission tomographic scans of cerebral blood flow using (^{123}I)iodoamphetamine in epilepsy. In: Proc. III World Congr. Nucl. Med. and Biol. Raynaud C (ed), Pergamon Press, p 139, 1982.

12. Podreka I, Höll K, Dal-Bianco P, Mamoli B, Roszucky A, Angelberger P, Anwendungsgebiet von [123]J-Amphetamin (IMP)- Studien in der Neurologie. In: Radioaktive Isotope in Klinik und Forschung. Höfer R, Bergmann H (eds), Verlag Egermann, Wien S 3, 1984.

13. Holman BL, Zimmerman RE, Shapiro JR, Kaplan ML, Jones AG, Hill TC, Biodistribution and dosimetry of N-isopropyl-p-(-[123]J) iodoamphetamine in the primate. J. nucl. Med. 24:922, 1983.

14. Biersack HJ, Zschalitz L, Klünenberg H, Breuel HP, Reske SN, Oehr P, Winkler C, Radiojod-markiertes fenetyllin (Captagon): ein neues Radio-diagnostikum für die Hirnszintigraphie? NucCompact 15:13, 1984.

15. Biersack HJ, Klünenberg H, Friedrich G, Hartmann A, Reichmann A, Oehr P, Winkler C, 123J-N-(sec.butyl)-p-Jodamphetamin: ein neues Radiopharmakon für die Hirnszintigraphie. NucCompact 15:124, 1984.

16. Lafrance ND, Wagner HN, Whitehouse P, Corley E, Duelfer T, Decreased accumulation of isopropyl-iodoamphetamine (I-123) in brain tumours. J. nucl. Med. 22:1081, 1981.

17. Moretti JL, Askienazy S, Raynaud C, Mathieu E, Sanabria E, Cianci G, Bardy A, Leponcin-Lafitte M, Brain single photon emission tomography with isopropyl-amphetamine I-123: Preliminary results. In: Proc. III World Congr. Nucl. Med. and Biol. Raynaud C (ed), Pergamon Press, p 135, 1982.

RADIOLABELLED SCHIFF BASES IN BRAIN STUDIES

A.D. VARVARIGOU, E. CHIOTELLIS, G. EVAGELATOS

INTRODUCTION

The development of Tc^{99m}-radiopharmaceuticals for positive brain scanning is today one of the main goals of radiopharmacy (1,2). The ability of a drug to penetrate the blood brain barrier (BBB) depends on different factors (3,4). High lipophylicity combined with low protein affinity is demanded to ensure that a substance is able to leave blood-stream and enter the lipid of the endothelial cell plasma membranes (4,5). Different chemical structures have been tested (2) for the preparation of Tc^{99m}-radiopharmaceuticals that would fulfil the above demands.

The present study refers to the preparation of a series of lipophylic Schiff bases, o-aminophenyl derivatives, and the investigation of their brain uptake in rats in combination with lipophylicity and protein binding studies. I^{131}-antipyrine is used as the reference radiopharmaceutical (6).

MATERIAL AND METHODS

Synthesis. The Schiff bases were synthesized by heating 0.1 mol of o-aminophenol and 0.1 mol of the respective amine in methanol for 30 min. After removal of the solvent the Schiff bases remained as coloured solids recrystallized from warm methanol. The melting points are presented in table 1.

Labelling procedures. The Schiff base (0.5-1 mmol) was dissolved in 3 ml of chloroform. A solution of stannous chloride, containing 0.2 mg $SnCl_2$ in 0.1 ml of methanol was added, followed by a small quantity of pertechnetate in saline. The mixture was agitated for some minutes and consequently extracted with water. The organic layer was evaporated to

132

TABLE 1

Biodistribution in rats 2 min. p.i.

Compound	Melting point °C	p.c.	Blood	Brain	Liver
Antipyrine		4.80	0.816±0.42	0.661±0.06	0.706±0.36
Benzylidene o-aminophenol	200-201	11.30	4.180±0.95	0.223±0.04	3.856±1.25
p-methoxy-benzylidene o-aminophenol	87-89	4.80	4.770±1.23	0.348±0.08	5.721±2.46
p-dimethylamino-benzylidene o-amino-phenol	118-119	5.00	1.683±0.61	0.104±0.01	2.183±0.78
p-nitro-benzylidene o-aminophenol	161-163	2.20	5.090±1.31	0.300±0.16	4.314±1.20
p-naphthyl-benzylidene o-aminophenol	69-70	29.30	4.033±0.61	0.211±0.06	3.548±1.95
Salicylidene o-aminophenol	188-189	12.60	4.791±0.29	0.430±0.07	4.067±1.14
5-chloro-salicylidene o-aminophenol	183-185	17.70	1.524±0.10	0.113±0.00	2.365±0.44
Pyridinyl o-aminophenol	75-77	5.60	1.935±1.15	0.117±0.07	4.088±2.09

dryness and the remaining solid was dissolved in methanol.

A final solution of the complex in 10-50% methanol and prepared for further studies.

The radiochemical purity of the Tc^{99m}-complexes was determined by Instant Thin Layer Chromatography (ITLC) using saline acetonitrile/water 3/1, methanol and chloroform as solvent systems.

Lipophylicity studies. A quantity of 0.1 ml of the final purified solution of the Tc^{99m}-complex was added to a mixture of 2 ml of octanol and 2 ml of 0.05N phosphate buffered saline pH: 6.8. The mixture was agitated vigorously and samples of the 2 layers were weighted and counted. The octanol-to-buffered saline partition coefficients were normalized to a constant weight of solvent. The values are presented in table 1.

Protein binding studies. The protein affinity of the labelled Schiff bases was determined by equilibrium dialysis 0.5 ml of the solution of the complex was equilibrated with plasma in a dialysis tube, emersed in phosphate buffered saline. Samples of the buffered solution were withdrawn at predetermined time intervals and counted in comparison with blind samples. The degree of protein binding was expressed as a function of time. Fig 1 and 2 represent the protein binding curves of the Tc^{99m}-labelled Schiff bases in comparison to I^{131}-antipyrine.

Animal studies. Female Wistar rats, weighing 150 - 200 g were used. 0.1 ml of the final solution, containing 0.3-2 mg of the labelled Schiff base, was injected into the femoral vein of the preanesthetized animal. The rats were sacrificed by freezing them in liquid nitrogen.

Samples of the main organs were selected, weighted and counted. The percent dose per gram of organ was calculated.

RESULTS AND DISCUSSION

Chromatographic studies showed a 60-70% yield of labelling. After purification practically all the remaining radioactivity was in the complex form and only negligible amounts of pertechnetate could be detected. In the saline the labelled

134

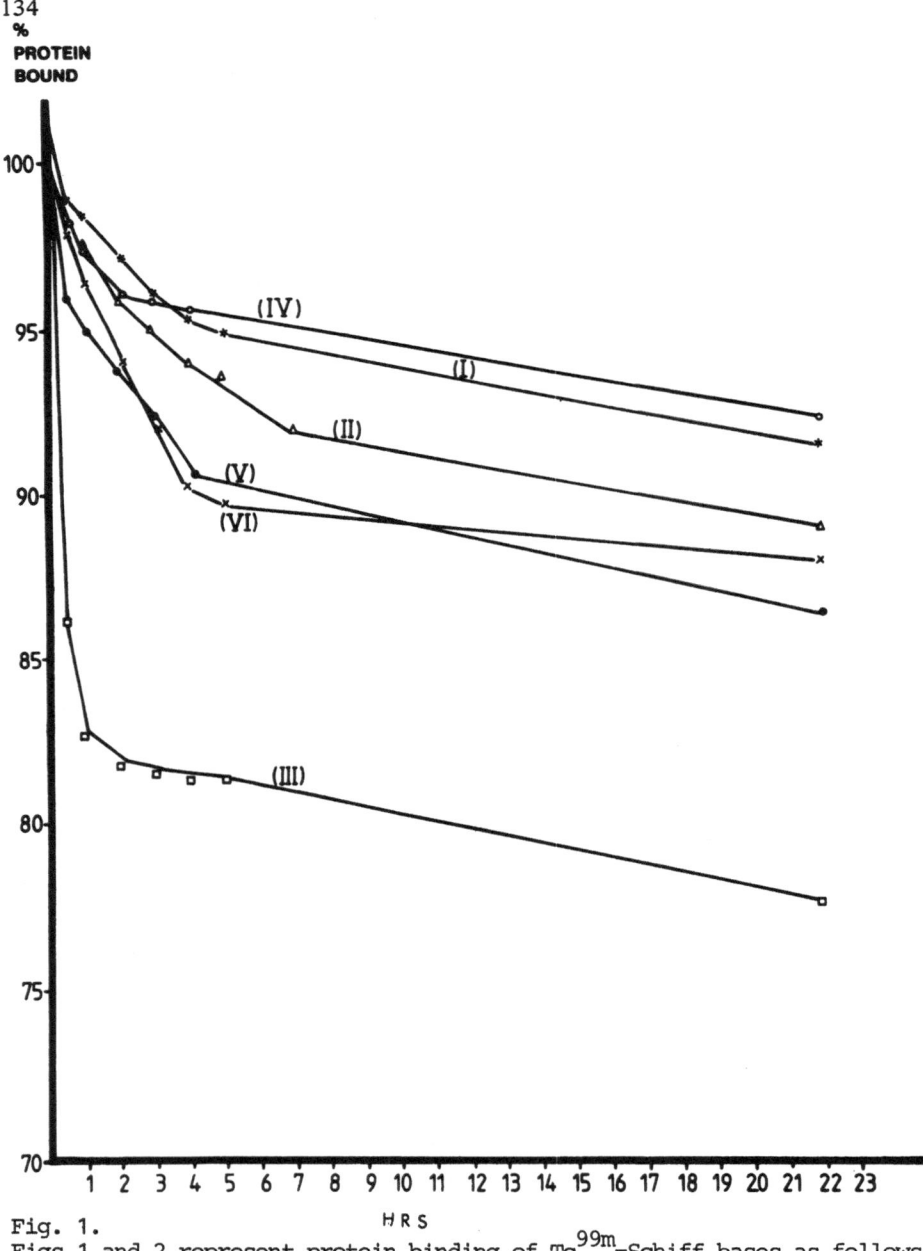

Fig. 1.
Figs 1 and 2 represent protein binding of Tc^{99m}-Schiff bases as follows:
(I)   p-dimethylamino-benzylidene o-aminophenol
(II)   p-methoxy-benzylidene o-aminophenol
(III)   naphtyl-benzylidene o-aminophenol
(IV)   benzylidene o-aminophenol
(V)   p-nitro-benzylidene o-aminophenol
(VI)   pyridinyl-benzylidene o-aminophenol
(VII)   p-chloro-benzylidene o-aminophenol
(VIII)   salicylidene o-aminophenol

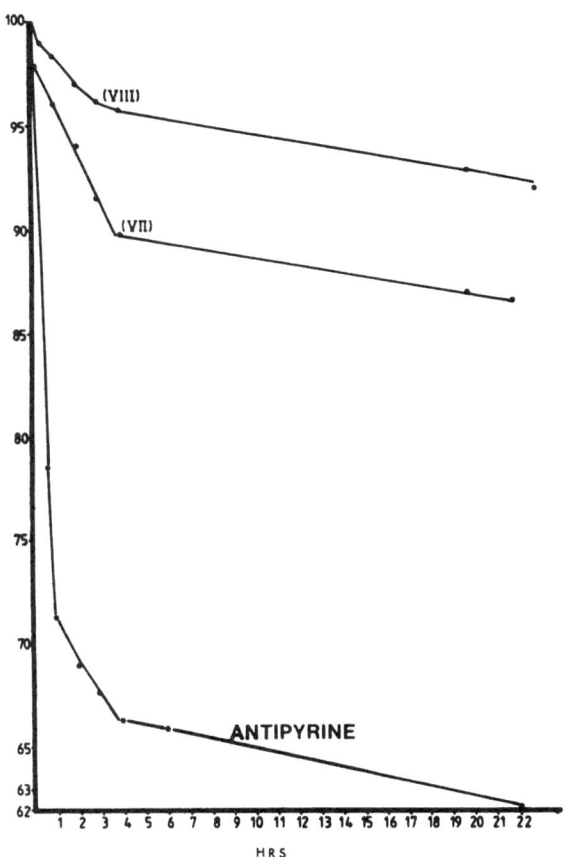

Fig. 2 (see legend of fig 1).

compounds remained at the origin while in chloroform they
moved to the front. In methanol and acetonitrile: water Rf
values were 0.8-1.0.

In table 1 the partition coefficient of the labelled
compounds as well as blood, brain and liver uptake 2 min p.i.,
are reported in comparison to I^{131}-antipyrine. Although in
most cases the partition coefficient of the Tc^{99m}-chelates
showed higher values than I^{131}-antipyrine, the brain uptake
was lower and the blood-clearance slower. From the protein
binding curves it is obvious that practically all Schiff
bases under study presented high affinity for blood-proteins.
This eliminated the possibility to leave blood-stream and

TABLE 2

p-Methoxy-benzylidene o-aminophenol biodistribution in rats

Organ	2 min	5 min	15 min	30 min
Blood	4.770±1.23	3.061±0.41	2.693±0.33	1.937±0.84
Brain	0.348±0.08	0.103±0.01	0.127±0.03	0.106±0.03
Liver	5.721±2.46	4.027±0.36	4.932±1.42	5.090±2.13
Kidneys	1.451±0.24	3.177±0.23	6.490±0.82	6.298±3.95
Stomach	0.263±0.10	0.213±0.00	0.458±0.15	0.663±0.23
Intestines	0.392±0.06	0.230±0.06	0.460±0.34	3.251±1.04
Spleen	1.257±0.13	1.232±0.27	1.957±0.45	1.807±0.60
Muscle	0.282±0.09	0.078±0.03	0.123±0.01	0.200±0.09

enter into the brain cells. The in vivo kinetics of p-methoxy-benzylidene o-aminophenol from 2 to 30 min showed higher brain uptake 2 min p.i. (table 2). Blood-clearance was slow; the blood-concentration changed from 4.770 at 2 min to 1.937 at 30 min p.i. The chelates were excreted both by the hepato-biliary system and the kidneys.

Concluding one can say that low protein binding and fast blood-clearance combined with high lipophylicity seem to be indispensable characteristics for radioactive substances as possible radiopharmaceuticals for positive brain scanning.

REFERENCES

1. Oldendorf WH, Need for new radiopharmaceuticals. J. nucl. Med. 19:1182, 1978.

2. Loberg MD, Corder EH, Fields AT, Callery PS, Membrane transport in Tc-99m-labelled radiopharmaceuticals. I. Brain uptake by passive transport. J. nucl. Med. 20:1181, 1979.

3. Oldendorf WH, Lipid solubility and drug penetration of the blood-brain barrier. Proc. Soc. exp. Biol. Med. 147:813, 1974.

4. Oldendorf WH, Blood-brain barrier permeability to drugs. Ann. Rev. Pharm. 14:239, 1974.

5. Kung HF, Blau M, Regional intracellular pH shift: A proposed new mechanism for radiopharmaceutical uptake in brain and other tissues. J. nucl. Med. 21:147, 1980.

6. Uszler MJ, Bennett LR, Mena I, Oldendorf WH, Human CNS, Perfusion scanning with ^{123}I-Iodoantipyrine. Radiology 115:197, 1975.

BIODISTRIBUTION AND METABOLISM OF
RADIOPHARMACEUTICALS

SOME RECENT PROGRESS IN THE DEVELOPMENT AND APPLICATION
OF RADIOPHARMACEUTICALS LABELLED WITH ^{11}C AND ^{18}F

V.W. PIKE

INTRODUCTION

Positron emission tomography (PET) (1) has gained importance
in clinical research because it enables pathophysiology to be
investigated quantitatively in vivo. Advances in the application of PET now depend very much on the progressive development of radiopharmaceuticals labelled with positron emitting
radionuclides. The available radionuclides include ^{15}O /$t_{\frac{1}{2}}$ =
2 min), ^{13}N ($t_{\frac{1}{2}}$ = 10 min), ^{11}C ($t_{\frac{1}{2}}$ = 20 min) and ^{18}F ($t_{\frac{1}{2}}$ =
110 min),which are produced with a cyclotron, and ^{68}Ga ($t_{\frac{1}{2}}$ =
68 min) and ^{82}Rb ($t_{\frac{1}{2}}$ = 1.3 min), which are obtained from
portable generators. Of these radionuclides ^{11}C and ^{18}F are
the most useful for the preparation of organic radiopharmaceuticals. This is not least because it is often possible to
make use of one or other of these radionuclides to label a
target compound without causing a change in bioactivity. Moreover the half-lives of ^{11}C and ^{18}F, unlike those of ^{15}O and
^{13}N, do not impose over severe limits on the durations of
radiosyntheses.

This chapter discusses some recent progress in the development of radiopharmaceuticals labelled with ^{11}C or ^{18}F and
their application in PET for the study of regional myocardial
metabolism, regional myocardial blood-flow, cardiac output,
drug pharmacokinetics and brain dopamine systems.

STUDIES OF REGIONAL MYOCARDIAL METABOLISM

Fatty acids are the prefered energy source of healthy
myocardium. Indeed about two thirds of cardiac energy requirements are normally met by fatty acid oxidation. Fatty acid
metabolism is complex (fig 1). The essential features are

142

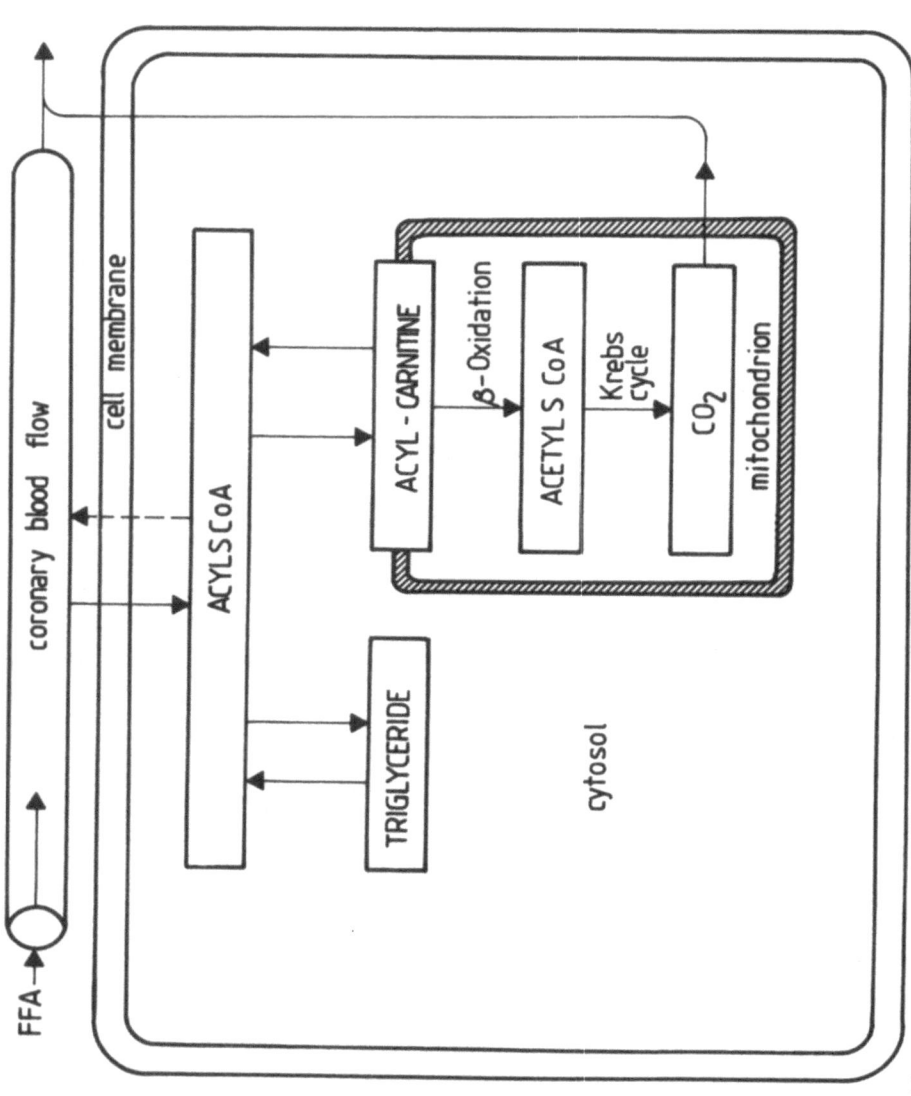

Fig. 1. Free fatty acid (FFA) metabolism.

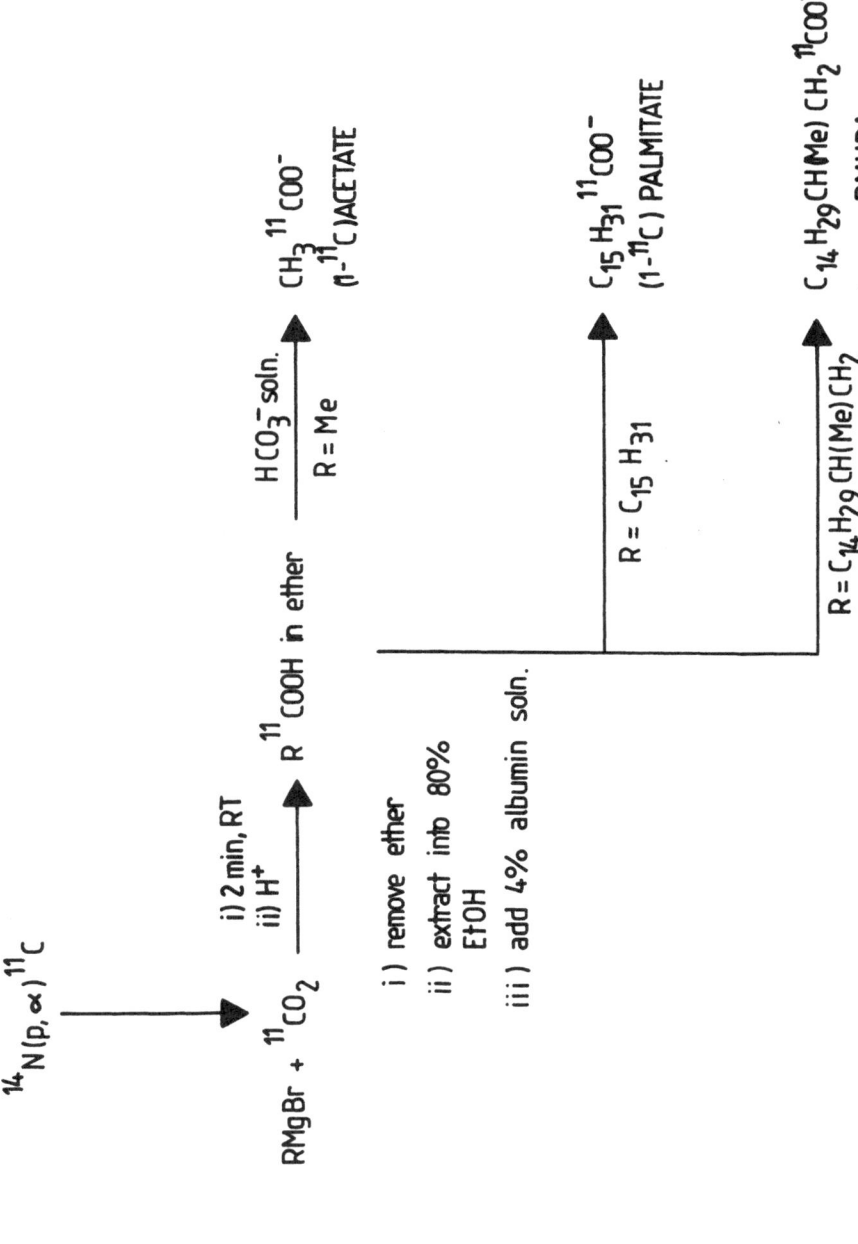

Fig. 2. The radiosyntheses of (1-¹¹C)palmitate (3), (1-¹¹C)acetate (7) and BMHDA (11).

entry of fatty acid into cytosol, probably by passive diffusion, activation by conversion into acylSCoA and then either
reversible esterification, mainly to triglyceride, or oxidation to carbon dioxide. Oxidation itself involves transport of
acylSCoA into mitochondria via the carnitine shuttle, β-oxidation to acetylSCoA and finally oxidation to carbon dioxide in
the Krebs cycle. It was early realized that natural fatty acids
labelled with ^{11}C or ^{18}F might be useful probes for the investigation of regional myocardial metabolism by PET.

Much work has been carried out with $(1-^{11}C)$palmitate, which
is conveniently prepared via the (^{11}C)carbonation of penta-
decylmagnesium bromide with cyclotron-produced (^{11}C)carbon
dioxide (fig 2) (2,3). After an intravenous injection of
$(1-^{11}C)$palmitate in the dog there is a high and very rapid (ca
1 min) uptake of radioactivity into normal myocardium (4).
Subsequent clearance of radioactivity is biexponential, after
correction for physical decay, and is characterized by a fast
early phase ($t_{\frac{1}{2}}$ = 2-7 min) and a slow late phase ($t_{\frac{1}{2}}$ = ca 36
min). The fast phase of radioactivity clearance largely re-
presents the egress of the catabolite (^{11}C)carbon dioxide in
the venous coronary blood-flow and is related to fatty acid
oxidation, whereas the slow phase of radioactivity clearance
largely represents "(^{11}C)lipid washout" and is related to the
turnover of esterified $(1-^{11}C)$palmitate (4). These relationships have some value for the external evaluation of myocardial
metabolism in vivo. Thus, for example, the analysis of clearance curves can provide measures of the ratios of esterification to direct oxidation in normal and ischemic myocardium (4).
Measures of the myocardial uptake of $(1-^{11}C)$palmitate are also
of value, because regional deficiencies in uptake correlate to
infarct size (5). Nevertheless, as a result of the participa-
tion of $(1-^{11}C)$palmitate in all fatty acid metabolism, the
interpretation of data from the use of $(1-^{11}C)$palmitate in PET
studies on patients can be complex or even equivocal. Attempts
have now been made to develop ^{11}C-labelled radiopharmaceuticals
that provide information on only limited aspects of fatty acid
metabolism.

<u>Studies with (1-^{11}C)Acetate</u>. Acetate, a short chain analogue
of palmitate, bypasses the early stages of fatty acid metabolism, such as β-oxidation, and is thought to enter mitochondria
directly for oxidation in the Krebs cycle (fig 1). Preliminary
investigations (6), using (1-^{14}C)acetate in dogs, indicated
that (1-^{11}C)acetate would have value for PET studies of regional myocardial metabolism in man. Consequently, a procedure was
developed for the preparation of (1-^{11}C)acetate via the (^{11}C)
carbonation of methylmagnesium bromide with cyclotron-produced
(^{11}C)carbon dioxide (fig 2) (7). The utility of this radiopharmaceutical has since been evaluated by means of PET in dog
and man.

The uptake of (1-^{11}C)acetate into normal myocardium of man
is both high and rapid (< 2 min) and provides clear emission
scans of myocardium in which the left ventricular wall is
clearly distinguished from the septum (7). In many subjects
the right ventricular wall is also differentiated. Subsequent
clearance of radioactivity from myocardium is monoexponential
after correction for physical decay (8). The clearance of
radioactivity is significantly faster for subjects at exercise
($t_{\frac{1}{2}}$ = 7.8 min) than for subjects at rest ($t_{\frac{1}{2}}$ = 12 min). For
patients with angina and coronary artery disease who are at
rest the uptake of radioactivity into myocardium is uniform
and the rate of clearance of radioactivity matches that in
healthy subjects. However, for the same patients at exercise,
the clearance of radioactivity from healthy myocardium ($t_{\frac{1}{2}}$ =
7.9 min) is faster than that from ischemic myocardium ($t_{\frac{1}{2}}$ =
10 min). Such difference allow transiently ischemic regions
of myocardium to be easily identified by their retained activity on emission scans taken shortly (12 min) after the injection of (1-^{11}C)acetate (7-9). Such studies (7-9) indicate that
disturbances arising in ischemic myocardium are prolonged
beyond the disappearance of electrocardiographic and sympto-
matic evidence.

PET studies of dogs injected intravenously with (1-^{11}C)
acetate have shown that the rates of radioactivity clearance
from myocardium are related to metabolism, presumably to the

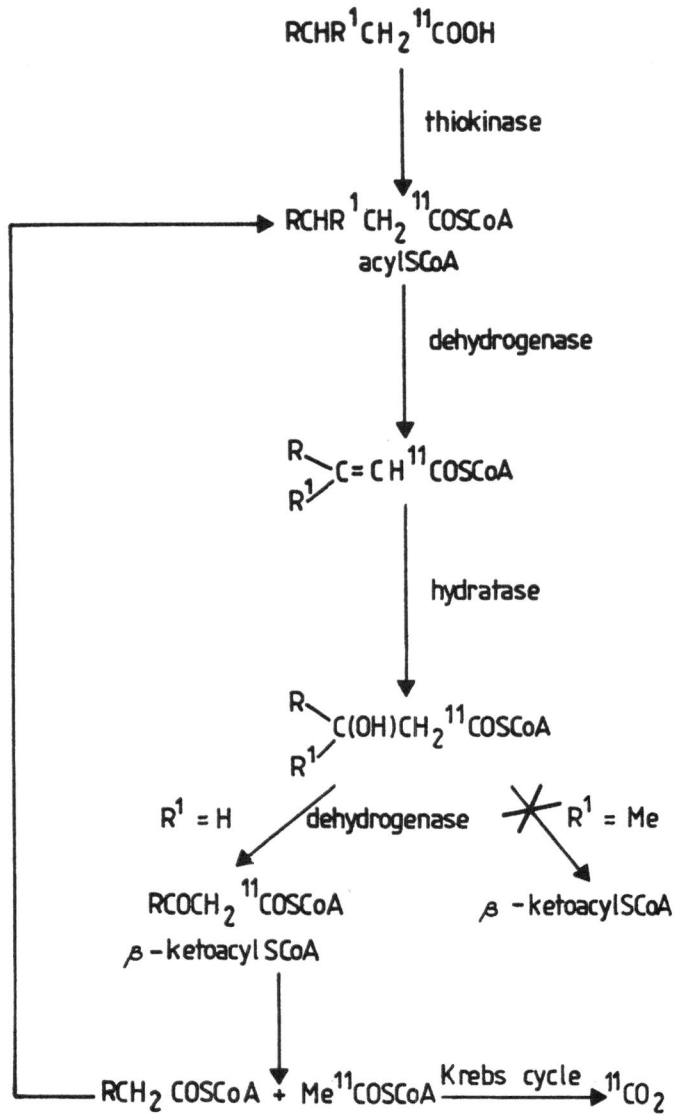

Fig. 3. Comparison of the β-oxidation of $(1-^{11}C)$palmitate $(R = C_{13} H_{27}, R' = H)$ with the supposed metabolism of BMHDA $(R = C_{14} H_{29}, R' = Me)$.

function of the Krebs cycle (10). Thus during electrical pacing, when myocardial blood-flow and oxygen consumption are increased, the rate of radioactivity clearance is also increased, whereas during dipyridamole infusion, when blood-flow increases dramatically without change in oxygen consumption, the rate of radioactivity clearance is unchanged. These results

imply that the use of $(1-^{11}C)$acetate with PET has great
potential for the evaluation of the effect of drugs and other
interventions on regional myocardial function in man.

Studies with D,L-3-Methyl-$(1-^{11}C)$heptadecanoate (BMHDA).
A recent approach to the development of a radiopharmaceutical
for the investigation of myocardial metabolism by PET has been
to prepare a ^{11}C-labelled compound that follows fatty acid
uptake only. This implies that such a radiopharmaceutical
should be subject to the early stages of fatty acid metabolism
but not undergo complete oxidation to (^{11}C)carbon dioxide.
Accordingly, Livni et al (11) have developed the radiopharmaceutical, D,L-3-methyl-$(1-^{11}C)$heptadecanoate (BMHDA), a fatty
acid analogue which is unable to form a β-ketoacylSCoA, an
intermediate in β-oxidation (fig 3). The radiosynthesis of
BMHDA is analogous to that of $(1-^{11}C)$palmitate (fig 2). De Landsheere et al (12,13) have studied BMHDA in detail by PET in dogs.

After an intravenous injection of BMHDA, the arterial
concentration decreases to 10% within 10 min and to 5% within
18 min. The difference between arterial and venous radioactivity concentrations is zero after 3-5 min and remains so for
at least 40 min. The uptake of radioactivity into myocardium
is rapid. Thus peak extraction is 40% at 3 min and overall
extraction is 25%. Thereafter the decay-corrected concentration of radioactivity in myocardium is stable. Since the
concentration of radioactivity in myocardium to that in background increases from 7 to 12 between 5 and 20 min after
injection, excellent images of myocardium are obtained on
serial emission scans. This study (12) therefore supports the
notion that BMHDA behaves as a non-oxidisable fatty acid
analogue.

In a series of experiments (13) in which myocardial blood-
flow was reduced by arterial occlusion or increased by the
drug dipyridamole, it was found that the myocardial uptake of
BMHDA is proportional to blood-flow at values below normal,
whereas uptake increases progressively less rapidly with blood-
flow at higher values. In other experiments (13) myocardial
oxygen consumption was decreased by the drugs, propanolol and

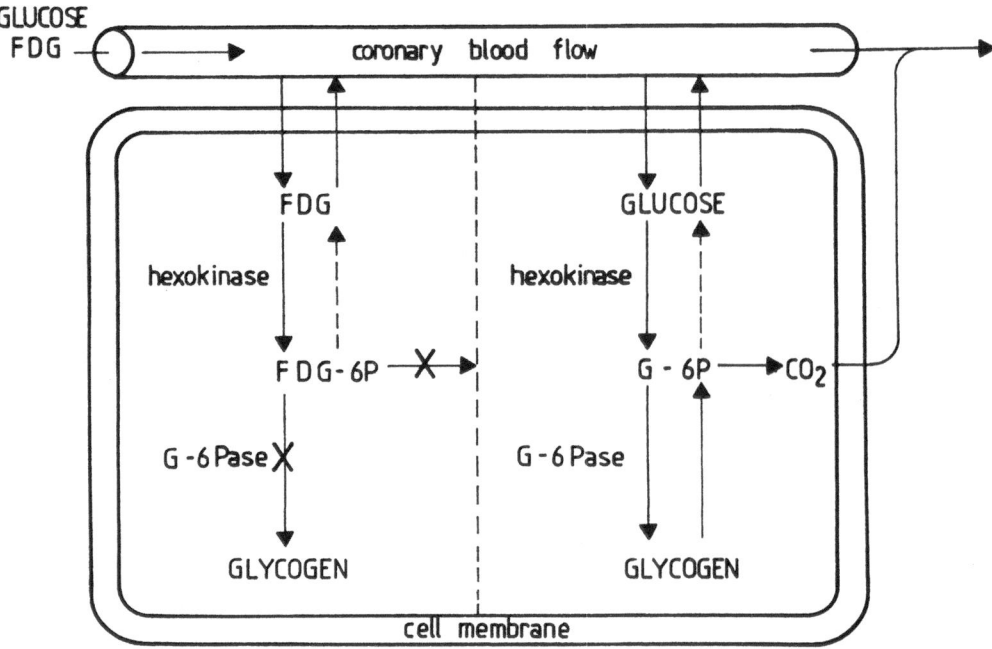

Fig. 4. A comparison of the metabolism of FDG with that of glucose.

and verapamil, or increased with electrical pacing. The myocardial uptake of BMHDA was found to be sensitive to these
changes. If however fatty acid levels are sharply reduced and
glucose greatly increased by glucose-insulin-K^+ infusion, the
extraction of BMHDA is reduced in step with the reduction in
natural fatty acid extraction, monitored using ^{14}C-or ^{3}H-
labelled palmitate (13). Thus BMHDA would appear to mark
fatty acid availability.

Clearly BMHDA may prove valuable for PET studies of regional myocardial fatty acid metabolism in man. In particular the
kinetics of BMHDA uptake are likely to prove useful for the
study of myocardial fatty acid utilization, ischemia and
infarction.

Studies with $\underline{D}$ -(^{11}C)Glucose. Though fatty acids are the
preferred substrates for cardiac energy production under
certain circumstances myocardium makes greater use of other
substrates, such as glucose. These circumstances include,

during ischemia, during glucose-insulin-K^+ infusion and after a heavy carbohydrate meal. For this reason there has been some interest in the study of myocardial glucose metabolism by PET (14,15). These studies have used 2-(^{18}F)fluoro-2-deoxy-$\underline{D}$-glucose (FDG), an analogue of natural glucose that is unable to undergo metabolism beyond intracellular conversion into its 6-phosphate (fig 4). The value of FDG is that its uptake in man can be correlated to glucose uptake. By the use of FDG alone, however, it is not possible to differentiate between glucose uptake for glycolysis and glucose uptake for glycogen formation. Differentiation should be possible by using (^{11}C) glucose, since (^{11}C)glucose that acts as a substrate for glycogen formation is expected to be retained in myocardium, whereas (^{11}C)glucose that acts as a substrate for glycolysis will be cleared from myocardium as (^{11}C)carbon dioxide (fig 4). This concept is now being applied to investigate whether the myocardial accumulation of FDG observed in anginal patients during recovery from ischemia (15) represents repletion of glycogen stores or not. $\underline{D}$-(^{11}C) Glucose is prepared for these studies by photosynthesis in unicellular green algae, Scenedesmus obtusiusculus Chod, with (^{11}C)bicarbonate as substrate (16). The radiosynthesis (fig 5) has been adapted from that reported by Ehrin et al (17). Early results indicate that $\underline{D}$ - (^{11}C) glucose will be a useful complement to FDG for the study of myocardial glucose metabolism in patients with ischemic heart disease. For example, normal subjects injected with $\underline{D}$-(^{11}C) glucose, soon after a heavy carbohydrate meal, show a significant uptake and retention of radioactivity not only in the liver but also in the myocardium (16).

STUDIES OF REGIONAL MYOCARDIAL BLOOD-FLOW AND CARDIAC OUTPUT

Fundamental to the study of metabolism is the study and measurement of blood-flow, since the uptake of a metabolic tracer is often a complex function of both blood-flow and metabolism. For this reason many radiopharmaceuticals, including rubidium-82 cation, (^{13}N)ammonia and (^{68}Ga)albumin microspheres, have been applied to the measurement of myocardial

150

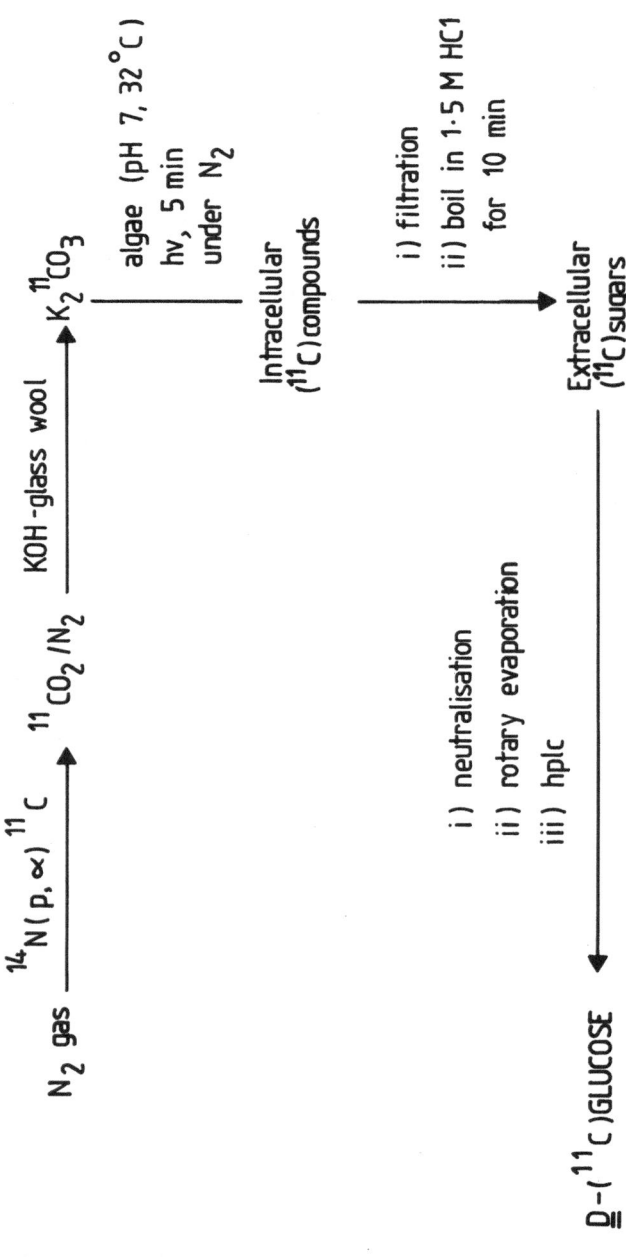

Fig. 5. Preparation of Δ-(11C)glucose via photosynthesis in algae, according to Sohanpal et al (16), as adapted from Ehrin et al (17).

blood-flow by PET. Diffusible markers of blood-flow, such as rubidium-82 cation and (^{13}N) ammonia, are less than ideal because they are incompletely extracted and therefore recirculate, and also because they participate in metabolism; their attraction is that they may be administered intravenously. In principle, labelled microspheres can provide pure measures of blood-flow, since they are completely trapped in capillary beds on first pass and cannot participate in metabolism. Nevertheless, the use of (^{68}Ga) albumin microspheres has several disadvantages in practice. Thus, because of the energetic mode of decay (β^+ = 1.9 MeV, 89%; EC 10%) and relatively long half-life (68 min) of ^{68}Ga, the activity of (^{68}Ga) microspheres that is administered to a patient must be quite low (50 - 100 MBq) for the radiation doses to critical organs to be acceptable, and also rapid serial measurements are impossible. Furthermore, there is some evidence that the bonding between ^{68}Ga and an albumin microsphere can be unstable in vivo (18). For these reasons, Turton et al (19) have developed the preparation of (^{11}C) microspheres for the accurate measurement of regional myocardial blood-flow and cardiac output in man by PET. The method of preparation involves the (^{11}C) methylation of commercial albumin microspheres (15 μm diameter) with (^{11}C) iodomethane, itself prepared from cyclotron-produced (^{11}C) carbon dioxide (fig 6).

It has been established that the bond between ^{11}C and a microsphere is stable in vivo; less than 1% of the ^{11}C leaks from the microspheres during the first hour after administration (19). Thus serial emission scans of dog myocardium, taken after the administration of (^{11}C) microspheres into the left atrium, reveal a rapid distribution of radioactivity into myocardium according to blood-flow and no subsequent changes (19). The ratio of the radioactivity in myocardium to that in background is >12 measured by PET and hence excellent images of myocardium are obtained (19). In dogs, measurement of regional myocardial blood-flow obtained by the use of (^{11}C) microspheres and PET correlate well, over a wide range of flow, with measurements obtained by the use of gamma-emitting (^{46}Sc)

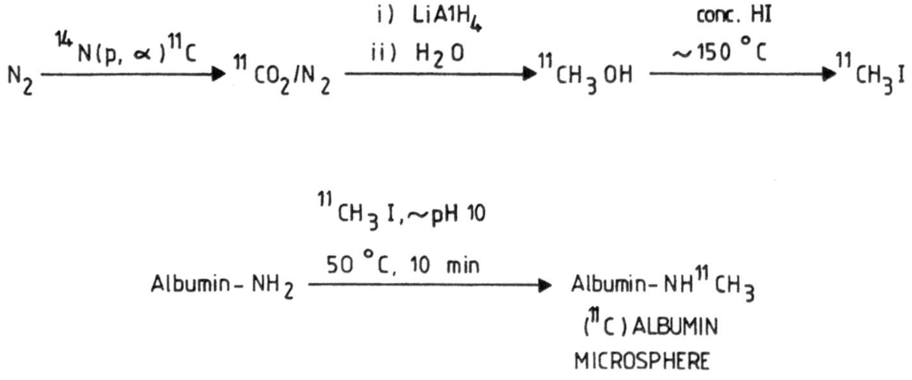

Fig. 6. The preparation of (^{11}C)albumin microspheres, according to Turton et al (19).

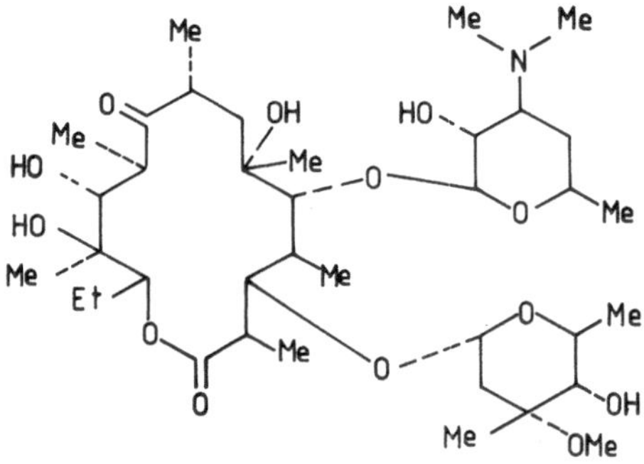

Fig. 7. The structure of the antibiotic, erythromycin A.

carbon microspheres and ex vivo well-counting (20). The correspondence in measurements is not quite one to one because with PET there is a reduced efficiency of count recovery from thin objects, such as the left ventricular wall (18).

Currently (^{11}C)microspheres are being used to study regional myocardial blood-flow and cardiac output in patients (20). For these studies (^{11}C)microspheres are administered into the left ventricle via a cannula from the left femoral artery, during a routine diagnostic catheterization. A timed-with-drawal of the cardiac output is taken from the left femoral artery, and well-counted to provide an input function. Division of a PET measurement of the radioactivity in any region of interest by the input function gives a measure of blood-flow to that region in ml min^{-1} g^{-1}.

Since ^{11}C decays by pure positron emission (β^+ = 1.0 MeV; 100%) and with a short half-life (20 min) quite high activities (ca 200 MBq) of (^{11}C)microspheres may be administered. To date 11 patients have been studied. These patients show no adverse physical symptoms or ECG changes as a result of the use of (^{11}C)microspheres (21).

Of course the requirement to administer (^{11}C)microspheres by catheter, either into the left atrium or left ventricle, in order to bypass entrapment in the pulmonary capillaries, limits their general applicability. Nevertheless, the use of (^{11}C) microspheres should prove valuable as a reference procedure in the evaluation of less invasive techniques for the measurement of myocardial blood-flow such as the use of rubidium-82 cation.

PHARMACOKINETIC STUDIES WITH (N-METHYL-^{11}C)ERYTHROMYCIN A

Of fundamental importance to the action of antibiotics is the rate of penetration and concentration achieved in infected tissue. Erythromycin A (fig 7) is one of the best known of the medicinally important macrolide antibiotics. Because of the lack of non-invasive techniques, the rate of penetration and the concentration of erythromycin A achieved in human pneumonic lung had until recently remained unknown. These measurements have now been obtained through the application of PET.

Pike et al (22) developed a fast method for labelling erythromycin A with ^{11}C, involving the reductive methylation of N-demethylerythromycin A with (^{11}C)formaldehyde, itself prepared from cyclotron-produced (^{11}C)carbon dioxide (fig 8). The desired (N-methyl-^{11}C)erythromycin A is chemically and

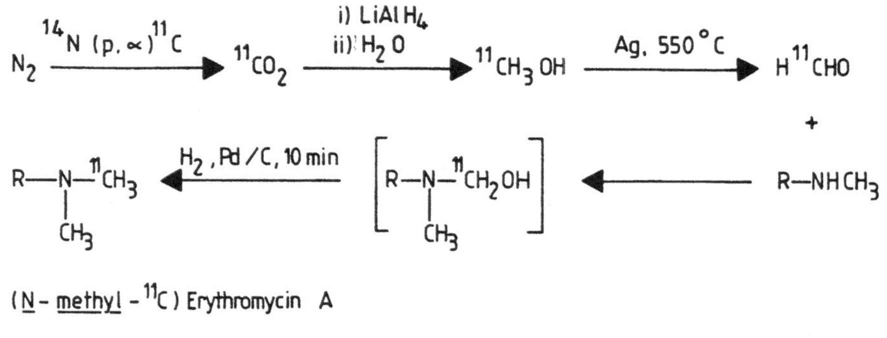

154

(N- methyl - ^{11}C) Erythromycin A

Fig. 8. The radiosynthesis of (N-methyl-^{11}C)erythromycin A, according to Pike et al (22). (R = erythromycin A residue, R-NHCH$_3$ = N-demethylerythromycin A).

radiochemically purified by high pressure liquid chromatography and formulated for intravenous injection as the lactobionate salt.

(N-methyl-^{11}C)Erythromycin A was used to compare the uptake and local concentration of erythromycin A in the pneumonic and unaffected lungs of five patients with lobar pneumonia (23). In order to obtain the regional distribution of the extravascular concentration of erythromycin A in lung, transaxial emission scans of the uptake of (N-methyl-^{11}C)erythromycin A were corrected for lung density by using an external ring source of positron-emitting ^{68}Ga (24) and for blood-volume by using (^{11}C)carbon monoxide to label the blood-pool. The mean extravascular concentrations obtained during the first hour after the intravenous injection of a pharmacological dose of erythromycin A lactobionate (270 mg) were found to be similar in pneumonic and unaffected lung (ca 6 µg/g) Such a concentration, which is above the minimum inhibitory concentrations of many sensitive organisms, is reached within 10 min of injection and is maintained throughout the period of the measurement (60 min).

This study has provided what is probably the first measurement of the concentration of an antibiotic at its site of

action in man, and illustrates the largely unexploited potential of PET for the investigation of drug pharmacokinetics in
vivo.

STUDIES OF DOPAMINE SYSTEMS

Dopamine (3,4-dihydroxyphenylethylamine) is a well-known
neurotransmitter that is implicated in many neuropsychiatric
disorders. For example, Parkinson's disease is associated
with a deficiency of dopamine in brain. The immediate metabolic
precursor to dopamine is L-dopa (L-3,4-dihydroxyphenylalamine).
L-Dopa, unlike dopamine, is able to cross the blood-brain
barrier and for this reason has become an important drug in
the therapy of Parkinson's disease. Recently Garnet et al (25)
succeeded in preparing L-(^{18}F)fluorodopa, a fluoro-analogue
of L-dopa, and by means of PET demonstrated its uptake into
the striatum of normal human brain, a region active in dopamine turnover and rich in dopamine receptors.

There is evidence that populations of dopamine receptors
are higher than normal in schizophrenics (26), though this
may be because receptors increase as a result of neuroleptic
therapy (27). Spiperone, a butyrophenone, is well-known to be
a good ligand for dopamine receptors. Recently Wagner et al
(28) prepared a ^{11}C-labelled derivative of spiperone, namely
2-(^{11}C)methyl-spiperone, and reported its localization in the
basal ganglia of normal human brain.

At the MRC Cyclotron Unit, London, both 2-(^{11}C)methyl-
spiperone and L-(^{18}F)fluorodopa are being used to study
Parkinson's disease and untreated schizophrenia. For these
studies, Turton et al (29) have developed a method for the
preparation of 2-(^{11}C)methyl-spiperone (fig 9), which, like
that of Wagner et al (28), involves the N-methylation of
spiperone with (^{11}C)iodomethane. The method produces (2-^{11}C)
methyl-spiperone in 12% radiochemical yield, decay-corrected
from cyclotron-produced (^{11}C)carbon dioxide, and with a
specific activity of 20 - 40 GBq/µmol. The L-(^{18}F)fluorodopa
is prepared according to a method developed by Firnau et al
(30), which involves the direct fluorination of L-dopa. This

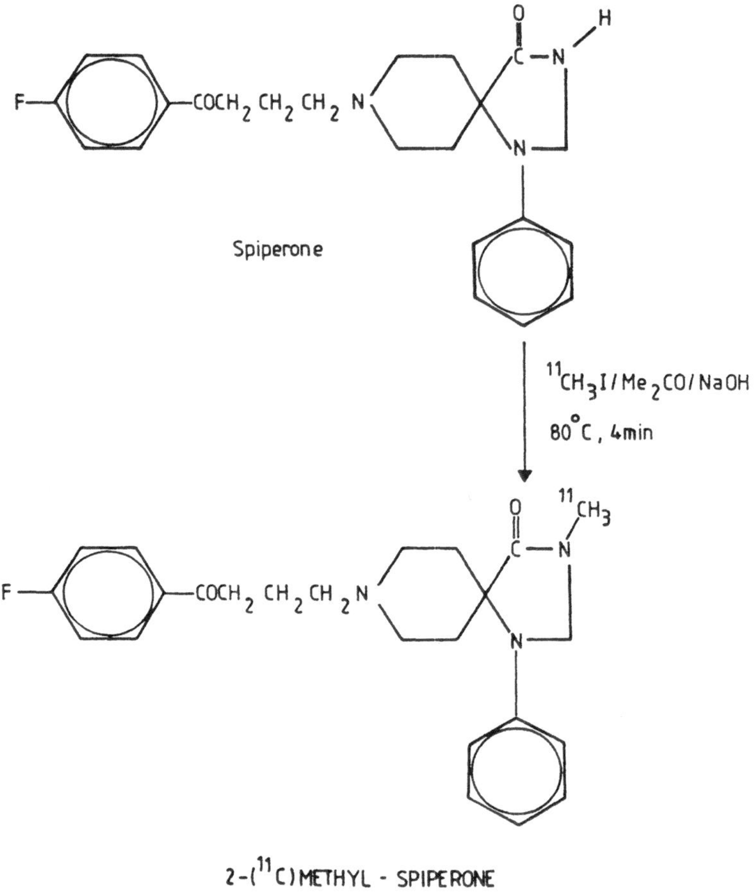

Fig. 9. The radiosynthesis of 2-(^{11}C)methyl-spiperone, according to Turton et al (29).

route produces predominantly the desired 6-(^{18}F)fluoroisomer with the 2- and 5-(^{18}F)fluoroisomers as impurities.

It is expected that the combined use of these radiopharmaceuticals will yield valuable information on both the pre- and post-synaptic dopaminergic systems of brain in relation to Parkinson's disease and schizophrenia. In particular, it should be possible to measure the distribution, storage and rate of turnover of dopamine with L-(^{18}F)fluorodopa and the distribution and concentrations of dopamine receptors with 2-(^{11}C)methyl-spiperone.

CONCLUSION

The advances described in this chapter serve to show the increasing power of PET for the investigation of pathophysiology and drug pharmacokinetics in vivo. This power stems, not only from the quantitative nature of PET, but also from the opportunities that continue to be taken in the development of positron-emitting radiopharmaceuticals that can closely monitor some aspect of physiology.

ACKNOWLEDGEMENTS

Most of the studies described in this chapter originate from the PET programme at the MRC Cyclotron Unit. As such they have involved the active collaboration of numerous radio-chemists, medical physicists and clinicians. I would like to express my thanks to all of these colleagues, all of whom may be identified as being associated with particular projects from the bibliography to this chapter. Also I would like to express my thanks to Mr. D.D. Vonberg, Dr D.J.Silvester, Mr. J. Clark and Mr. T. Jones for their invaluable support and encouragement.

158

REFERENCES

1. Phelps ME, Hoffman EJ, Mullani NA, Ter-Pogossian NM, J. nucl. Med. 16:210, 1975.

2. Welch MJ, In: Yearbook of Nuclear Medicine, Quinn III, J, (ed), Yearbook Medical, Chicago 4, pp 6-18, 1969.

3. Pike VW, Eakins MN, Allan RM, Selwyn AP, J. Radioanal. Chem. 64:291, 1981.

4. Schelbert HR, In: Computed Emission Tomography, Ell PJ, Holman BL (eds), Oxford Medical Publications, Oxford University Press, pp 91-133, 1982.

5. Ter-Pogossian MM, Klein MS, Markham J, Roberts R, Sobel BE, Circulation 61:242, 1980.

6. Selwyn AP, MacArthur C, Allan R, Pike V, Jones T, Proc. 8th Eur. Congr. Cardiology, p 194, 1980 (abstract).

7. Pike VW, Eakins MN, Allan RM, Selwyn AP, Int. appl. Radiat. Isot. 33:505, 1982.

8. Allan RM, Pike VW, Fox K, Maseri A, Selwyn AP, Eur. J. Nucl. Med. 6:A3, 1981 (abstract).

9. Selwyn AP, Allan RM, Pike V, Fox K, Maseri A, Cardiology, 47:481, 1981 (abstract).

10. Allan RM, Pike VW, Maseri A, Selwyn AP, Clin. Sci. 62:3p, 1982 (abstract).

11. Livni E, Elmaleh DR, Levy S, Brownell GL, Strauss WH, J. nucl. Med. 23:169, 1982.

12. De Landsheere C, Wilson R. Shea M, Pike V, Elmaleh D, Livni E, Jones T, Maseri A, Selwyn A, Circulation, 68:supp III-139, 1983 (abstract).

13. De Landsheere C, Shea M, Wilson R, Pike V, Elmaleh D, Livni E, Jadv A, Sohanpal SK, Jones T, Maseri A, Selwyn A, Eur. Heart J. (in press) (abstract).

14. Phelps ME, Selin C, Huang SC, Robinson G, MacDonald N, Schelbert MR, Kuhl DE, J. nucl. Med. 19:1311, 1978.

15. Camici P, Kaski JC, Shea MJ, Selwyn AP, Jones T, Maseri A, Circulation, 68:supp III-324, 1983 (abstract).

16. Sohanpal SK, Pike VW, Camici P, Nucl. Med. Comm. 24:238, 1984 (abstract).

17. Ehrin E, Westman E, Nilsson SO, Nilsson JLG, J.Lab. Comp. Radiopharm. 17-453, 1980.

18. Wisenberg G, Schelbert HR, Hoffman EJ, Phelps ME, Robinson GD, Selin CE, Child J, Skorton D, Kuhl DE, Circulation, 63:1248, 1981.

19. Turton DR, Brady F, Pike VW, Selwyn AP, Shea MJ, Wilson RA, De Landsheere CM, Int. J. appl. Radiat. Isot. 35:337, 1984.

20. Pike VW, Turton DR, Brady F, Deanfield J, De Landsheere CM, Shea MJ, Wilson RA, Maseri A, Selwyn AP, Nucl. Med. Comm. 24:257, 1984 (abstract).

21. Selwyn AP, Personal communication.

22. Pike VW, Palmer AJ, Horlock PL, Perun TJ, Freiberg LA, Dunnigan DA, Liss RH, Int. J. appl. Radiat. Isot. 35:103, 1984.

23. Wollmer P, Pride NB, Rhodes CG, Sanders A, Pike VW, Palmer AJ, Silvester DJ, Liss RH, Lancet 2:1361, 1982.

24. Rhodes CG, Wollmer P, Fazio F, Jones T, J. Comput. Assist. Tomogr. 5:783, 1981.

25. Garnet ES, Firnau G, Nahmias C, Nature 305:137, 1983.

26. Owen F, Cross AJ, Crow TJ, Longden A, Poulter M, Riley GJ, Lancet 2:223, 1978.

27. Burt DR, Creese I, Snyder SH, Science 196:326, 1977.

28. Wagner Jr, HN, Burns HD, Dannals RF, Wong DR, Langstrom B, Duelfer T, Frost JJ, Ravert HT, Links JM, Rosenbloom SB, Lukas SE, Kramer AV, Kuhar MJ, Science 221:1264, 1983.

29. Turton DR, Pike VW, Cartoon M, Widdowson DA, J. Lab. Comp. Radio-pharm. (in press) (abstract).

30. Firnau G, Chirakel R, Garnett ES, J. nucl. Med. (in press).

RADIOPHARMACEUTICALS SUITABLE FOR CARDIAC EMERGENCY STUDIES

H.W. PABST, R. BAUER

A variety of different isotopes are used in cardiac studies.
The most important isotopes are summarized in table 1. This
table comprises short lived positron emitting cyclotron
products, like C^{11}, N^{13}, O^{15} and F^{18}, ultra short lived
isotopes like Kr^{81m} and Au^{195m}, In^{111} to be used in labelling
platelets and leucocytes, I^{123} to be used in metabolic studies,
and of course the most commonly applied isotopes Tc^{99m} and
Tl^{201}.

The short lived cyclotron products and their applications
are shown in table 2. Various fatty acids, amino acids and
glucose are labelled with C^{11}, N^{13} and F^{18} to investigate
myocardial metabolism and its pathological alterations. Left
ventricular function is assessed by inhalation of O^{15} labelled
CO_2, which is converted to radioactive water in the lung, thus
providing a compact bolus of activity to reach the left heart.
Due to the short half life between 20 and some 100 min, those
investigations can only be performed near a cyclotron site at
certain times when the isotopes are produced and available.

Kr^{81m} has a half life of only 13 sec and is useful in
studies of the right ventricular function. Au^{195m} has a half
life of 31 sec and can be used for multiple first pass investigations of both the right and left ventricular function.
Both isotopes are obtainable as generator products from a
Rb^{81} and a Hg^{195} mother with nearly 5 and 10 hours half life,
respectively (table 3). Those generators are expensive and
can be used only for a short space of time. Therefore, these
isotopes and the before mentioned positron emitters are un-
likely to be available and applicable in cardiac emergency
studies.

Table 1

Isotopes used in cardiac studies

Isotope	T 1/2	rad.	keV
C–11	20 m.	β^+	511
N–13	10 m.	β^+	511
O–15	2 m.	β^+	511
F–18	110 m.	β^+	511
Kr–81m	13 s	γ	190
Tc–99m	6 h	γ	140
In–111	2.8 d	EC,γ	247,173
I–123	13 h	EC,γ	159
Au–195m	31 s	γ	262
Tl–201	73 h	EC,γ	167,135 65–82

Table 2

Short lived cyclotron products

metabolic studies:

C–11 fatty acids	20 min
C–11, N–13 amino acids	20, 10 min
F–18 glucose	110 min

left ventricular function:

$$O-15-CO_2 + H_2O \rightleftharpoons CO_2 + O-15-H_2O$$

Table 3

Ultra short lived isotopes (generator products)

Rb-81   4.7 h

Kr-81m   13 s, 190 keV

right ventricular function

Hg-195   9.5 h

Au-195m   31 s, 262 keV

left (right) ventricular function

Table 4

Long lived cyclotron products

I-123 fatty acids   (13h, 159 keV)

     metabolism

TI-201   (73h, 167, 135, 65-82 keV)

     myocardial perfusion

     infarction, ischemia

The application of the long lived cyclotron products I^{123} and Tl^{201} to investigations of the heart is summarized in table 4. Metabolic studies are performed using I^{123} labelled fatty acids, but these investigations are usually of no interest in cardiac emergency patients. The myocardial perfusion is assessed by using Tl^{201}, demonstrating stress induced hypoperfusion and myocardial infarcts. Thus, Tl^{201} is widely applied in the diagnosis of coronary artery disease. One of the most important applications is the demonstration of vital myocardium, when the myocardial function is suppressed due to a persistent ischemia, causing severe wallmotion anomalies to be seen in contrast or radionuclide ventriculography.

The most important isotope to be used in cardiac emergency studies is Tc^{99m}. Common applications are listed in table 5. Left and right ventricular function can be assessed using pertechnetate or Tc^{99m} labelled human serum albumin "HSA" or autologous reds cells "RBC". Whereas pertechnetate can only be applied to first pass studies, labelled human serum albumin and red cells are retained in the intravasal space (1). ECG-triggered heart studies can be recorded for a couple of hours, especially when using red cells and the heart function can be assessed over a period of up to 10 hours. Stress induced myocardial ischemia, myocardial infarcts and global pump failure can be diagnosed and both regional and global heart function can be investigated.

Tc^{99m} labelled polyphosphates highlight myocardial infarcts in positive contrast. Tc-labelled Di-Methyl-Phosphino-Ethane demonstrates myocardial perfusion. Those two radiopharmaceuticals are of no importance in cardiac emergency studies.

Cardiac emergency means acute pump failure, the reason of which sometimes can not be revealed by non-invasive investigations. Since the patients are severely ill, an invasive heart catheterization is not performed on account of its considerable inherent risk. On the other hand, radionuclide ventriculography can be performed without risk for the patient, demonstrating morphology, position, size and shape of the heart and its 4 cavities, and demonstrating global and regional

Table 5

Tc−99m in heart studies

Tc−99m−TcO$_4^-$
Tc−99m−HSA
Tc−99m−RBC
   left (right) ventricular function
   (first pass, EKG gated)

Tc−99m polyphosphates
   infarct imaging

Tc−99m−DMPE
   myocardial perfusion

Table 6 **Radionuclide ventriculography
in cardiac emergency**

left heart infarction

   aneurysm
   perforation
   rupture of papillary muscle
   pericardial effusion

right heart infarction

polytrauma

   aneurysm of aorta
   rupture of pericardium

complications after surgery

lung embolism

function of both ventricles as well. Because global and regional heart function are the most important parameters to be
known to the refering cardiologist, radionuclide ventriculography is the scintigraphic investigation of choice in cardiac
emergency.

Some indications of RNV in cardiac emergency are listed
in table 6. Most commonly, pump failure will be due to left
heart infarction accompanied by an aneurysm of the myocardium,
a myocardial perforation, rupture of a papillary muscle or a
pericardial effusion causing a heart tamponade. An isolated
infarction of the right ventricular myocardium is not very
common. But it is very important to diagnose a massive right
heart infarction correctly due to its therapeutic implications. Polytraumatized patients can come into cardiac emergency with an aneurysm of the aorta or a luxation of the
heart following a pericardial rupture. Finally, complications
after heart surgery and hemodynamic restrictions caused by
massive lung embolism may result in cardiac emergency (2).

In radionuclide ventriculography studies, we record both
the first pass and ECG-triggered studies after equilibration
of the tracer. Especially in situations with probable atypical
morphology, a combination for both studies is very useful.
During the first pass, 36 images showing the tracer passage
(cf fig 3a and 4a), (3,7), ECG-triggered representative cycles
of the right and the left heart and time activity curves are
recorded (cf fig 8). During equilibrium representative cycles
with 16 images are obtained, showing the heart from different
views (4).

Each scan is complemented by amplitude and phase images
computed by a Fourier analysis (5). The diastolic, systolic,
amplitude and phase images together with phase histograms are
given in fig 1 for the anterior view, above, and the left
anterior oblique view, LAO 40, below. The amplitudes correlate
with the change of volume, indicating the amount of ventricular and atrial contraction. The phases demonstrate the co-
herence of contraction and relaxation during the heart cycle
(3). Usually, the change of volume of both ventricles is highly synchronized, which is demonstrated by the sharply peaked

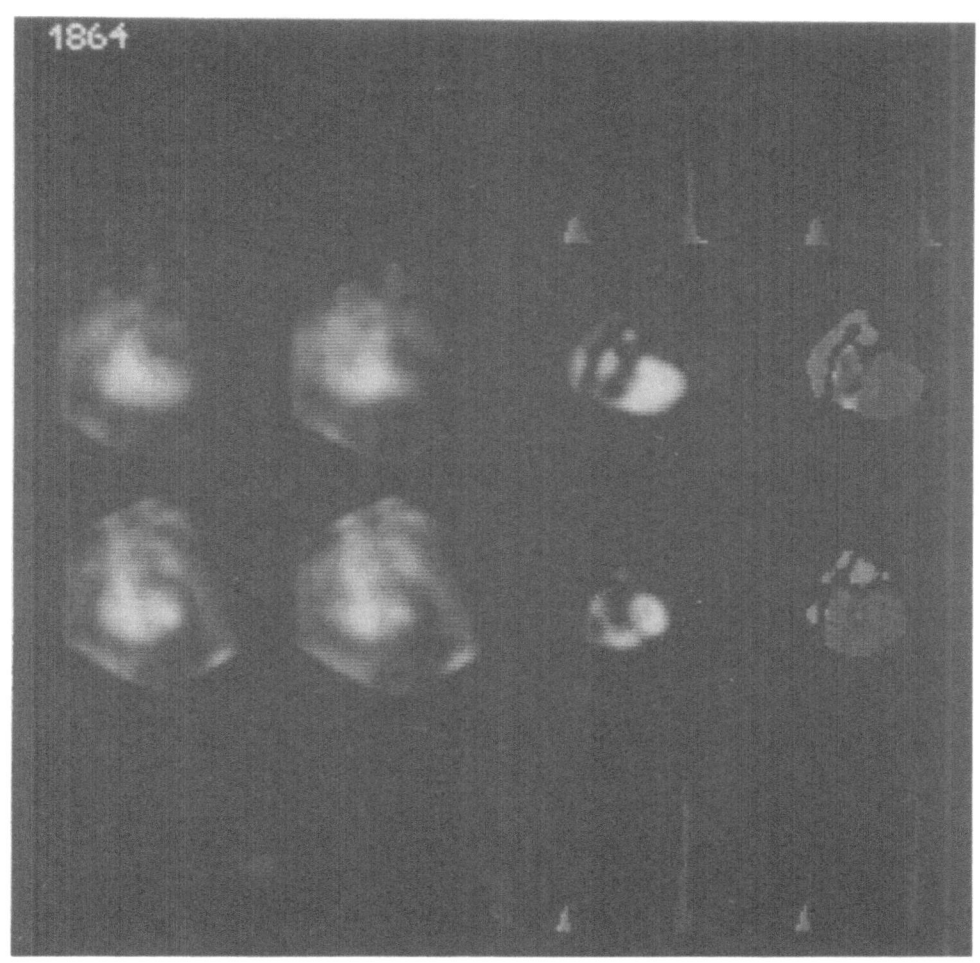

Fig. 1. Diastolic, systolic, amplitude and phase images and phase histograms of a healthy patient, recorded in anterior (above) and LAO 40 view (below).

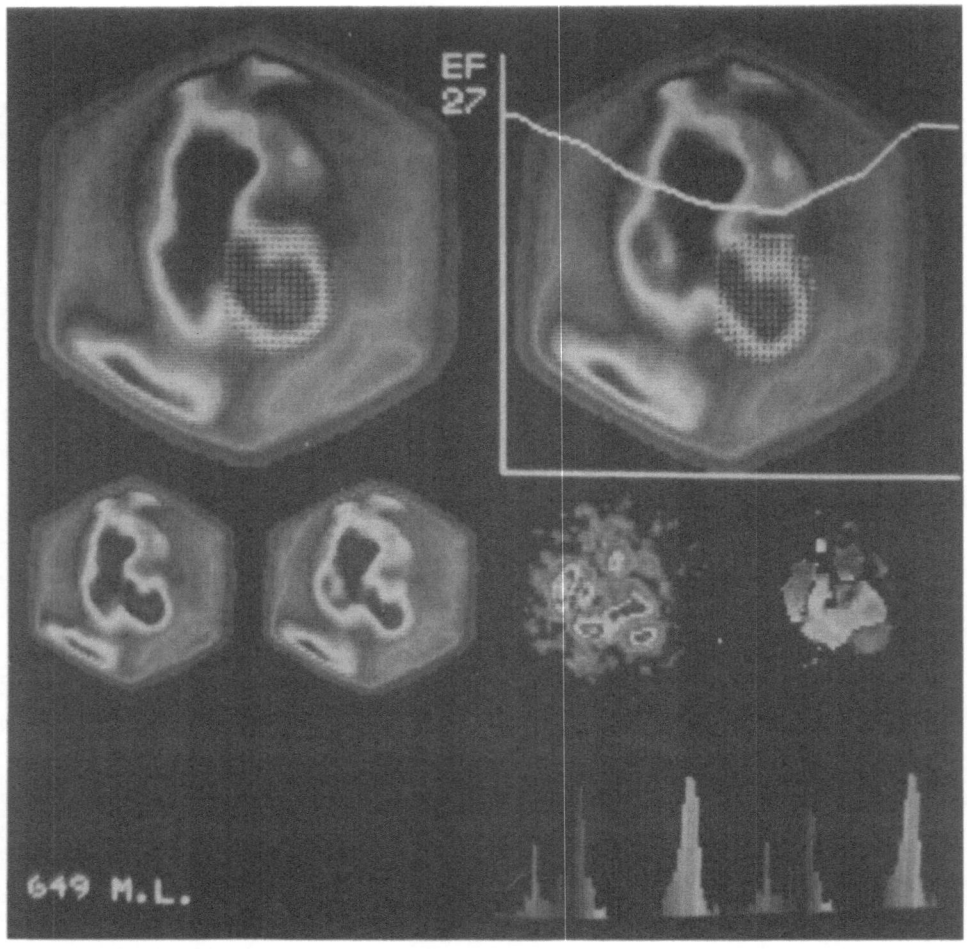

Fig. 2. Aneurysm of the left ventricle. Above: enddiastolic and end-systolic image with ROI's and time activity curve. Below: enddiastolic, endsystolic, amplitude and phase image and phase histograms.

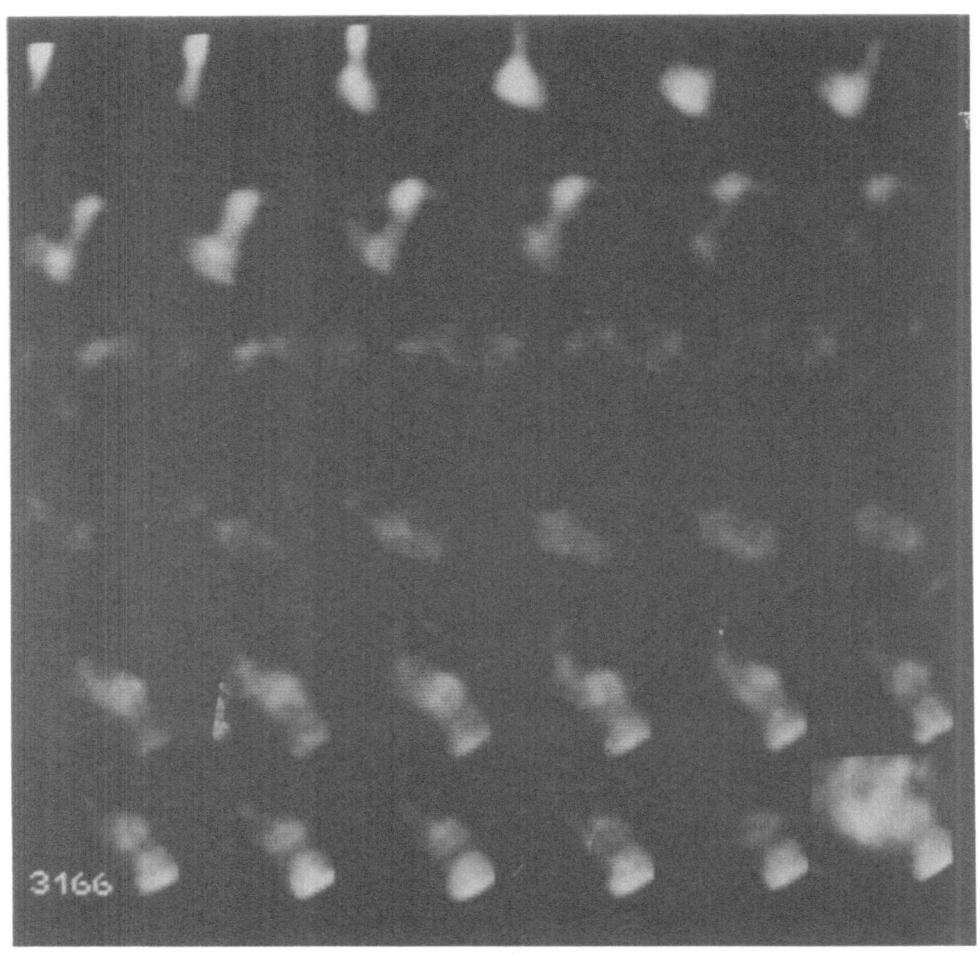

Fig. 3a. 36 Images of the first pass of a patient with a huge
aneurysm of the left ventricle.

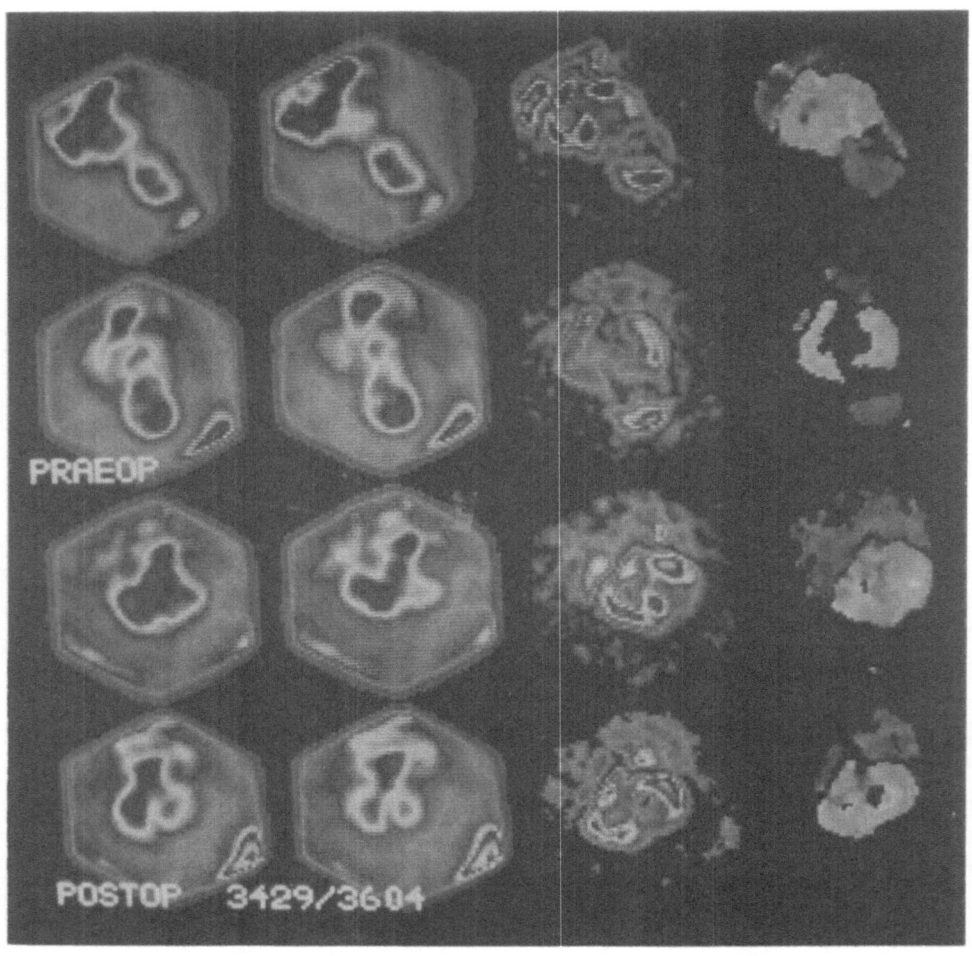

Fig. 3b. Diastolic, systolic amplitude and phase images prior to and following aneurysmectomy, recorded in anterior and LAO 40 view (upper and lower rows, respectively).

red phase histograms.

A patient with heart failure due to a large aneurysm of the left ventricle is demonstrated in fig 2. The ejection fraction is reduced to 27%. It is derived from a background corrected time activity curve of a diastolic and a systolic region as shown in the upper quadrants (6).

The phase image reveals by the blue phases the extent of the aneurysm, the area of the aneurysmatic region, comprising the apex and the antero-lateral wall. The amplitude image indicates the amount of volume change: from the nearly equal red colour of the amplitudes of both the basal vital myocardium and the aneurysm it becomes evident that the aneurysm reduces markedly the left ventricular output. Whereas the left vital myocardium is contracting, the aneurysmatic sac is widening, causing a severe reduction in stroke volume of every beat.

Fig 3a demonstrates a patient with a huge false aneurysm due to a perforation of the myocardium covered only by the pericardium. This image shows the first pass with right atrium and ventricle, the lungs and the left heart. Following the influx of tracer into the left ventricle, a large sac below the ventricle is filled with activity, remaining there when the ventricle itself is emptying again. Fig 3b shows the situation after equilibration of the tracer, the columns giving the diastolic, systolic, amplitude and phase images in anterior and LAO 40 view pre- and postoperatively. Preoperatively, shown above, the sac of the false aneurysm is seen, moving paradoxically as indicated by the amplitudes and phases. The next day, the diagnosis was proven by contrast ventriculography and the patient had aneurysmectomy shortly afterwards. Postoperatively, shown below, heart function has much improved, only the scar is akinetic.

Fig 4a shows the first pass of a patient with a perforated septal wall following myocardial infarction. When the activity returns to the left heart, the right ventricle does not empty further, in contrary its activity increases slightly, whereas the right atrium is not seen any more. These findings

172

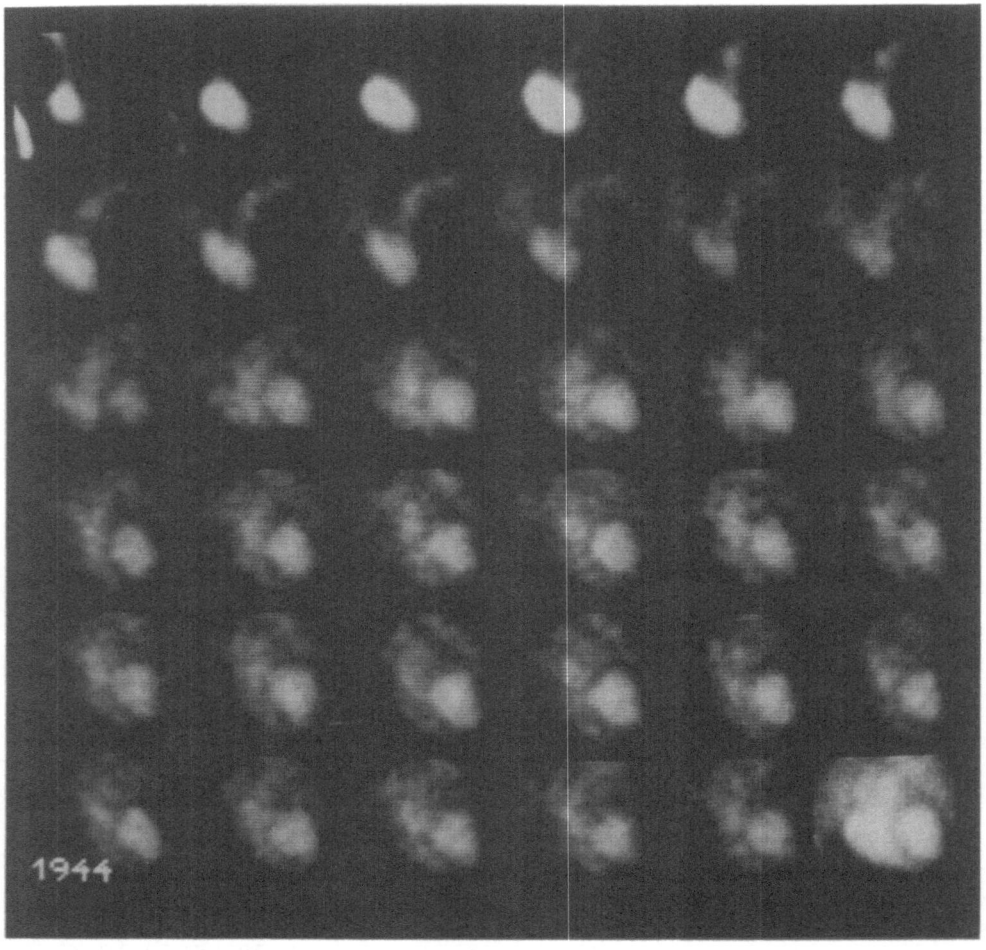

Fig. 4a. First pass study of a patient with ventricular septal defect due to an extended anteroseptal infarction and left to right shunt.

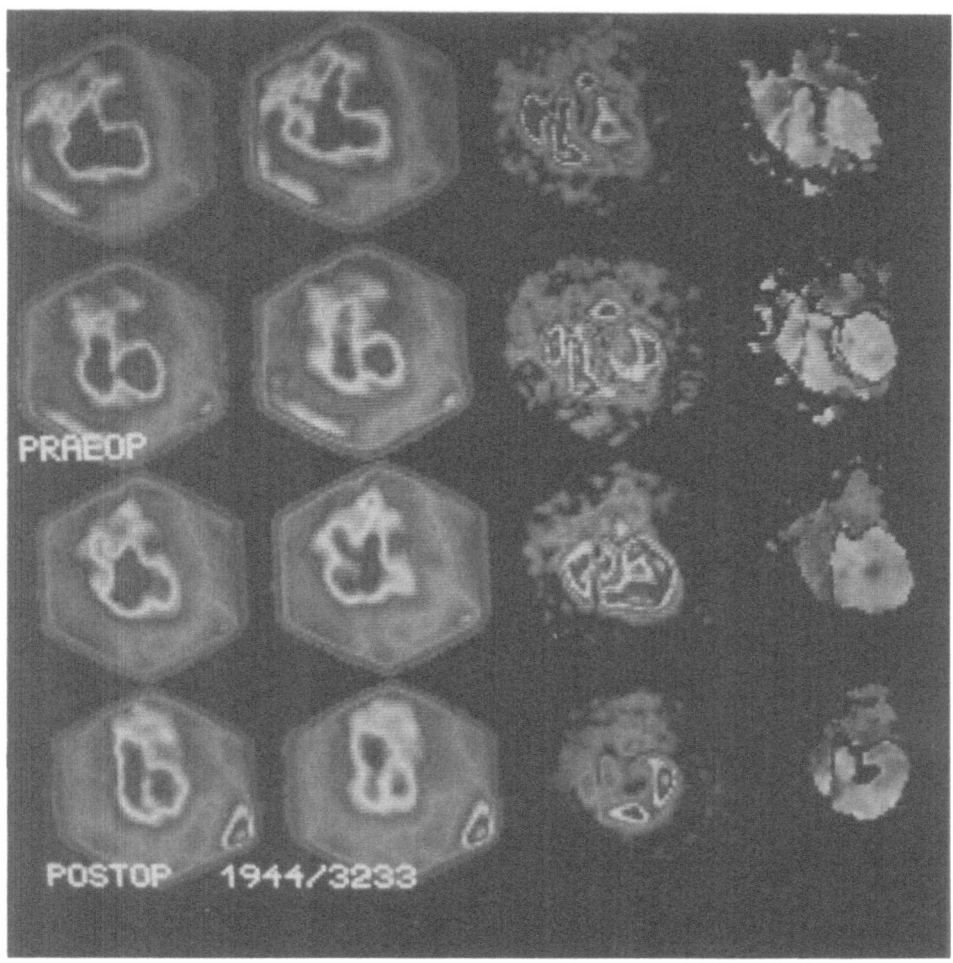

Fig. 4b. Diastolic, systolic, amplitude and phase images prior to and following heart surgery in anterior and LAO 40 view (upper and lower rows, respectively).

174

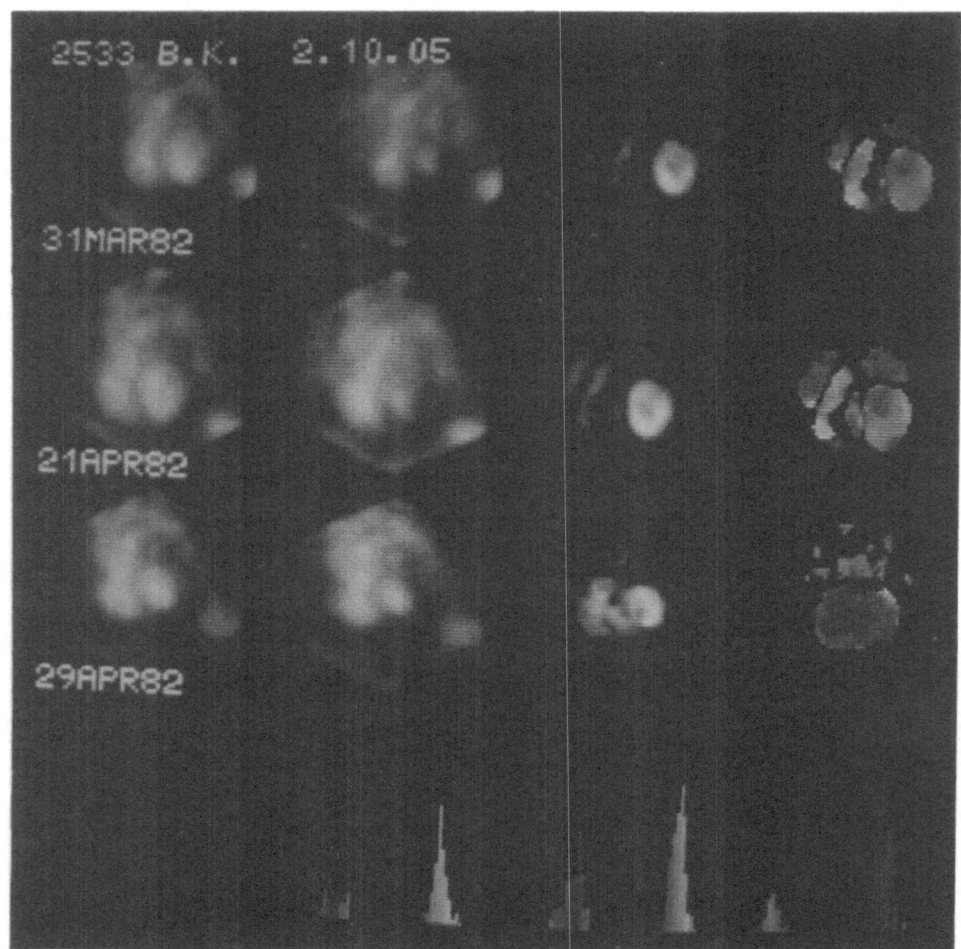

Fig. 5. Diastolic, systolic amplitude and phase images and phase histograms of a patient with mitral insufficiency. Follow-up pre- and postoperatively.

demonstrate a large left-to-right shunt due to a ventricular
septal defect. Right and left ventricular function was assessed by EKG gated radionuclide ventriculograms, as given in fig
4b.

Again, enddiastolic, endsystolic, amplitude and phase
images are shown pre- and postoperatively. The right ventricle
has an unusual high concentration amplitude due to the shunt
volume. The septal wall is moving paradoxically, depicted by
the green en blue colours. The septal defect is outlined by
the green phases. After surgery and closing the defect by a
dacron prosthesis, both ventricles have reduced in size, the
left ventricle is contracting more rigorously than the right
one, except for the akinetic septum. Whereas prior to surgery
the lungs and the liver were overloaded by blood due to a
beginning right heart failure, the situation has normalized
afterwards, as can be seen when comparing the respective
images.

A case of an acute mitral regurgitation due to a myocardial
infarction and rupture of a papillary muscle is shown in fig 5.

Preoperatively, both ventricles are enlarged, and the enddiastolic volume increased within 3 weeks. Nevertheless, the
left ventricular function was sufficient, and despite the age
of the patient, being 78 years, he had a left heart catheter
and surgery. After insertion of an artificial valve, heart
function has normalized as shown in the lower row. With
respect to the age of the patient, he certainly would not have
had invasive diagnostics and surgery, if radionuclide ventriculography would not have proven a sufficient left heart function.

A right heart infarction is difficult to diagnose by non-
invasive means, whereas it can be easily demonstrated by
radionuclide ventriculography as demonstrated in fig 6. Scintigraphy reveals a normal sized left ventricle and an enlarged
right ventricle. Right ventricular ejection fraction is reduced
to 34% in contrast to the normal or even slightly elevated
left ventricular ejection fraction of 70%. Right ventricular
contraction is markedly retarded and depressed, as indicated
by the phase and amplitude images.

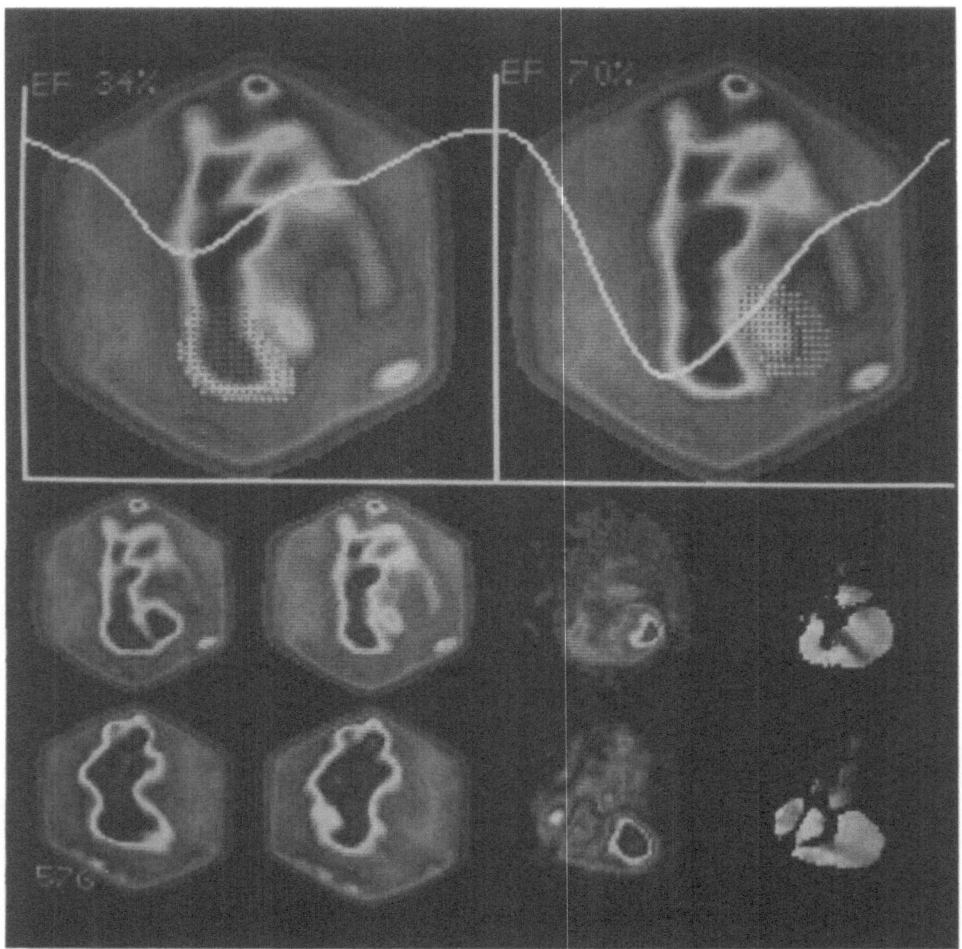

Fig. 6. Systolic images of a right heart infarction with superimposed time activity curves of the right and left ventricle (above). Diastolic, systoli, amplitude and phase images in LAO 40 and anterior view are given below.

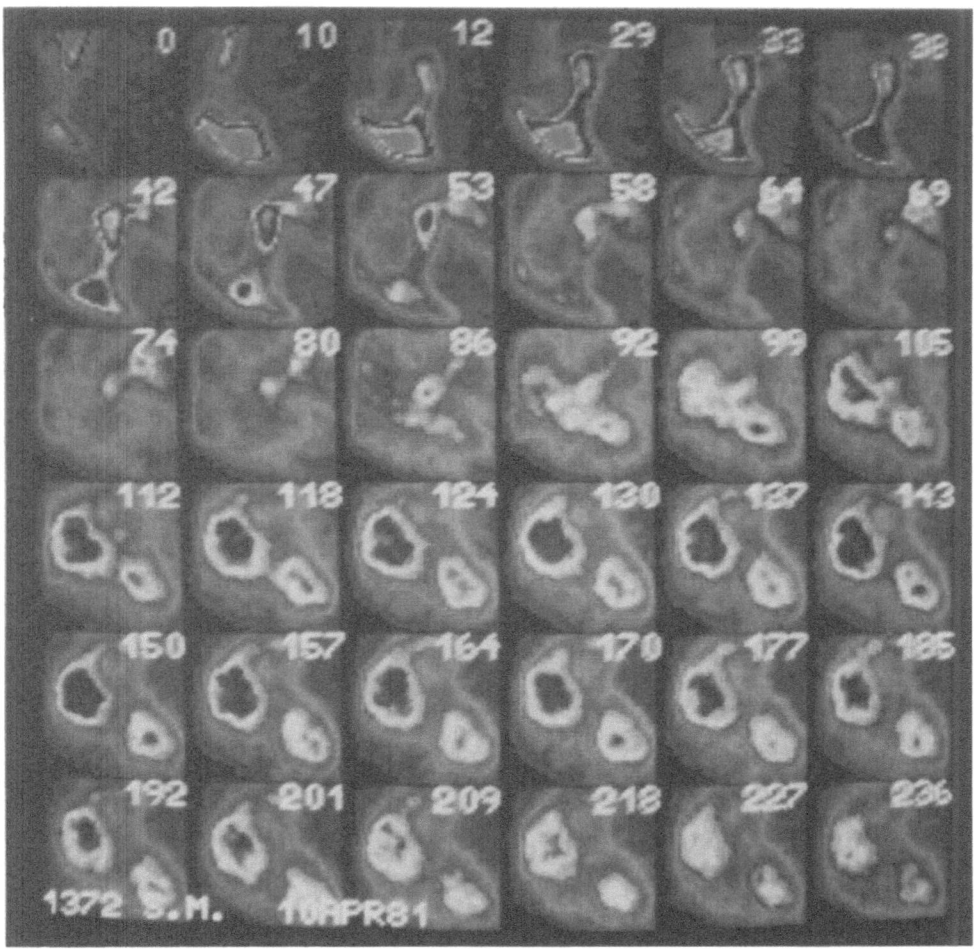

Fig. 7a. First pass of a patient with a traumatic rupture of the aorta ascendens and aortic regurgitation.

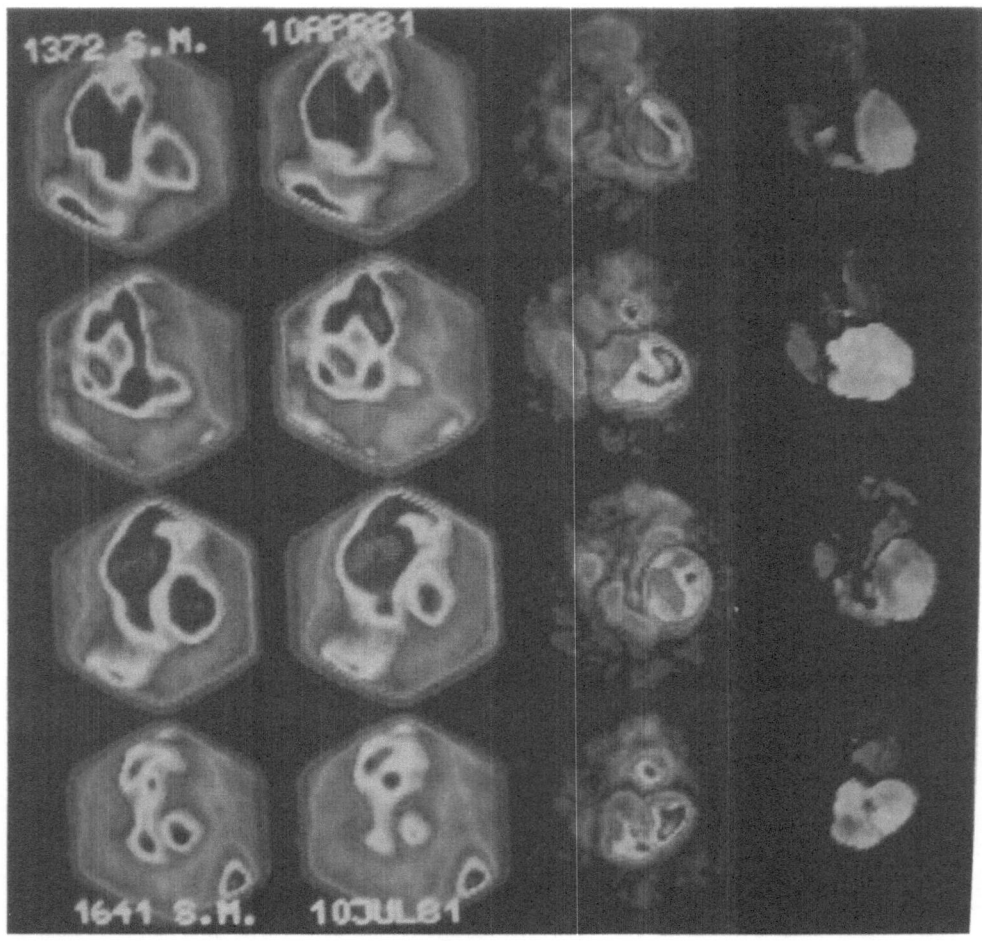

Fig. 7b. Diastolic, systolic, amplitude and phase images in anterior view (above) and LAO 40 view (below) prior to and following surgery aortic valve replacement and implantation of a dacron conduit.

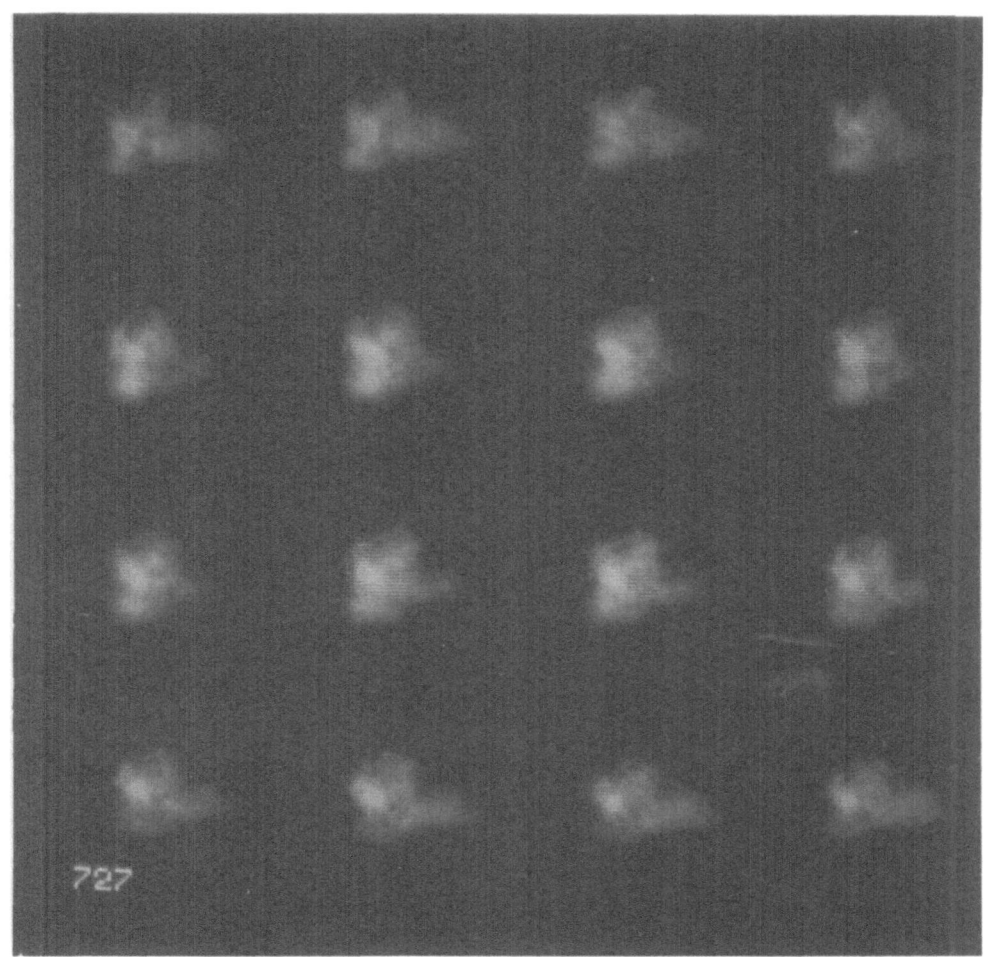

Fig. 8. ECG gated representative cycles of the right heart, represented in blue, and of the left heart, given red, of a patient with luxation of the heart.

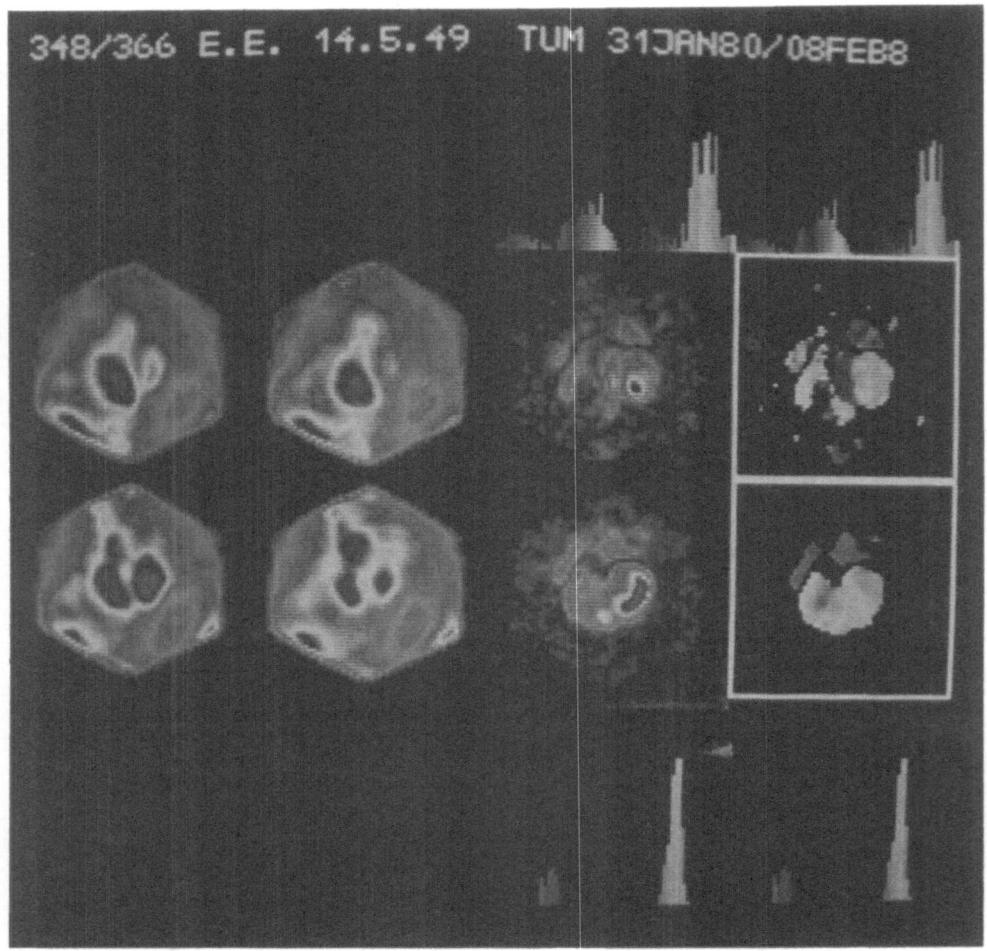

Fig. 9. Diastolic, systolic amplitude and phase images and phase histograms during acute lung embolism (above) and after successful therapy (below).

It is clinically important to differentiate between left and right heart infarction, because of different therapeutic requirements. In this patient, volume was substituted and the cardiac shock could be overcome.

A typical complication of heavy car accidents or of a fall from a great high is a traumatic aneurysm of the aorta, as shown in fig 7a.

In the first pass, the vena cava superior and the pulmonary artery are widely separated. Immediately following the onset of the left heart phase, the aneurysmatic enlarged aorta is filled. Radioactivity is maintained for a long period of time due to aortic regurgitation. The volume of this aneurysm was estimated to be three times the left ventricular volume.

Fig 7b gives the results pre- en post surgery, in anterior and LAO 40 view. Prior to surgery, the left ventricle is enlarged, and the aneurysm shows a systolic pulsation as indicated by the phases. After surgery, heart function has normalized.

A rare case is a traumatic rupture of the pericardium with subsequent luxation of the heart, as demonstrated in fig 8. Both of the right and the left heart cycle, obtained from the first pass, are given in blue and red. The right ventricle projects over the left one, a finding not to be discovered after equilibration of the tracer.

In patients with massive lung embolism, heart function can be severely reduced, as demonstrated in fig 9. The heart is shown in LAO 40 view, above immediately following embolism, below 8 days later. On account of the increased pressure in the pulmonary circulation, the right ventricle is enlarged, and the complete right ventricular contraction is out of phase. The right heart output and consequently the left heart output is reduced, as can be seen from the small left ventricular volume. Thus, the reduced systemic blood-flow was causing a cardiogenic shock. 8 days later, the patient had recovered and the cardiac situation had completely normalized: both ventricles are normal in size, shape and contraction pattern.

The examples shown underline the importance of radionuclide ventriculography in patients with cardiac emergency. The

182

morphological and functional information as provided by the scintigraphic investigation is often very useful in the diagnosis and for the further treatment of patients with heart failure. Because Tc^{99m} is commonly available, labelled HSA or RBC will be the radiopharmaceutical of choice in these cases.

REFERENCES

1. Bauer R, Halusczynski I, Langhammer H, Bachmann W, In vivo/in vitro labeling of red blood cells with 99m-Tc. Eur. J. Nucl. Med. 8:218, 1983.

2. Pabst HW, Bauer R, Nuklearmedizinische Diagnostik beim kardinalen Notfall. Nukl. Med. suppl. 19:191, 1981.

3. Bauer R, Pabst HW, Sauer E, Ein interaktives Rechenprogramm zur Bestimmung globaler Parameter der Herzfunktion aus der Radionuklid-ventrikulographie. Systeme und Signalverarbeitung in der Nuklear-medizin. Pöppl SJ, Pretschner DP, (eds), Springer Verlag, Berlin, Heidelberg, B27, pp 177-186.

4. Bauer R, Sauer E, Langhammer H, Pabst HW, Parametric images of amplitudes and phases in analysing regional heart function. Nukl. Med. suppl. pp 80-83, 1982.

5. Adam WE, Geffers H, Sigel H, Bitter F, Kampmann H, Strauch M, Wasser-mann B, Evaluation of left ventricular function by radionuclide-angiography. Herz, 2:195, 1977.

6. Bauer R, Sauer E, Truckenbrodt R, Langhammer H, Pabst HW, Sebening H, Wirtzfeld A, Blömer H, Die linksventrikuläre Herzfunktion in Ruhe und unter Ergometerbelastung. Herz, 5:159, 1980.

7. Pabst HW, Bauer R, Sauer E, Optimale Datenaufnahme und – auswertung bei der Herzbinnenraumszintigraphie - Vergleich von first pass (mit Zeitaktivitätskurven und repräsentativen Zyklen) und Aufnahmen in steady state. Systeme und Signalverarbeitung in der Nuklearmedizin. Pöppl SJ, Pretschner DP, (eds), Springer Verlag, Berlin, Heidelberg, B 27, pp 59-67, 1981.

THE PHARMACOKINETICS OF Tc^{99m}-DIETHYL IDA IN HYPER-FERREMIC MICE

C. SAWAS-DIMOPOULOU, C. SOULPI, N. TOUBANAKIS

INTRODUCTION

Iron excess may potentiate diseases affecting the liver. Hepatic cirrhosis of thalassaemia major is characterized by iron particles or aggregates deposition in parenchymal and reticuloendothelial cells especially in lysosome as haemosiderin or ferritin or in cellsap as ferritin (1,2). Most thalassaemic patients have however normal liver function tests until "end-stage disease" is reached (3). In idiopathic haemochromatosis, the enormous quantities of iron, in the order of 20-60 g, accumulate in the liver as a result of increased intestinal absorption and produce hepatic structural changes. In the early stages, portal zone fibrosis is observed with deposition of iron in the periportal liver cells and to a lesser extent in the Kupffer cells (4). Surprisingly, biochemical tests show little disturbance except for a positive BSP test (5). That would suggest a peculiar sensitivity to iron overload of the important bile excretory pathway including organic anions such as BSP, conjugated bilirubin, dyes and IDA derivatives. The purpose of the present study was to investigate the effect of hyperferremia on the pharmacokinetics of Tc^{99m}-diethyl IDA.

MATERIAL AND METHODS

Male mice SWR/De, 2½ months old were used. Jectofer, a micromolecular complex of iron sortibol and critic acid (Astra chemicals and pharmaceuticals, N.V. Holland) were injected intra-peritoneally once daily for 3 days. The total dose of iron received by each mouse was equal to 525 µg. Control mice received identical volumes of 0.18% citrate in

isotonic solution (0.1 ml per 20 g body weight). One to 2
hours after the last injection of Jectofer, a biodistribution
study of Tc^{99m}-diethyl IDA was performed. The radiopharmaceutical was injected into the tail vein. The experimental
animals were sacrificed at 2,3,4,5,10,15,30 and 60 min after
the i.v. injection. Aliquots of blood, the gallbladder, urine
and various organs were weighed and measured for their radioactivity content. The results were expressed as a percentage
of the injected dose. The means of controls and iron injected
animals were compared by the Student's t test.

Tissue distribution of iron was studied by injection of
1 μCi of Fe^{59} (ferric citrate) into the tail vein of mice,
1 min after the i.p. injection of 250 μg iron as Jectofer.
The animals were sacrificed 1 hour after the injection of
Fe^{59}. The radioactivity in blood, urine and various organs was
measured and the percent dose was calculated by reference to
a standard.

RESULTS

Table 1 shows the biodistribution of Fe^{59} co-administered
with a dose of 250 μg Fe as Jectofer. One hour after the injection of Fe^{59} the higher concentration of radioactivity is
found in the liver (23%). The effect or iron overload on the
biodistribution of Tc^{99m}-diethyl IDA is shown in table 2 and
figs 1-6.

The rate of Tc^{99m}-diethyl IDA disappearance from the blood
of hyperferremic mice was slower than that of controls. The
differences between the means were significant ($p < 0.05$) at
all the times between 2 and 60 min after injection. Analysis
of the liver time activity curves obtained in control and
hyperferremic animals (fig 2) shows that the shape of the
curve of treated mice is significantly distinct to that of
controls except for the initial uptake phase which does not
show significant differences between the 2 groups of mice.
The downslope portion of the curve regresses much faster in
controls than in iron-overloaded mice. Thus half-time of
liver elimination of radioactivity, measured on the downslope

Table 1. Biodistribution of Fe^{59} (Ferric citrate) in mice 1 hour after the administration of 250 μg iron

	% dose per organ*
Blood	6.28 ± 2.15
Liver	23.55 ± 2.55
Gallbladder	0.02 ± 0.01
Kidneys	4.79 ± 1.21
Stomach	0.76 ± 0.18
Intestine + faeces	4.12 ± 0.35
Spleen	0.98 ± 0.33
Muscle	6.15 ± 3.02
Bone marrow	8.55 ± 2.28
Urine	5.08 ± 1.62
Heart	0.39 ± 0.09
Lungs	0.55 ± 0.09
Pancreas	1.51 ± 0.14

*mean of 6 values ± 1 s.d.

from the t.max., is 0,8 min in controls and 2.7 min in hyperferremic mice. The hepatic clearance is delayed in hyperferremic mice. Thus, in control animals the percent dose in liver is 24.0 ± 0.9% at 2 min and 11.8 ± 0.6% at 3 min compared to 21.6 ± 2.1% at 2 min and 20.9 ± 1.3% at 3 min in iron treated mice. One hour after injection, liver concentration is still 4.8 ± 0.6% in hyperferremic mice compared to 0.9 ± 0.2% in controls. The gallbladder content did not show significant differences in controls and treated animals. The cumulated excretion of radioactivity into intestine was, however, significantly reduced in iron-treated mice to 36.0 ± 2.2% at 3 min and 49.6 ± 2.3% at 60 min compared to 45.9 ± 2.1% and 70.9 ± 2.2% in controls. Urine excretion was significantly increased in treated mice and reached 19.5 ± 1.7% at one hour compared to 7.1 ± 1.4% in normal mice.

186

Table 2. Biodistribution of Tc^{99m}-diethyl IDA in hyperferremic mice

% Dose per organ*

Time after injection	2 min	3 min	4 min	5 min	10 min	15 min	30 min	60 min
Blood of control mice	8.87 ± 0.33	4.72 ± 0.50	3.02 ± 0.41	2.26 ± 0.36	1.78 ± 0.31	1.60 ± 0.21	0.98 ± 0.26	0.51 ± 0.21
Hyperferremic mice	13.59 ± 1.69	8.92 ± 1.06	7.32 ± 0.61	6.23 ± 0.93	4.31 ± 0.70	3.60 ± 0.62	2.80 ± 0.48	2.44 ± 0.36
Liver of control mice	24.02 ± 0.97	11.80 ± 0.61	7.01 ± 1.32	4.86 ± 0.62	3.07 ± 0.41	2.71 ± 0.28	1.89 ± 0.31	0.96 ± 0.21
Hyperferremic mice	21.62 ± 2.09	20.91 ± 1.27	14.21 ± 2.27	11.53 ± 1.52	7.42 ± 1.21	5.50 ± 0.97	5.56 ± 0.79	4.80 ± 0.60
Gallbladder in control mice	2.52 ± 0.42	2.72 ± 0.51	2.46 ± 0.32	2.12 ± 0.43	1.76 ± 0.38	2.01 ± 0.39	6.38 ± 0.52	2.61 ± 0.39
Hyperferremic mice	1.89 ± 0.38	2.12 ± 0.44	1.92 ± 0.51	1.88 ± 0.37	1.58 ± 0.45	2.47 ± 0.41	6.82 ± 0.46	2.75 ± 0.45
Intestine of control mice	27.52 ± 2.81	45.89 ± 2.13	53.46 ± 1.67	56.66 ± 1.18	62.51 ± 1.36	65.51 ± 1.67	69.20 ± 2.21	70.99 ± 2.26
Hyperferremic mice	26.20 ± 2.21	36.02 ± 2.21	40.54 ± 2.12	42.81 ± 2.81	46.81 ± 2.24	47.76 ± 1.45	48.82 ± 2.80	49.68 ± 2.32
Urine of control mice	0.22 ± 0.03	0.89 ± 0.25	1.10 ± 0.20	1.27 ± 0.31	1.46 ± 0.31	6.70 ± 1.21	6.98 ± 1.36	7.08 ± 1.46
Hyperferremic mice	0.30 ± 0.11	2.50 ± 0.35	4.42 ± 0.61	5.91 ± 1.07	13.31 ± 1.84	17.65 ± 1.67	19.21 ± 2.17	19.63 ± 1.73

* mean of 5 values ± 1 s.d.

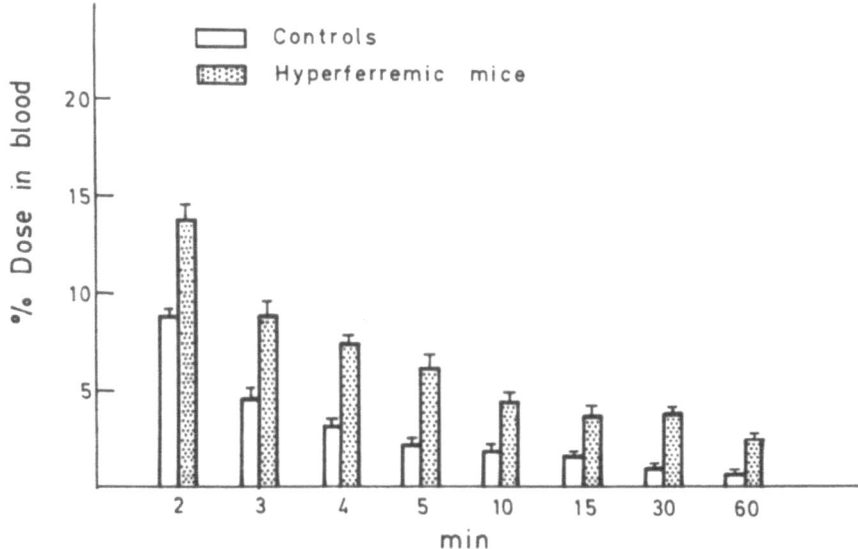

Fig. 1. Effect of iron administration on the blood clearance of Tc^{99m}-diethyl IDA in mice treated with Jectofer and in controls.

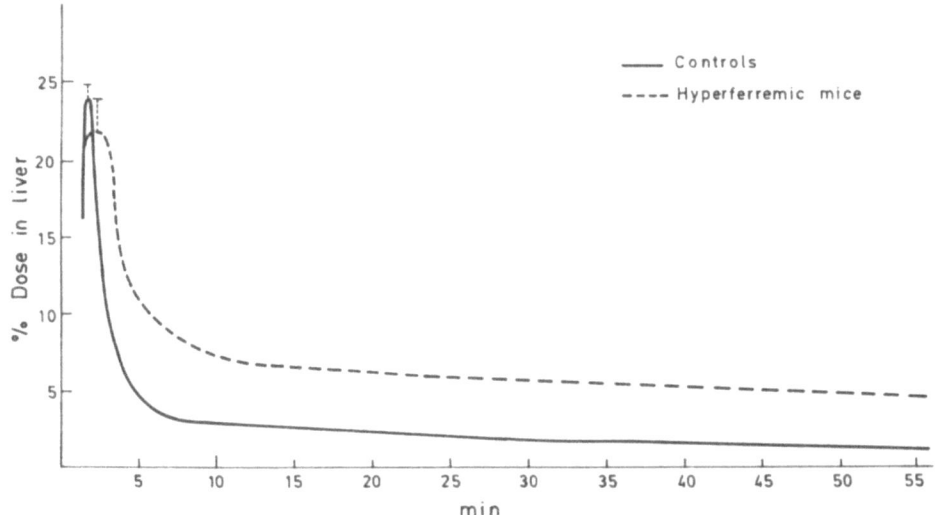

Fig. 2. Liver time-activity curves of Tc^{99m}-dietyl IDA in mice which received iron (------) and in controls (——).

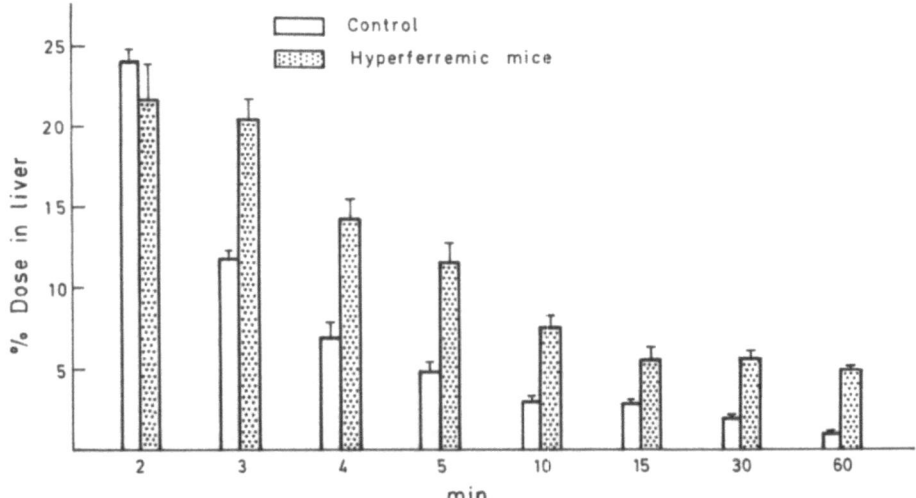

Fig. 3. Effect of iron on the liver concentration of Tc^{99m}–diethyl IDA in mice treated with Jectofer and in controls.

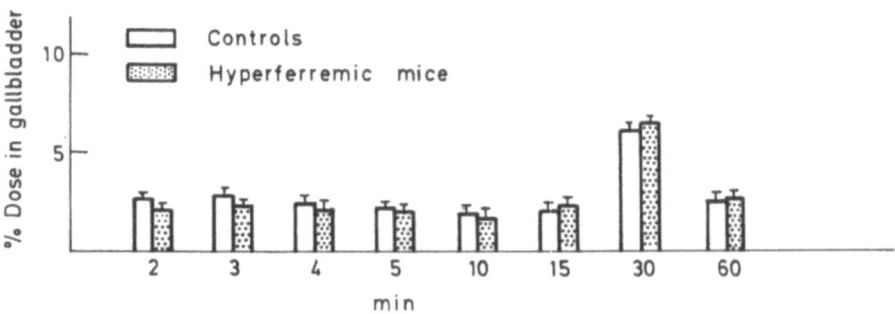

Fig. 4. The gallbladder radioactivity content at various time after the injection of Tc^{99m}-diethyl IDA in controls and mice injected with Jectofer.

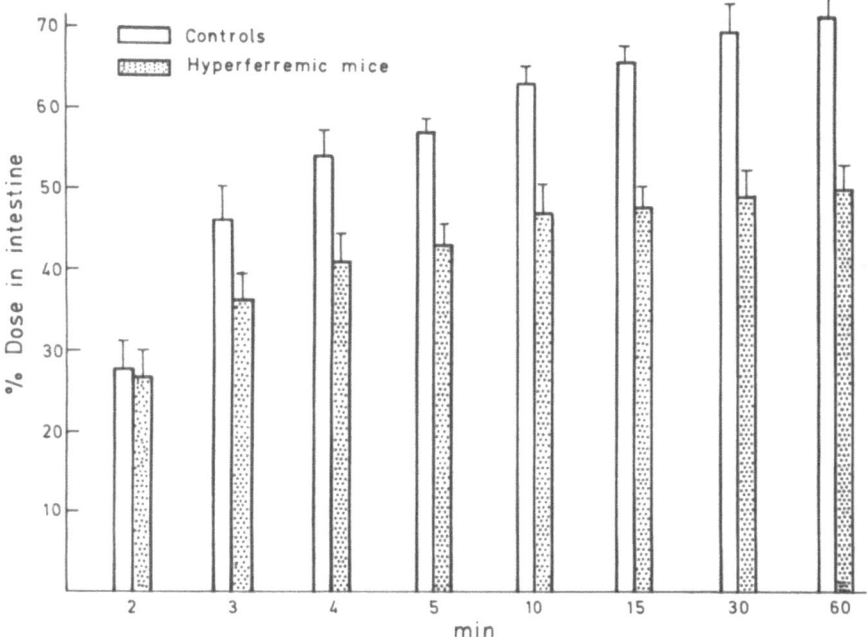

Fig. 5. Effect of the injection of Jectofer on the excretion of radio-activity from Tc^{99m}-diethyl IDA into the intestine of mice.

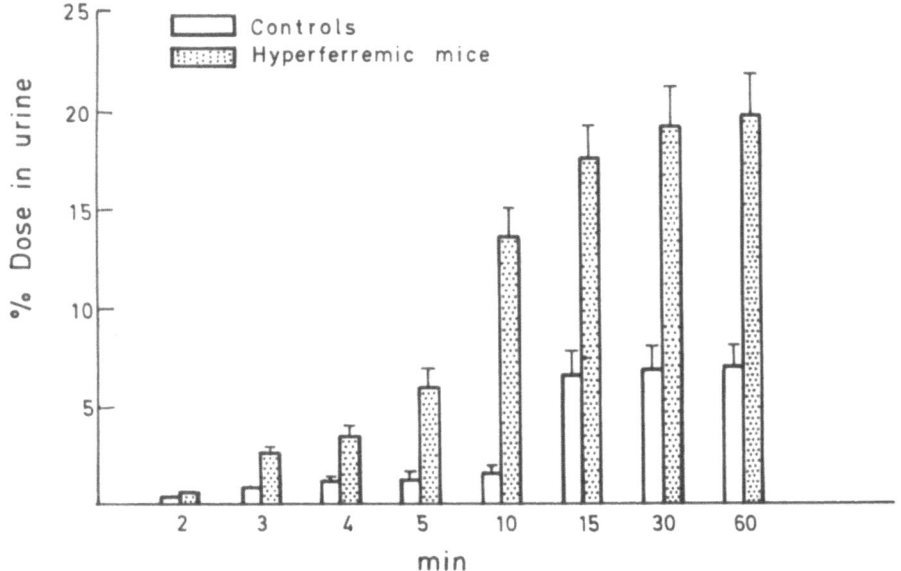

Fig. 6. Effect of the injection of Jectofer on the excretion of radio-activity from Tc^{99m}-diethyl IDA in urine of mice.

DISCUSSION

The pharmacokinetic study of Tc^{99m}-diethyl IDA showed that iron overload induces in mice a delayed blood-clearance, a subnormal initial liver uptake, a delayed elimination of radioactivity from the liver, a decreased biliary excretion of radioactivity into testine excretion. Similar effects were observed by other authors when BSP was infused to rats at saturating doses (6). A significant decrease in the rate constant of biliary excretion of Tc^{99m}-diethyl IDA has also been shown in moderately jaundice patients with serum bilirubin concentration above 15 μmol/l (7).

Tc^{99m}-diethyl IDA transport is of course a rather complex phenomenon and it might be difficult to provide an "a priory" formal explanation of the mechanism by which iron overload induces a decreased rate of biliary excretion and a significant increase of urine excretion. However, these important modifications of the normal pattern of excretion of Tc^{99m}-diethyl IDA, together with the fact that in cases of iron overload biochemical tests show little disturbance except for a positive BSP test suggest that both Tc^{99m}-diethyl IDA and BSP are reliable means to detect early changes of the hepatobiliary function. Experiments made by other authors after saturation of the dye anion pathway by BSP (6) supported the suggestion of a transport system common to Tc^{99m}-diethyl IDA and BSP. Present results would suggest that this common transport system is especially sensitive to iron-induced changes in liver.

In our experiments the dose of iron administered daily was largely in excess of the total iron binding capacity in plasma which has been estimated as 3.5 μg Fe for a mouse of 25 g (8,9). Study of the Fe^{59}-distribution (table 1) showed that the excess iron is mainly concentrated in the liver (23% of the injected dose one hour after the injection). Thus at the time of the distribution study of Tc^{99m}-diethyl IDA, there is evidence for an overdeposition of iron in the liver.

Studies in rats injected with Jectofer showed that iron overload produces in the liver dense lysosomes containing

large aggregates of iron like haemosiderin (10). Similar
observations have been made in patients with iron overload
(11). It has been suggested that the functional iron pool of
the cell plays an important role in toxicity because that form
of iron may activate certain enzymes and induce peroxidation
of membrane lipids (12-14). These processes might influence
many specific cellular constituents as membrane, vacuoles,
cisternae of the endoplasmic reticulum, golgi vesicles and
lysosomes which are all involved in the basic mechanisms of
iron uptake, distribution and excretion (15). A great deal of
subtle cell damage may, thus, be induced by iron overload
through the above pathway. According to the hypothesis presented by Suchy et al (16), both smooth endoplasmic reticulum and
the golgi apparatus are involved in bile acid transport in
rat liver. So, there is a high probability for a toxic effect
of iron on the intracellular pathway of Tc^{99m}-diethyl IDA.

Some reports were refering to the ability of some compounds
to bind iron, in vivo, in the Fe(II) and Fe(III) form (17,18).
Bone scan abnormalities have thus been described as a result
of the interaction of Tc^{99m}-phosphates with iron dextran
complex. The low concentration of radioactivity in the stomach
of mice throughout our experiments (1.19% at one hour) are
however an indirect evidence of the absence of free pertechnetate. Furthermore, the pharmacokinetics of Tc^{99m}-ferritin
studied by Nadkarni et al (19) show significant differences
of those of Tc^{99m}-diethyl IDA in the present study. Thus, in
the 30 min period after injection, 65% of the administered
dose of Tc^{99m}-ferritin was found in the liver compared to
5.56% after Tc^{99m}-diethyl IDA injection. Moreover, the excretion of Tc^{99m}-ferritin in the liver was 6.39% and that in
urine 5.9% compared to 48.82% and 19.21% respectively after
Tc^{99m}-diethyl IDA injection. These striking differences can
not support the hypothesis of a dissociation of Tc^{99m}-diethyl
IDA by the presence of iron and a complex formation with
ferritin.

It is thus suggested that iron-induced increase of urine
excretion and decrease in biliary excretion are likely due to

a dominant toxic effect of iron on the mechanism of Tc^{99m}-diethyl IDA excretion more than to a direct interaction of iron with the radiopharmaceutical. The sensitivity of the pathway of transport of organic anions to iron would be of interest as a means of detection of early changes induced by iron overload. The above results justify studies in man on the ability of hepatobiliary pharmaceuticals to detect early functional deficiencies in patients suffering of iron overload.

REFERENCES

1. Iancu TC, Neustein HB, Landing BH, The liver in thalassaemia major ultrastructural observations. Symposium on Iron Metabolism. Ciba Found. Symp. London, (new series) 51, pp 293:316, 1976.

2. Sherlock S, Diseases of the liver and biliary system. Blackwell Sci. Publ. 5th ed. pp 461:473, 1975.

3. Peters TJ, Selden C, Seymour CA, Lysosomal disruption in the pathogenesis of hepatic damage in primary and secondary haemochromatosis. Symposium on Iron Metabolism. Ciba Found. Symp. London, (new series) pp 317-329, 1977.

4. Scheuer PJ, Disturbances of iron and copper metabolism: Liver biopsy interpretation. Baillière, Tindall and Cassell, London, 2nd ed. pp 121:126, 1973.

5. Kleckner MS, Kark RM, Baker LA, Chapman AZ, Kaplan E, Moore TJ, Clinical features, pathology and therapy of haemochromatosis. J. Amer. Med. Ass. 157:1471, 1955.

6. Fritzberg AR, Whitney WP, Klingensmith WC, Hepatobiliary transport mechanism of Tc-99m-diethyl IDA. In: Radiopharmaceuticals II. Proc. Sec. Intern. Symp. on Radiopharm. Soc. Nucl. Med., New York, Sodd VG, Allen DR, Hoogland DR, et al (eds), Seattle, pp 577-586, 1979.

7. Coenegracht JM, Oei TL, Van Breda Vriesman PJC, The influence of bilirubin, alcohol and certain drugs on the kinetics of Tc-99m-diethyl IDA in human. Eur. J. Nucl. Med. 8:140, 1983.

8. Gams RA, Webb J, Glickson JD, Serum inhibition of in vitro Ga-67 binding to L 121_0 leukaemic cells. Cancer Res. 35:1422, 1975.

9. Hammersley PAG, Taylor DM, Path MRC, The effect of the administration of iron on Gallium-67 citrate uptake in tumours. Brit. J. Radiol. 53:563, 1980.

10. Arborgh BAM, Glaumann H, Erickson JLE, Studies on iron loading of rat lysosomes: Effects on the liver and distribution and fate of iron. Lab. Invest. 30:664, 1974.

11. Bessis M, Caroli J, A comparative study of haemochromatosis by electron microscopy. Gastroenterology 37:538, 1959.

12. Peters TJ, Shio H, Acid hydrolase activities and lysosomal integrity in liver biopsies from patients with iron overload. Clin. Sci. Mol. Med. 50:75, 1976.

13. Golberg L, Martin LE, Batchelor A, Biochemical changes in tissues of animals injected with iron. 3. Lipid peroxidation. J. biol. Chem. 83:291, 1962.

14. Hunter FE, Gebicki JM, Hoffsten PE, Weinstein J, Scott A, Swelling and lysis of rat liver mitochondria induced by ferrous ions. J. biol. Chem. 238:828, 1963.

15. Trump BF, Valigorsky JM, Arstila AU, Mergner WJ, Kinney TD, The relationship of intracellular pathway of iron metabolism to cellular iron overload and the iron storage diseases. Cell sap and cytocavitary network pathways in relation to lysosomal storage and turnover of iron macromolecules. Amer. J. Path. 72:295, 1975.

16. Suchy FJ, Balistreri WF, Hung J, Miller P, Carfield SA, Intracellular bile acid transport in rat liver as visualized by electron microscope autoradiography using a bile acid analogue. Amer. J. Physiol. 245: G681, 1983.

17. Van Antwerp JD, Hall JN, O'Mara RE, et al, Bone scan abnormality produced by interaction of Tc99m-diphosphonate with iron dextran (Imferon). J. nucl. Med. 16:577, 1975.

18. Buyn H, Rodman SG, Chung KE, Soft-tissue concentration of Tc99m-phosphates associated with injections of iron dextran complex. J. nucl. Med. 17:374, 1976.

19. Nadkarni GD, Noronha CPD, Sewatkar AB, Deshpande UR, Ganatra RD, Studies on Tc-99m-labelled liver ferritin: Hepatobiliary behaviour in rats. J. nucl. Med. 21:1177, 1980.

SUBCELLULAR DISTRIBUTION OF Tc^{99m}-Sn-PHYTATE IN THE LIVER OF RATS

C. DASSIOU

INTRODUCTION

Various radiocolloids are used for hepatosplenic imaging, the two most in use being Tc^{99m} sulfur colloid and Tc^{99m} tin-phytate.

The purpose of these studies was to investigate the subcellular components in which these radiocolloids are mainly localized, in order to show if the two Tc^{99m} radiocolloids present similar subcellular distribution, or whether some biochemical differences could be observed.

In this preliminary work, we studied the subcellular distribution of Tc^{99m} tin-phytate (inositol hexaphosphate) in the liver of rats.

MATERIAL AND METHODS

A total of 12 rats (Wistar albino rats) from both sexes were used in groups of two in each experiment. They were fed the standard rat diet. All rats were maintained and kept in an Animal House (temp. 21° C and relative humidity 55%) and each group belonged to the same litter. At 60 days old the body weights were 160-180 gram. A dose of 600-700 µCi of Tc^{99m} tin-phytate (NRC "Democritos" production) was injected in a volume of 0,5 ml intravenously in the dorsal vein of the tail. 30 min after the injection the rats were sacrificed. The liver was immediately removed, weighed and put in chilled sucrose solution 0.25 m. The average liver weight was 8-9 gram. For subcellular fractionation a 5 gram piece was used.

In order to minimize autolytic processes during centrifugal fractionation and other necessary manipulations all steps were carried out at low temperature: 4°-6° C. The liver was rinsed

and homogenised with sucrose 0.25 m in an Omnimixer for 1 min
at low speed (3000 rpm). In the sucrose solution Tris 0.05 m
was added. The fractionation of the different subcellular
components was carried out by different centrifugations using
sucrose gradient (1,2).

Homogenates were submitted to differential centrifugation
using a Sörvall RC-5B refrigerated superspeed centrifuge, and
a Beckman L_5-75 ultracentrifuge, according to Hageboom and
Pezzuto. Final pellets of the different fractions (nuclei-
debris, mitochondria, cytosol and microsomes) were resuspended
in a standard volume of 5 ml KCL 1.15%.

Radioactivity was measured in 1 ml aliquots, using a well
type single channel scintillation counter.

RESULTS

The subcellular distribution of Tc^{99m}-Sn-phytate in the
rat liver, 30 min after intravenous injection gave the following values (relative radioactivity expressed as % to the whole
homogenate, as it is shown in table 1.

In the nuclei-debris fraction the percentage of radioactivity was 26% in mitochondrial fraction 7.5%, in cytosol 16%
and in microsomes 5%. A similar distribution was obtained in
another group on which 72 days old rats were used: in nuclei-
debris fraction 20%, in mitochondrial fraction 6%, in cytosol
12% and in microsomal fraction 5%. Some very early experiments
are made using Tc^{99m} sulfur colloid, indicating a different
distribution of radioactivity in the subcellular liver components (table 2). The relative radioactivity was: nuclei-debris
fraction 29%, mitochondria 24%, cytosol 26% and microsomes
13%.

DISCUSSION

Many studies have been made to describe the organ scinti-
scanning distribution of the Tc^{99m} colloidal hepatosplenic
imaging agents. We thought it to be of great interest to study
the subcellular localization of these colloids.

These studies were begun after some observations were made

on scintigraphic imaging of rat livers intoxicated by overdoses
of the aminoacid methionine.

As it is well known some aminoacids have been used as
supplement to foods in order to promote growth etc., especially in animals. Aminoacid intake, however, given in excess
produces undesiderable results. In rats fed with an overdose
of methionine (3) (by another research group in NRC "Democritos") we performed some preliminary scanning of the liver
of methionine intoxicated rats. For this purpose we have used
both Tc^{99m} colloids. The results were interesting because
scintigrams with phytate show the overall liver tissue
apparently normal and scintigrams with sulfur colloid indicated
some absence of localization of the colloid in the liver.

With this in mind we performed the above mentioned studies.
Our preliminary results indicate that phytate colloid is
strongly bound in the nuclei fraction and cytosol, and less
in mitochondria and microsomes. More experiments are needed
especially with sulfur colloid, to clarify the liver subcellular components in which the two colloids are preferably
bound.

This work was carried out with the help of Miss Desp
Xatjipetrou. Also I wish to thank the Biological Department of
the NRC "Democritos" and the Radiochemical Lab. of Radioisotope
Department, who allowed me to use their facilities for the
above studies.

198

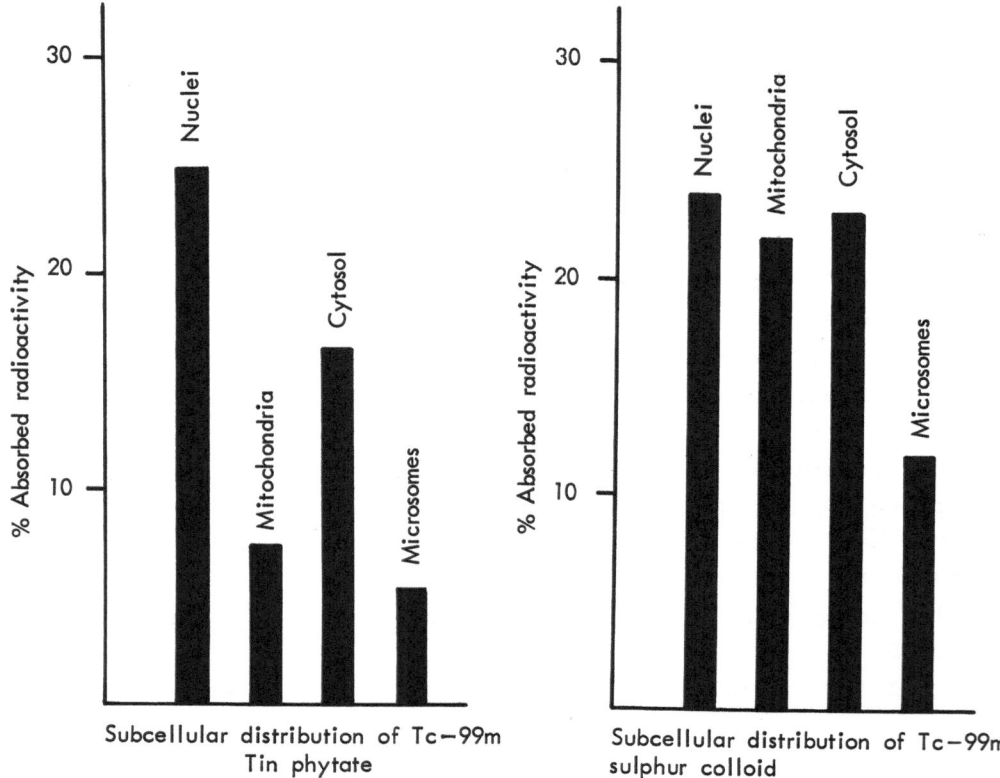

Subcellular distribution of Tc—99m
Tin phytate

Subcellular distribution of Tc—99m
sulphur colloid

LITERATURE

1. Pezzuto JM, Lea MA, Yang CS, Binding of metabolically activated Benzo
   (a) pyrene to nuclear macromolecules. Cancer Res. 36:3647, 1976.

2. Fundamentals of drug metabolism and drug disposition, Mandel and Way,
   La Du (eds), 1972.

3. Dassiou C, Drouliskos NJ, Liver scanning with radiopharmaceuticals in
   rats given high level of methionine. 2nd Int. Symp. of Radiopharmacology, Chicago, September 1982 pp 8-12.

TREATMENT OF THYROID DISORDERS BY ^{131}I

P. PFANNENSTIEL

INTRODUCTION

The therapeutic action of ^{131}I can be employed whenever destruction of thyroid cells is desired, and the main use is still in the treatment of hyperthyroidism, i.e. Graves' disease and autonomy of the thyroid gland associated with thyrotoxicosis. Furthermore, ^{131}I treatment provides a valuable agent in patients with differentiated thyroid carcinomas, particularly with papillary and follicular adeno carcinomas. In European endemic goiter areas ^{131}I is also used in euthyroid patients with large goiters (1,2), who are more than 35 years old; both diffuse and nodular goiters can be decreased markedly by ^{131}I therapy (3).

In all instances the task of the therapist is to produce a predictable dose of radiation from a known amount of ^{131}I. My own interest in this field originated 20 years ago when I was a trainee in clinical investigation at the Medical Division of the Oak Ridge Institute of Nuclear Studies (now Oak Ridge Associated Universities) in Tennessee, USA, and I have had an active interest in this subject since then (4).

Although considerable progress has been made in providing more accurate physical input data, evidently the chief factors limiting the accuracy of radiation dose calculations are not physical but biological. Therefore, I would like to devote a major portion of this presentation to the biological aspects of ^{131}I dosimetry.

One of the main problems in radiobiology is the search for a quantitative relation between absorbed radiation dose and biological effects. For internally deposited radioactive isotopes, such relations are particularly difficult to assess (5,6).

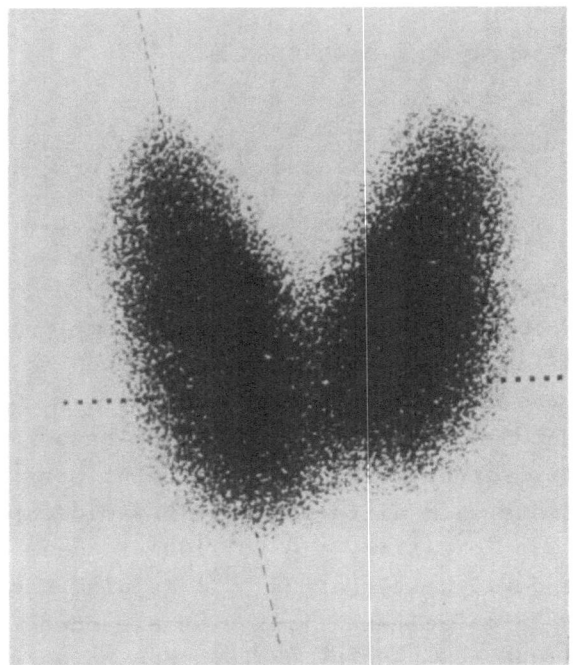

Fig. 1. Two dimensional image of a thyroid scintigram.

ESTIMATION OF THE IRRADIATED TISSUE VOLUME

The precise determination of the weight of tissue to be irradiated seems to me the most important factor. While in former years the mass of the thyroid gland was estimated by palpation and from planimetry of the two-dimensional scinti-gram (fig 1) of the thyroid gland the volume of the thyroid tissue is now determined from the ultrasonographic image providing length, breadth and depth of the gland by saggital and longitudinal views (fig 2).

The volume of each thyroid lobe is determined by the following formula describing each thyroid lobe as an ellipsoid:

$$V_{\text{thyroid lobe}} = \frac{4}{3} \pi \times \frac{\text{length}}{2} \times \frac{\text{breadth}}{2} \times \frac{\text{depth}}{2} \qquad (1)$$

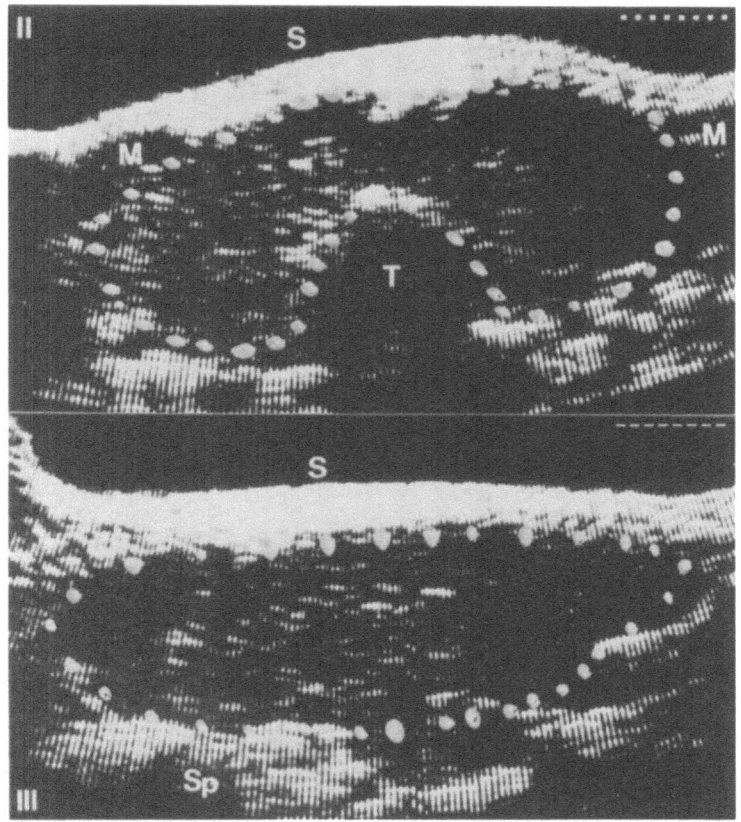

Fig. 2. Transverse and longitudinal ultrasonic images of the human thyroid gland.

Even this is a simplifying approximation, the method was shown to be reliable within ± 20% of the true weight when the results were compared with surgically removed thyroid glands of different sizes.

The mass of extrathyroidal metastases from thyroid cancer is very difficult to calculate (7,8). The estimation of the size by means of collimated scintillation counters using empirical formulas to calculate the weight from the area of the frontal projection, did not prove satisfactory in our experience. Therefore, during the course of radioiodine therapy of thyroid carcinoma, we have had to content ourselves with being mainly interested in measuring the amount of local

202

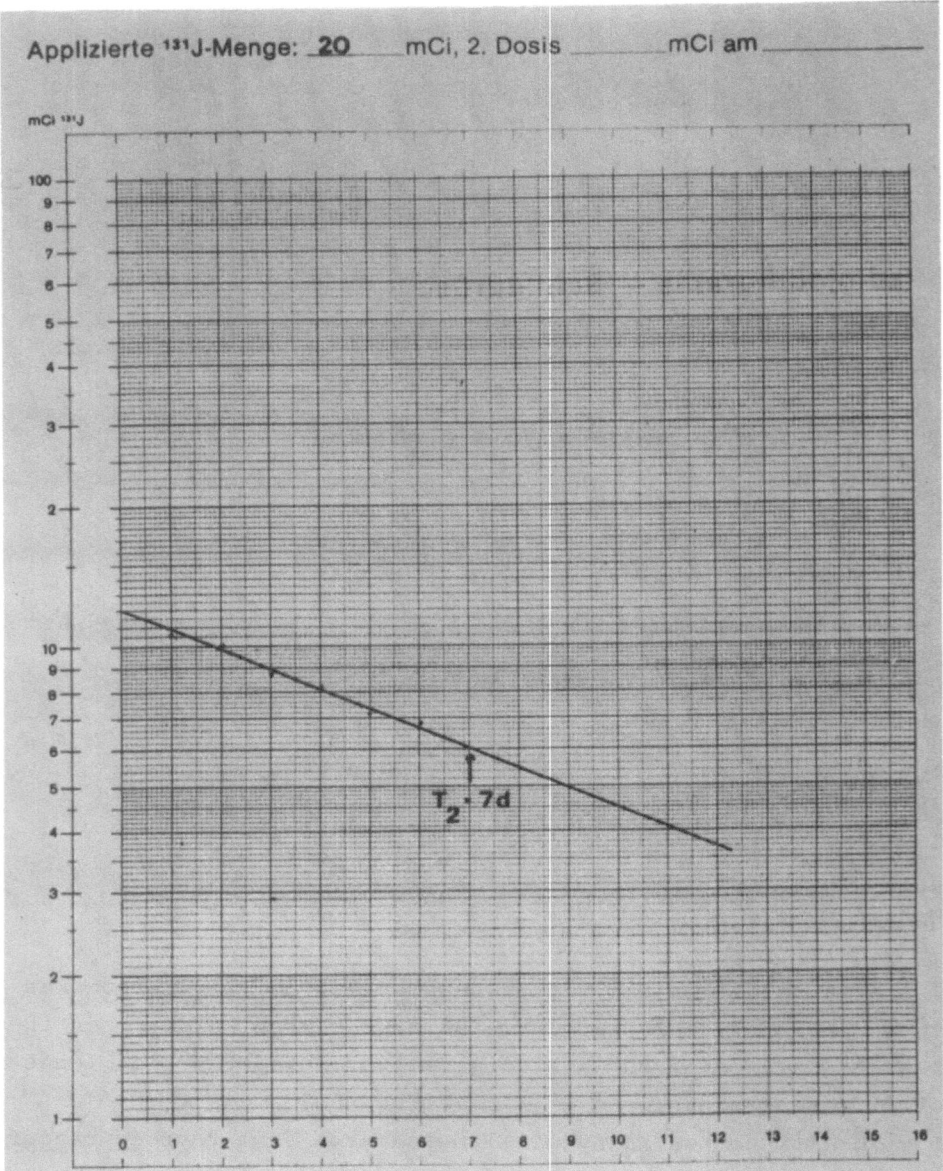

Fig. 3. Determination of the effective half-life after radioiodine treatment.

iodine retention to find how the degree of retention changes from dose to dose, thus indicating the progress of the treatment. Only in patients with lymph nodes in the neck area may ultrasonography help to determine the mass of the irradiated tissue (9).

QUANTITATIVE MEASUREMENTS OF ^{131}I RETENTION AND HALF LIFE

For the quantitative measurements of radioiodine retention in the thyroid and in extrathyroidal lesions, we obtain serial measurements by the following method (10,11):

The uptake of radioiodine is measured by a 2-inch sodium iodide scintillation counter shielded by a bore collimator on two succesive days prior the radioiodine treatment using a dose of 200 μCi ^{131}I. The turnover rate of ^{131}I within the thyroid gland is estimated by measuring the PB-^{131}I in percent of the given tracer dose per liter plasma 24 hours after the administration of the ^{131}I.

After the radioiodine treatment daily measurements with a similar device are performed. The measured radioactivity within the thyroid gland is plotted against the appropriate dates after the treatment. Except for the first few days after administration these curves are exponential (fig 3). By extrapolating the curves to the time of administration, the theoretical maximum ^{131}I uptake at zero time is estimated. The effective half-life (T_{eff}) can be found by simple inspection.

SIMPLIFIED ^{131}I DOSE FORMULAS

The absorbed radiation dose (rad) is then calculated by the classic expression (12):

$$\text{Dose(rads)} = 73.8 \; \overline{E}_{abs\beta+\gamma} \; \frac{\mu Ci}{g} \; T_{eff} \qquad (2)$$

where g is the estimated tissue mass in grams, and T_{eff} is the effective half-life in days. The average absorbed energy from the beta and gamma rays is, for ^{131}I 0.203 MeV, assuming an average beta energy of 0.187 MeV, allowing for complete

absorption of the beta dose, and assuming absorption of 0.016
Mev of the emitted gamma energy (12) from an uniformly distributed source in a small mass of tissue.

So for ^{131}I dosimetry, Eq (2) can be written as follows:

$$Dose(rads) = \frac{15^{\mu Ci\ ^{131}I}}{g}\ T_{eff} \qquad (3)$$

The following modification of Eq 3 permits the calculation of
the dose in millicuries required to produce a given number of
rads:

$$Dose(mCi\ ^{131}I) = \frac{rad \times gland\ weight\ (g)}{150 \times T_{eff} \times max\ ^{131}I\ uptake(\%)} \qquad (4)$$

With this formula, the amounts of ^{131}I to be given is calculated
for each patient individually to produce radiation dose in the
range of 5000 to 30000 rads to the thyroid tissue (13-16).

Admittedly, the accuracy of estimation of the effective
half-life from the pretreatment thyroid-uptake study with
measurements at 2,6, 24, and sometimes 48 hr after the ^{131}I
tracer dose may be questioned. After the administration of
the therapeutic dose, the ^{131}I uptake curve is determined and
the absorbed dose delivered to the gland is calculated. This
corresponds to the intended radiation dose with a maximal
error of ± 20%.

In thyroid cancer the actual irradiation dose received by
the tumour is estimated retrospectively by means of daily
external gamma-ray measurements; standard tumour doses of
100 mCi of ^{131}I in thyroid cancer are applied.

CALCULATED ABSORBED DOSES IN THYROID TISSUE

In all instances we can only hope to calculate a mean
total radiation dose. We recognize the serious objections to
the calculations since the distribution of the ^{131}I within
the tissue is not uniform (17). However, Anspaugh (18) has

shown theoretically that with ^{131}I applied to that normal
human thyroid gland over a resonable period of time, the absorbed dose is homogeneous even though the actual distribution of
^{131}I is not.

Therefore, our cross assessments, based on an assumed
homogeneous deposition of ^{131}I, are probably valid, although
the assumption of homogeneity is undoubtedly not correct.
Furthermore, different tissues have greatly varying sensitiv-
ities to radiation dosage. Crude as this method may seem, it
has given satisfactory, if not ideal, results.

Even though I have just indicated the serious limitations
of our measurements, these data still provide information that
is useful for the establishment of a rational administration
of the isotope and for the correct interpretation of the
patients clinical response, as we will see later.

TIME FACTOR AND ITS RELATION TO ABSORBED DOSE

I would like to discuss one potentially important biological aspect that seems to me to have been relatively neglected
in therapy with radioisotopes (19-23).

Experiences with conventional X-rays has shown that satisfactory results can usually be obtained in thyrotoxicosis with
a total X-ray dose to the thyroid of about 3000 rads (24). Why
then do we need to deliver a total radiation dose of the magnitude of 6000 rads to the thyroid using ^{131}I as a therapeutic
agent to yield the same biological effect?

To what extent the information gathered from exposure to
external radiation sources can be compared with that for
internal emitters is a matter of controversy. In fig 4 the
dose rates to the thyroid in a hypothetical case are shown
for internal and external irradiation.

The calculations are based on the assumption that the
total dosage to the thyroid would have to be the same from
^{131}I and from external irradiation.

Under the conditions chosen for this example, ^{131}I gives
the greater part of its irradiation to the thyroid in the
beginning of the treatment. Owing to physical decay and

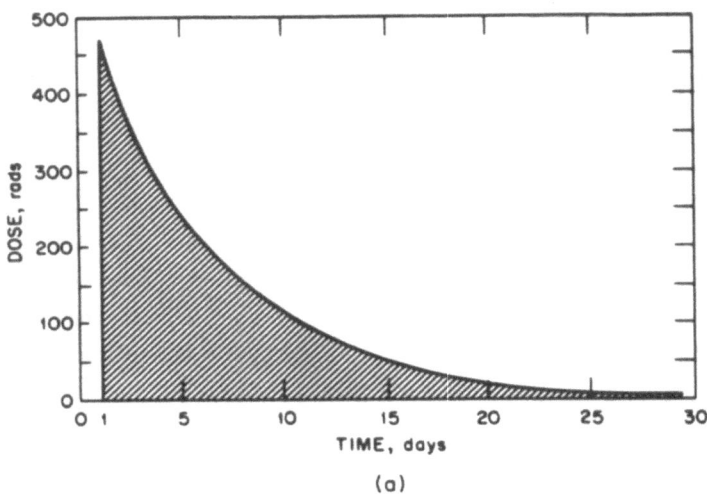

(a)

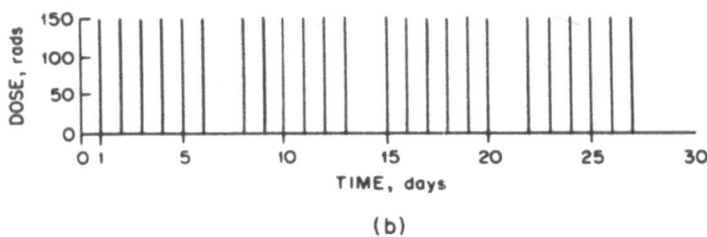

(b)

Fig. 4. Scheme of constantly decreasing dose rates in ^{131}I therapy in a hypothetical case of toxic goiter (A) compared with the short fractions of a constant dose rate in external radiation treatment (B). Total dose: 3000 rads.

excretion, the dose rate decreases as the irradiation proceeds. Thus, if the effective half-life is short, most of the planned dose is delivered in a short time; if the effective half-life is long, the final cumulative dose is reached more slowly and presumably with less biological effect. In external beam treatment the dose is delivered in short daily fractions of a constant dose rate.

Using this model, I would like to draw your attention to the importance of the time factor, which is well known to the radiotherapists but in my experience less to the nuclear specialists. A dose delivered in a short time is more potent than an equal dose delivered over a longer time; the differ-

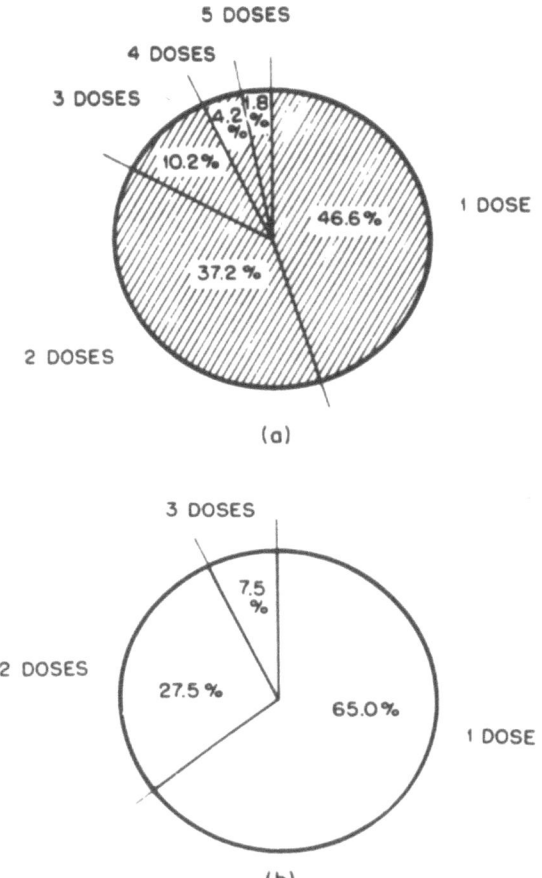

Fig. 5. Total number of treatments with ^{131}I (as a percent of total cases treated) required to control disease in toxic (a) and nontoxic (b) goiter patients.

ence arises from the greater possibilities of tissue recovery during longer irradiation periods. In addition to the uneveness of the concentration of radioisotopes the dose-rate-factor seems to me also important, the relatively slow radiation rate from the isotope allowing some repair.

Although research on dose-rate effects is extraordinarily complicated because of the many variables that must be considered, we can conclude from our clinical observations that the relation of dose effects between a protracted continous ^{131}I irradiation and a fractionated X-ray dose is about 1 : 2. Similar observations have been made by others (25,26).

A statistical evaluation of more than 300 cases treated with ^{131}I for benign thyroid disorders revealed, as is shown in fig 5, that approximately 80 to 90% of all cases were controlled with one or two doses of ^{131}I, with millicurie doses providing a mean of about 7000 rads in toxic and 10000 rads in nontoxic goiter patients. The formula used for dose calculation tended to keep the administered dose well below those in most published results (20) without altering unfavorably the end results (27,28).

CLINICAL RESULTS

A review of the medical and nuclear medicine records of our patients (29,23) revealed the following results:

The return to the euthyroid stage in the hyperthyroid patients was gradual. A weight gain was observed, tachycardia decreased, and the determinations of thyroxine and triiodothyronine in the serum showed values within the normal range.

In both toxic and nontoxic goiters, an appreciable decrease in the size of the goiter was achieved. Measurements of the neck circumference and repeated measurements of the thyroid size by ultrasonography revealed significant reduction in the mass of the goiter.

From these results it may be stated that in our experience the determination of the weight of the thyroid gland and the calculation of the ^{131}I dose by use of the simple formula enable more accurate dosages in the therapeutic application of ^{131}I, thus yielding satisfactory clinical results with only a low incidence of artificial myxoedema due to overdosage (30,31).

RADIATION HAZARDS FROM THE THERAPEUTIC USE OF [131]I

During ^{131}I therapy radiation is also delivered to the blood and to every other extrathyroidal tissue. Without entering into details considering physical and anatomical factors involved we can state that the calculation based on blood ^{131}I levels will be fairly presentative of the whole body irradiation (32).

Fig 6 shows a representative curve of the ^{131}I concentra-

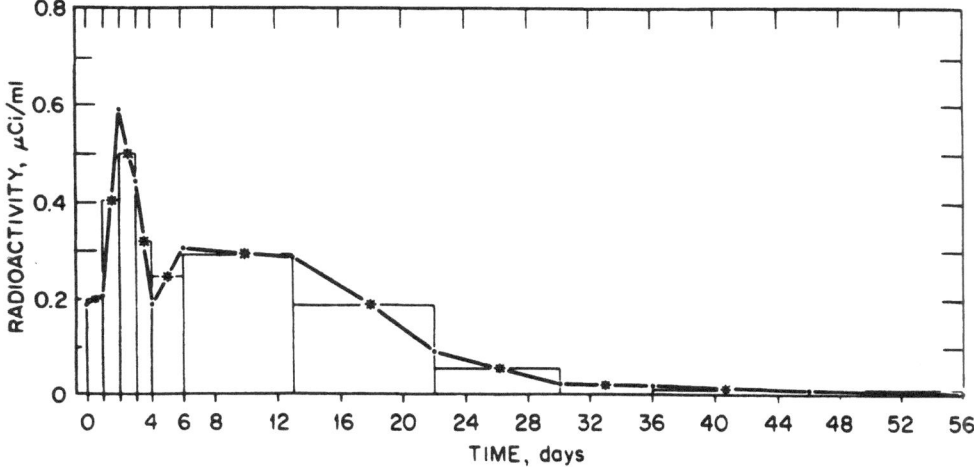

Fig. 6. Iodine[131]I blood concentrations from a representative case given 100 mCi of ^{131}I for metastasing thyroid cancer plotted against time after ^{131}I administration.

tion in whole blood against time in a patient treated with ^{131}I for thyroid cancer. In general, the concentration falls rapidly during the first one or two days as the ^{131}I is cleared from the thyroid and the kidneys. The irradiation of the blood from the protein-bound ^{131}I lasts up to several weeks. The area under this curve, as estimated by block counting, is used to calculate the whole body dose by the following equation:

$$\dot{D}(\text{rad/hr}) = 2.13 \; \bar{E}_{abs_{\beta+\gamma}} \quad \frac{\mu Ci}{g} \tag{5}$$

If we assume the beta radiation to the entire body to be half as high as that to the blood.

($\bar{E}_{abs}$ β = 0.187/2 = 0.093 MeV) and the total gamma energy absorbed to be as much as about 40% (i.e., $\bar{E}_{abs}$ γ = 0.061 MeV), then the generalized energy absorption is $\bar{E}_{abs}$ β+γ = 0.154 MeV.

For ^{131}I dosimetry, Eq 5 can be written:

$$\dot{D}(rad/hr) = 0.33 \ \frac{\mu Ci \ ^{131}I}{ml \ whole \ blood} \hspace{2cm} (6)$$

By multiplying the average ^{131}I concentration represented by each sample with the factor 0.33 and with the time in hours, the accumulated whole-body-radiation dose is calculated as a sum of all integrated areas under this curve. No contribution is included for the gamma dose from the ^{131}I present in the thyroid or in other local concentrations in tissue since this can be neglected for calculations of the degree of accuracy possible here.

The phrase "total-body-radiation" is again used somewhat loosely in the sence that it represents an average value. In fact, the radiation received per unit mass is again not constant. Since the blood-cell-forming bone marrow is distributed rather widely in the body, the radiation dose to this organ was assumed to be the same as that of the total body (33).

Table

Mean total-body radiation doses

Disease	No. of patients	^{131}I doses mCi	whole-body radiation doses	
			total rads	rads/mCi ^{131}I
Toxic goiter	8	6.9	6.29	0.84
Nontoxic goiter	13	16.1	4.33	0.28
Thyroid cancer	10	100.0	11.45	0.15
Malignant lymphoma	22	33.0	0.42	0.013

In table 1 the number of rads that would have been delivered by a dose of 1 mCi ^{131}I are given for three different disease groups. We can see that the resulting radiation doses to the blood depend upon the kind of disorders being treated

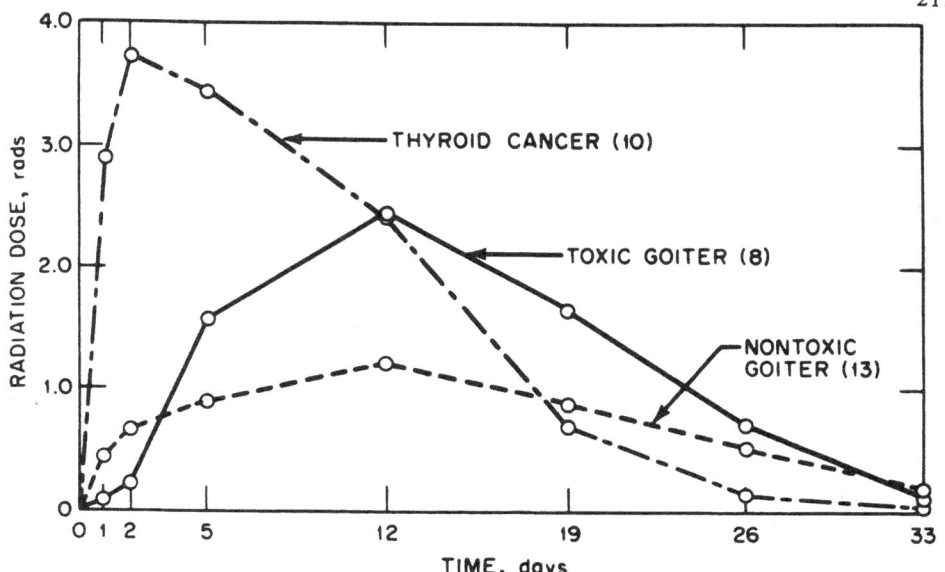

Fig. 7. Pattern of radiation dosages to the whole body in rads per day for three different states of thyroid disease.

since they determine the blood ^{131}I concentration.

In thyrotoxic patients about three to six times greater radiation doses are received per millicurie administered than in patients with nontoxic goiters or thyroid cancer. Even within any one disease group there is considerable variation in the levels of radioactivity in the blood per mCi given, and it is therefore impossible to predict the blood irradiation dose from the number of mCi of ^{131}I administered.

Fig 7 shows that, if the effective half-life is short, most of the dose is delivered in a short time; if the half-life is long, the final dose is absorbed more slowly. In most patients with thyroid cancer, most of the total radiation dose is delivered to the plasma, while the ^{131}I initially circulates as iodide. When the thyroid is normal or overactive, the dose of radio-iodi⌐ .s rem⌐ ⌐ed from the blood-stream more rapidly; so on⌐ . small prc ⌐ortion of the total dosage is given durin⌐ ⌐s early phase Thus the greater portion of the b⌐ dosage results fro⌐ the more protracted protein-bound ⌐I phase.

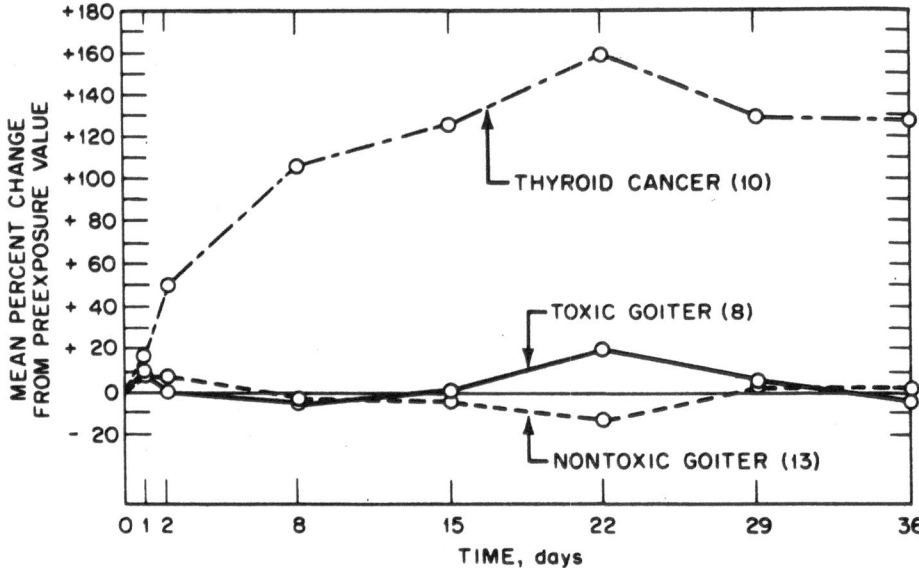

Fig. 8. Averages of the reticulocyte counts as related to the pretreatment value, which was taken as 100%, showing a significant increase in patients treated by 131I for thyroid cancer.

HEMATOLOGICAL RESPONSE TO TOTAL BODY IRRADIATION FROM 131I THERAPY

Intensive studies of the peripheral blood-cell elements have shown us that even at the initial high dose rate in thyroid cancer therapy (34) there is no effect on the proliferating cell systems (35-37) except for an increase of reticulocytes (fig 8). Under continuous exposure, proliferating cell systems presumably reach a new steady state. This is one of the most intriguing observations (38,39) in recent years. The tendency to reticulocytosis has been definitely established and it suggests that patients receiving a low total body 131I irradiation are able to maintain normal red-cell production from a depleted stem-cell population. There is perhaps an increase in cell production by the recognizable precursors (40-42).

CONCLUSIONS

There are several certainties in the preceding calculations. Our observations suffer quantitatively from retrospective analysis of clinical experiences rather than experiments. Nevertheless, they suggest that it is dangerous, in the assessment of radiation effects, to extrapolate data obtained with acute radiation exposure. Ideally we need to understand dose-rate effects sufficiently that we can predict the outcome for any type of dose rate from any type of ionizing radiation in man.

In ^{131}I therapy one has to assume that a continuous ^{131}I radiation with small dose rates is significantly less effective than a fractionated external irradiation with a high dose rate. Although there are many differences between therapeutic and diagnostic situations, it is interesting to study the time factor in its special application to routine diagnostic tests in nuclear medicine.

In my opinion further activities should be directed to an evaluation of dose rate as a factor in the biological response of man to incorporated ionizing radiations since the principle inaccuracies in dose estimation arise from uncertainties in the biological data on which practical calculations must be based. Actually what we need to know is whether the "pessimistic assumptions" made in practical clinical dosimetry owing to unknown parameters are justified.

214

REFERENCES

1. Horst J, Jores A, Schneider C, Strahlenbehandlung euthyreoter Strumen mit Radiojod 131-J. Dtsch. med. Wschr. 85:723 and 733, 1960.

2. Keiderling W, Therapie der Schilddrüse mit Radiojod. Ergeb. inn. Med. Kinderheilk. 8:245, 1957.

3. Keiderling W, Emrich D, Hauswaldt Ch, Hoffmann G, Ergebnisse der Radiojodverkleinerungstherapie euthyreoter Strumen. Dtsch. med. Wschr. 89:453, 1964.

4. Pfannenstiel P, Therapie von Schilddrüsenerkrankungen. 3. neu bearbeitete und erweiterte Auflage, 1982.

5. Emrich D, Pfannenstiel P, Dosimetrie und biologische Strahlenwirkungen. In: Nuklearmedizin, Funktionsdiagnostik. Emrich D (Hrsg), Thieme Verlag, Stuttgart, pp 73-80, 1971.

6. Pfannenstiel P, Probleme der physikalischen und biologischen Strahlendosimetrie nach therapeutischer Radionuklid-Inkorporation. In: Radioisotope in Pharmakokinetik und klinischer Biochemie. Hoffmann G, Ladner HA (Hrsg), Schattauer-Verlag, Stuttgart, pp 503-516, 1970.

7. Biersack HJ, Winkler C, (Hrsg), Neue Aspekte in Diagnostik und Therapie des Schilddrüsenkarzinoms. Schattauer-Verlag, Stuttgart, 1982.

8. Heinze HG, Die Radiojodtherapie maligner Schilddrüsentumore. Therapiewoche 30:6892, 1980.

9. Pfannenstiel P, Hoffmann G, Szintigraphische Kontrolle der Radiojodtherapie bei Struma maligna in Radioisotope in der Lokalisationsdiagnostik. Hoffmann G, Scheer KE (eds), Schattauer-Verlag, Stuttgart, pp 471-476, 1967.

10. Pircher FJ, Sitterson BW, Andrews GA, The ORINS linear scanner in diagnosis and treatment of thyroid carcinoma with Iodine-131. J. nucl. Med. 1:251, 1960.

11. Pochin EE, Cunningham RM, Hilton G, Quantitative measurements of radioiodine retention in thyroid carcinoma. J. clin. Endocr. 14:1300, 1954.

12. Loevinger R, Holt JG, Hine GJ, Internally administered isotopes in radiation dosimetry. Hine GJ, Brownell GL (eds), Acad. Press, New York, pp 801-875, 1956.

13. Heinze HG, Pickardt CR, Radiojodtherapie des autonomen Adenoms der Schilddrüse. In: Schilddrüse. Scriba PC, Rudorff KH, Weinheimer B (Hrsg), Georg Thieme Verlag, Stuttgart, New York, p 155, 1982.

14. Hoff HG, Reinwein D, Radiojodbehandlung der diffusen Hyperthyreose vom Typ des M. Basedow. Intern. Welt, p 264, 1980.

15. Schneider C, Crone-Münzebrock W, Radiojodtherapie der blanden Struma. In: Schilddrüse. Scriba PC, Rudorff KH, Weinheimer B (Hrsg), Georg Thieme Verlag, Stuttgart, New York, p 320, 1982.

16. Pfannenstiel P, Hoffmann G, Oehlert W, Bloedhorn H, Krieger P, Ergebnisse der Radiojodtherapie beim Schilddrüsenkarzinom. In: Verhandlungsberichte 76, Tagung der Deutschen Gesellschaft für innere Medizin. Bergmann Verlag, München, pp 489-492, 1972.

17. Myant NB, The problem of dosage in the treatment of thyrotoxicosis by 131-I. Minerva nucl. 8:87, 1964.

18. Anspauch LR, Special problems of thyroid dosimetry: Considerations of 131-I dose as a function of gross and inhomogeneous distribution. USAEC Report UCRL-12492, Lawrence Radiation Laboratory, Mar. p 25, 1965.

19. Hoffmann G, Pfannenstiel P, Therapie mit radioaktiven Substanzen in der inneren medizin. Med. Klin. 65:1019, 1970.

20. Hoffmann G, Pfannenstiel P, Therapeutische Anwendung offener Radio-nuklide. Der Krankenhausarzt 43:190, 1970.

21. Pfannenstiel P, Ermittlung der Strahlendosis und Beurteilung des Dosiseffektes nach Therapie mit Radiojod. Habilitationsschrift, Freiburg i. Br. 1969.

22. Pfannenstiel P, Determination of radiation dose and judgement of clinical results after radioiodine treatment. In: Medical radio-nuclides. Radiation dose and effects. Proc. Symp. Oak Ridge Assoc. Univ. December 1969. USAEC-Conference 69 12 12, Cloutier RJ, Edwards CL, Snyder WS (eds), US Atomic Energy Commission Div. of Technical Inform. pp 185-206, 1970.

23. Pfannenstiel P, Therapie mit offenen Radionukliden. Fortschr. Röntgenstr. 89:1294, 1971.

24. Zimmer EA, Zur Strahlentherapie der Hyperthyreosen. Strahlentherapie 74:473, 1944.

25. Berman M, Rall JE, Heslin J, Some physical considerations governing the choice of internally administered radioisotopes for therapy. Phys. med. Biol. 1:243, 1957.

26. Greig WR, Crooks J, McGregor AG, Clinical and radiobiological conse-quences of therapeutic irradiation (Abridged). Proc. roy. Soc. Med. 59:599, 1966.

27. Hagen GA, Quellette RP, Chapman EM, Comparison of high and low dosage levels of 131-I in the treatment of thyrotoxicosis. New Engl. J. Med. 277-559, 1967.

28. Smith RN, Wilson GM, Clinical trial of different doses of 131-I in treatment of thyrotoxicosis. Brit. med. J. 1:129, 1967.

29. Pfannenstiel P, Klinische Symptomatik und Ergebnisse der Radiojod therapie vor und nach Radiojodtherapie euthyreoter und hyper-thyreoter Strumen. In: Methoden und Ergebnisse der klinischen Nuklearmedizin in Diagnostik, Therapie und Forschung. Horst W (Hrsg), Schattauer Verlag, Stuttgart, New York, pp 879-887, 1971.

30. Beling U, Einhorn J, Incidence of hypothyroidism and recurrence following 131-I treatment of hyperthyroidism. Acta radiol. 56:275, 1961.

31. Pfannenstiel P, Hoffmann G, Graml G, Bloedhorn H, Erfolgsbeurteilung der Radiojodverkleinerungstherapie euthyreoter Strumen mit Hilfe elektronischer Datenverarbeitung. Therapiewoche 50:3308, 1970.

32. Seidlin SM, Yalow AA, Siegel E, Blood radioiodine concentration and blood radiation dosage during 131-I therapy for metastatic thyroid carcinoma. J. clin. Endocr. 12:1197, 1952.

216

33. Robertson JS, Godwin JT, Calculation of radioactive iodine beta radiation dose to the bone marrow. Brit. J. Radiol. 27:241, 1954.

34. Hoffmann G, Gehring D, Pfannenstiel P, Zur Frage der Beurteilung des Behandlungserfolges beim Schilddrüsenkarzinom. Nuklearmedizin IX:186, 1970.

35. Pfannenstiel P, Verhalten des peripheren Blutbildes und der Plasmaproteinfraktionen nach therapeutischer Radionuklidinkorporation. In: Strahlenschutz in Forschung und Praxis, Thieme Verlag, Stuttgart, pp 49-66, 1969.

36. Pfannenstiel P, Simon A, Heimpel H, Hoffmann G, Blood radiation dose and hematological findings during radioactive iodine therapy of hyperthyroidism euthyroid goitre and thyroid cancer. Acta Endocr. suppl. 119:212, 1967 (abstract).

37. Simon A, Pfannenstiel P, Heimpel H, Hoffmann G, Hämatologische Verlaufskontrollen in Beziehung zur Ganzkörperdosis nach 131-I-Inkorporation. In: Strahlenschutz in Klinik und Forschung, Thieme Verlag, Stuttgart, New York, pp 209-216, 1968.

38. Lajtha LG, Oliver R, Cell population kinetics following different regimes of irradiation. Brit. J. Radiol. 35:131, 1962.

39. Lamerton LF, Pontifex AH, Blackett NM, Adams K, Effect of protracted irradiation on the bloodforming organs of the rat. Part I: Continuous exposure. Brit. J. Radiol. 33:287, 1960.

40. Dienstbier Z, Arient M, Pospisil J, Postirradiation changes in the bone marrow and peripheral blood in effects of ionizing radiations on the haematopoietic tissue. Panel Proc. Vienna 1966, pp 60-68, International Atomic Energy Agency (STI/PUB/134), 1967.

41. Lewallen CG, Some observations on radiation dose to bone marrow during 131-I therapy of thyroid cancer. Amer. J. Roentgenol. Radium Ther. Nucl. Med. 89:618, 1963.

42. Pfannenstiel P, Die Bedeutung des Zeitfaktors für die Beurteilung von Strahlendosen in der Nuklearmedizin. In: Frontiers for Nuclear Medicine. Horst W (Hrsg), Springer Verlag, Berlin, Heidelberg, New York, pp 171-176, 1971.

EXTRANEOUS FACTORS AFFECTING
BIODISTRIBUTION

ALTERATIONS IN THE BIODISTRIBUTION OF RADIOPHARMACEUTICALS, CAUSED BY EXTRANEOUS INFLUENCES

M.G. WOLDRING

In a discussion on radiopharmaceuticals we should first concentrate on the differences between these and ordinary pharmaceuticals. In this way we gain insight into the special problems involved in the application of radiopharmaceuticals. Normally, pharmacy deals with therapeutic drugs and with the pharmacological response that is produced. Radiopharmacy is involved with diagnostic drugs. Because of their high specific radioactivity, radiopharmaceuticals have a negligible weight and a pharmacological or physiological response by the patient does not occur. It is for that reason that the biodistribution of those radiopharmaceuticals can be influenced by a number of factors.

Modifications in biodistribution can reduce the value of diagnostic nuclear medicine procedures, or worse, give rise to misleading results or to the necessity of revising dosimetric calculations.

As mentioned, the concentrations of radiopharmaceuticals are extremely small, and because they are radioactive, the preparations are not very stable. For instance, minute amounts of oxygen present during the preparation of some Tc^{99m} labelled radiopharmaceuticals may lead to the production of pertechnetate. This free pertechnetate will be taken up by the thyroid, stomach or salivary glands.

Results of administration of such inferior radiopharmaceuticals are usually predictable. Examples are:
- bone imaging with the presence of radioactivity taken up as colloid in the reticulo-endothelial system;
- bone imaging with the presence of small colloids bound to blood-proteins and leading to reduced clearance and a high

background;
- liver imaging with retention of radioactivity by the lungs
  caused by an excessive particle size;
- liver imaging with the presence of under-sized particles
  taken up by the bone-marrow;
- liver imaging with radioactivity in the kidneys, caused by
  the presence of soluble, reduced technetium in the blood;
- kidney imaging with uptake of radioactivity in the form
  of free pertechnetate by the gastro-intestinal tract and
  interpreted as left kidney radioactivity;
- kidney imaging with radioactivity in the liver caused by
  colloidal particles in the preparation and interpreted as
  right kidney activity;
- lung imaging with radioactivity present in the kidneys
  caused by soluble chelates in the radioactive preparation;
- lung imaging with asymmetric uptake and multiple foci of
  increased radioactivity caused by clumping of particles;
- lung imaging with perfusion defects caused by administration of too few radioactive particles.

Alterations in the biodistribution of radiopharmaceuticals
used in nuclear medicine also can be the result of an intended
pharmacological or physiological intervention. Such studies
are an extension of nuclear medicine procedures for obtaining
the desired diagnostic data and narrowing the differential
diagnosis. Many examples of this can be found in endocrinology,
especially in the diagnosis of thyroid disease. Other examples
are in the field of cardiology, where cardioactive drugs are
used. In nephrology, the introduction of the diuresis-renogram
enables differentiation of mechanical and functional obstructive uropathy, thus assisting in the decision to manage the
patient or not.

Another possibility is that the nuclear medicine study is
used to monitor the progress of a course of drug therapy. An
example of the effect of such a therapy is shown in fig 1.
Chemotherapeutic agents may have nonspecific effects, but
compromise bone-marrow reserves in the same way as radiation
therapy. A modern chemotherapeutic agent is Cis-platinum, an

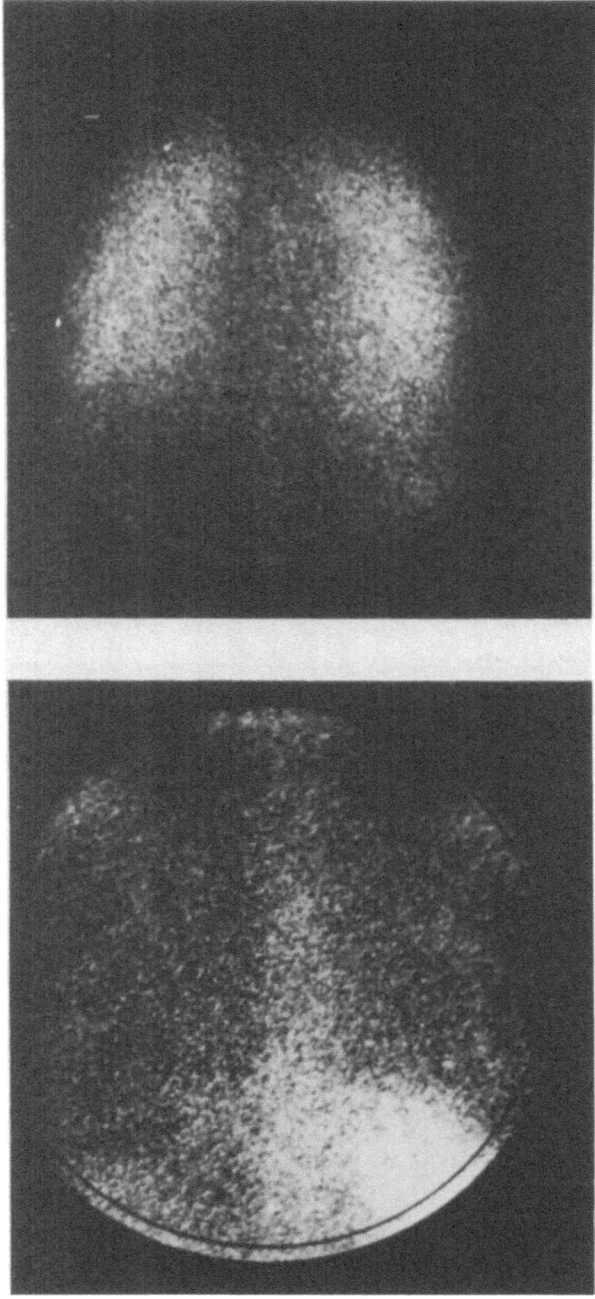

Fig. 1. In a patient with M. Boeck, diffuse uptake of radiogallium in the lungs is seen before treatment; after treatment with prednisolone a normal distribution pattern is seen (posterior view).

inorganic platinum-containing compound, particularly effective
against metastatic testicular carcinoma and carcinomata of
prostate and bladder. The compound is found mainly in the
liver after injection, but is also known to be nephrotoxic,
demonstrated by a disturbed hippuran accumulation. On the other
hand, as a result of patient medication, there is an increasing awareness of unexpected alterations in radiopharmaceutical
biodistribution.

We have to consider that not all medication modalities
involve the administration of different drugs, but the net
results of interaction with the radiopharmaceutical may be the
same: i.e. the radiopharmaceutical reflects a new process
secondary to the therapy (f.i. radiation therapy), which
possibly provides misleading information about the primary
disease of the patient. Causes of such alterations in the
biodistribution of the radiopharmaceutical by extraneous influences can be:

- drug interaction;
- interference from radiotherapy;
- interference from radiodiagnosis;
- interference from surgery;
- interaction between radiopharmaceuticals;
- radiopharmaceutical of inferior quality;
- false injection technique;
- unexpected pathophysiology.

An interaction between radiopharmaceuticals is the well-
known case of pertechnetate administration - f.i. for brain
scanning - after a previous bone scan. The result is that the
stannous iron from the bone imaging kit - remaining with the
red blood-cells - reduces the sodium pertechnetate, thus labelling the cells in vivo. The labelled cells are apparently not
able to penetrate possible blood-brain barrier defects. The
advice still basically applicable is that the use of radiopharmaceuticals containing stannous ions should be performed
after all other nuclear medicine studies requiring sodium
pertechnetate.

A typical drug interaction is illustrated by the administra-

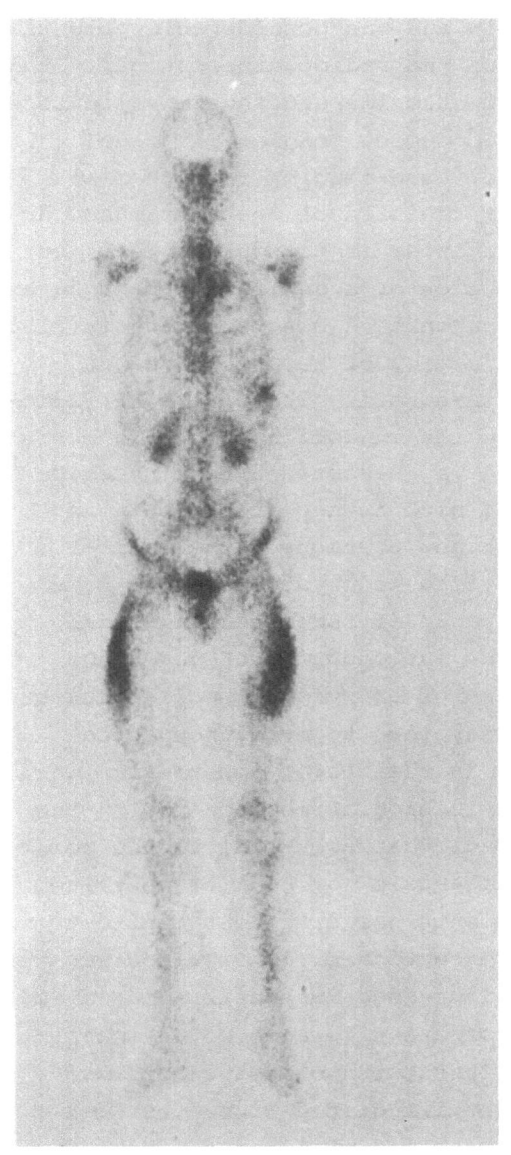

Fig. 2. Interference of intramuscular iron-dextran in bone-
imaging; local accumulation of
the radiopharmaceutical at the
injection sites.

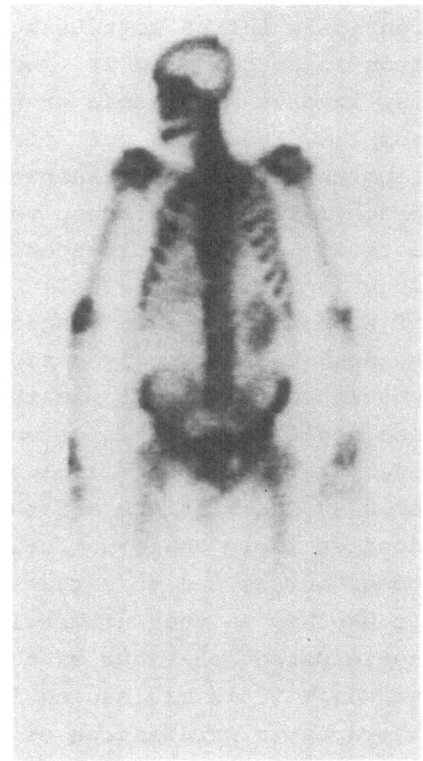

Fig. 3. Bone scan in a patient
with a scar due to gastrectomy.

tion of intramuscular iron-dextran. The excess body iron saturates the plasma-transferrin and has considerable potential to modify the biodistribution of the radiopharmaceutical. It prevents f.i. binding of indium chloride and thus invalidates plasma-space measurements or blood-pool imaging. It also results in local accumulation of bone-imaging radiopharmaceuticals in the soft tissue at the site of the intramuscular iron-injection (fig 2). The mechanism is not quite clear, but may involve hyperaemia or formation of a dextran-Tc-phosphate complex. Abdominal soft tissue uptake in bone scanning is also reported after subcutaneous injection of heparin, used as prophylaxis against deep vein thrombosis. The uptake of radioactivity exactly corresponds to the injection sites. In bone scanning increased renal uptake was reported after injection of Amphotericin B, a fungicide which is nephrotoxic. In bone scintigraphy normally a significant portion of the radiopharmaceutical is eliminated by the kidneys. Therefore bone imaging in general is often capable of demonstrating renal and pararenal abnormalities. The introduction of new drugs such as Cis-platinum and the use of existing drugs in greater dosages imply that the future may lead to more unexpected observations due to variations in the biology of the lesions. It may happen that alterations in biodistribution modify the anticipated behaviour of the radiopharmaceutical to the point at which it is misleading in diagnosis, or even of no value. Therapeutic irradiation of patients has different implications for the behaviour of radiopharmaceuticals. It is reported, that the uptake of radiogallium is increased in the irradiated soft tissue. A local effect of radiotherapy is also often seen in bone scintigraphy, f.i. in patients with breast carcinoma uptake of the tracer in the soft irradiated tissue is seen.

Radiographic contrast agents containing iodine are known to alter the thyroid gland uptake of radioactive sodiumiodide. Scintigraphic examinations after radiography also may result in focal defects appearing as cold areas on the scintigram because of the presence of barium sulphate. In the past, colloidal solutions of thoriumdioxide have been used as X-ray contrast medium. Its elimination is very slow and incomplete

and because of its long radioactive half-life the accumulation
is dangerous. The phenomenon of this effect of thorotrast is
named thorotrastosis; scintigraphy with Tc^{99m}-colloid shows
longterm sequelae including cirrhosis of the liver. Nowadays,
it is considered, that the use of thorotrast is never justified.

In surgery, gallium citrate localizes markedly in operative
sites as do bone-seeking radiopharmaceuticals to a lesser
degree. We have noted on occasion the uptake of technetium-
methylene-diphosphonate (MDP) in patients with a scar due to
gastrectomy (fig 3). Similar findings can be anticipated, i.e.
after pneumectomy, but also in trivial "surgical" lesions such
as i.m. injections of antibodies as well as pressure lesions
on skin or other physiotherapeutic effects.

Misadministration of radiocolloid may cause a troublesome
clumping of the colloidal particles with subsequent entrapment
in the vasculature of the lungs. Mixing the colloid i.e. with
some blood during intravenous injection causes such clumping;
the excessively large particles are retained by the lungs.
The possibility of an inadvertent extravenous injection also
causes modifications in the distribution pattern of the radiopharmaceutical. The nature of the altered distribution depends
upon the physiology of the localization of the specific radiopharmaceutical. It is one of the many artefacts that must be
born in mind to explain the occasional perplexing image.

Finally causes of totally abnormal biodistribution can be:
unexpected pathology or pathophysiology of the patients. There
are numerous examples of this unexpected biodistribution in
for instance oncology, hepatology or urology. Examples are
shown in fig 4 and fig 5.

Interactions secondary to drug- or treatment effects or
drug toxicity on radiopharmaceutical distribution seem to be
very important in the field of nuclear medicine imaging. In
conventional pharmaceutical practice, there is a growing
realization of the importance of drug interaction or drug
incompatibilities. The same applies for the application of
radiopharmaceuticals on the understanding, that its biodistribution can be influenced by concomitant drug administration and
other treatment modalities. The identification and recording

226

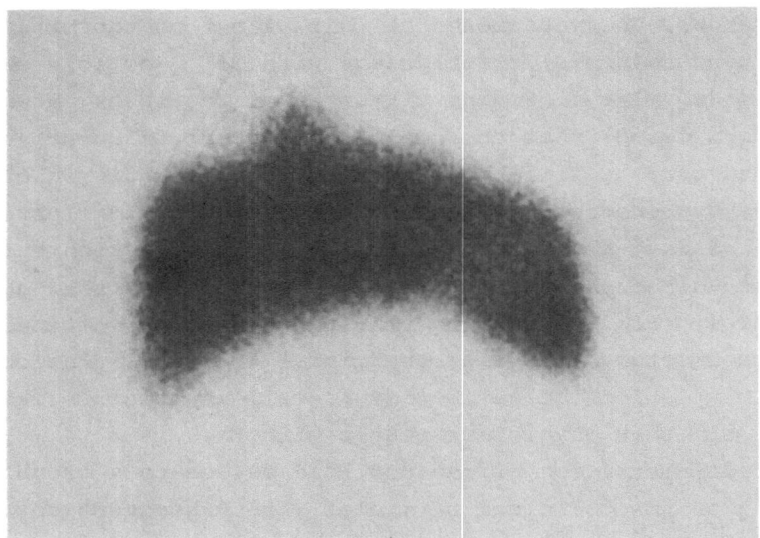

Fig. 4. Liver scan with a herniation of a small part of the liver through the diaphragm.

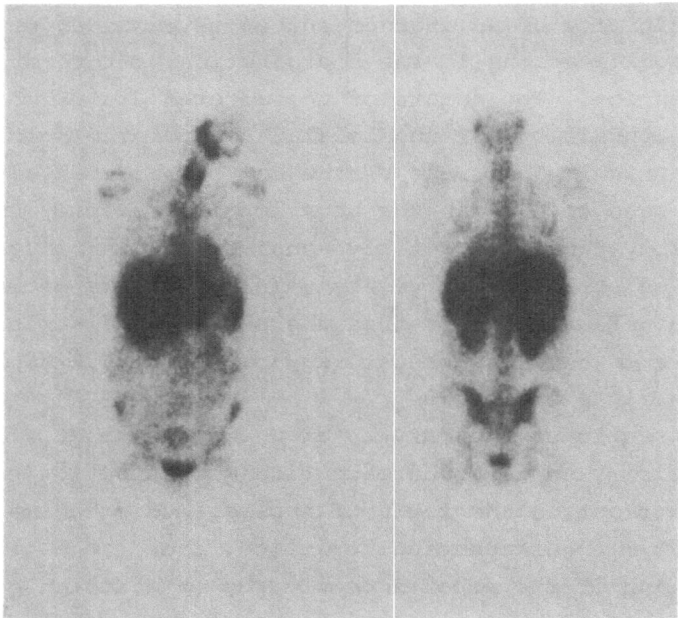

Fig. 5. Bone scan in a patient with amyloidosis: minor uptake in bone; the radioactivity is localized in amyloid in liver, spleen, uterus, kidneys, in the mouth, thyroid and gastro-intestinal tract.

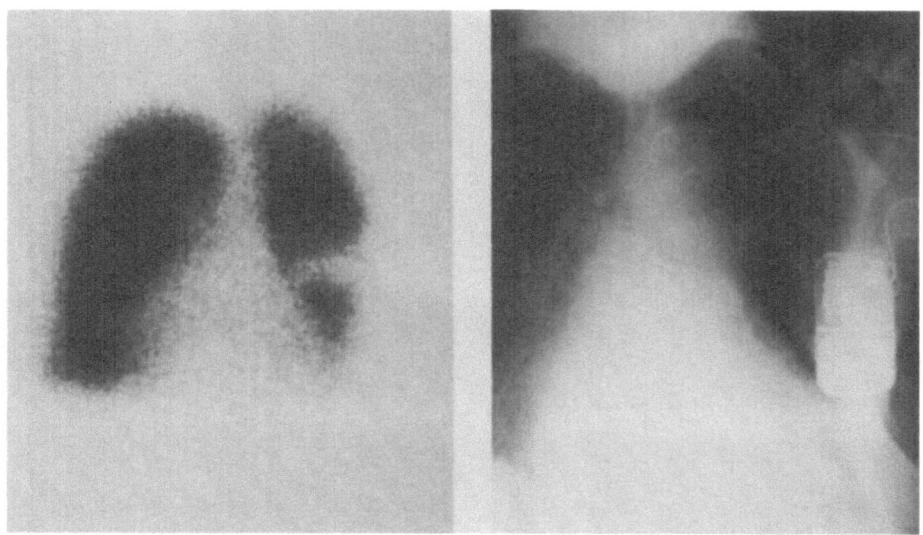

Fig. 6. A pacemaker, with the corresponding shadow - cold area - on the lungscintigram.

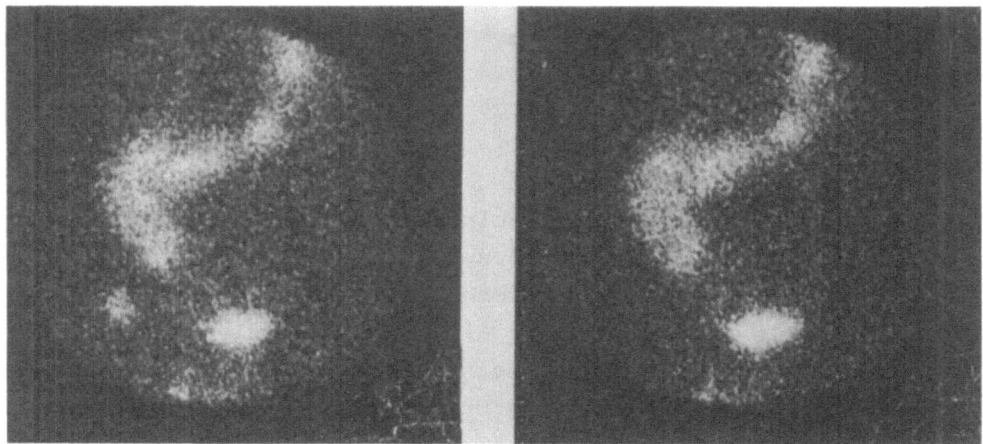

Fig. 7. Whole body scintigram shows gastro-intestinal tract and bladder plus a hot area (left). A contamined 131I handkerchief is removed (right).

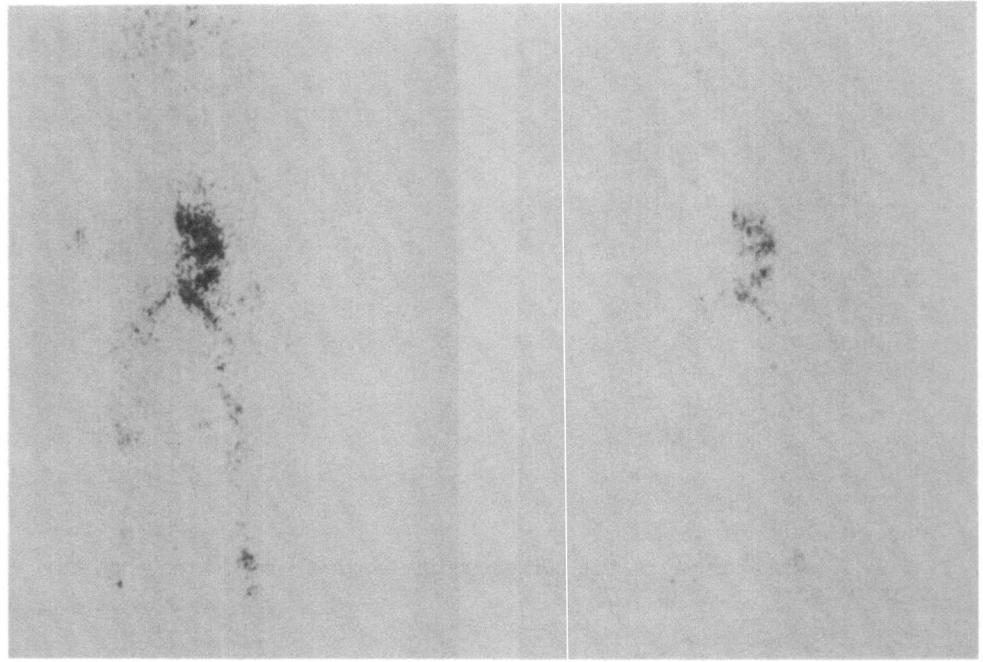

Fig. 8. Whole body scintigram of an older patient 10 days after ^{131}I-therapy, radioactive urine artefacts are seen (left). Contaminated clothes are removed (right).

of interfering interactions seems to be a potential function for the nuclear pharmacist.

Apparent alterations in the biodistribution of the radio-pharmaceutical may have totally different causes, for instance from iatrogenic and other changes. We have mentioned already that the presence of barium sulphate after a radiographic examination causes cold focal defects. But cold areas may also appear in the presence of watches, batteries of a hearing-aid or a built in pace-maker (fig 6). False positive Thallium scintigrams and also -liver scintigrams are reported in female patients because of overlying breast tissue producing a signif-icant absorption of photon, thus simulating defects. On the other hand, artefacts in the form of hot areas are also not exceptional, especially in the application of iodine-131 for

whole body scintigraphy or iodine therapy, where contaminated
areas occur. Fig 7 shows a whole scintigram where a contamined
handkerchief is present. Fig 8 shows a scintigram of a man
with contamined clothes 10 days after I^{131}-therapy using 150
mCi. After removal of the clothes a normal image is seen.
These last figures do not exactly represent an abnormal radiopharmaceutical biodistribution, but indeed they belong to the
unusual images.

THE EFFECTS OF DRUGS AND THERAPEUTIC PROCEDURES ON THE
BIODISTRIBUTION OF SKELETAL REAGENTS

P.H. COX

INTRODUCTION

Technetium labelled phosphate complexes have proved to be
extremely sensitive agents for the detection of pathophysiological changes in bone. As a result skeletal scintigraphy has
become the method of choice to screen patients for the early
detection of disease (1).

The precise mechanism whereby Technetium complexes
localize in bone has proved to be difficult to define (2) but
there is little doubt that bone uptake is affected by many
factors which can influence the interpretation of scintigrams.
Of these the effect of drugs and other forms of therapy is of
considerable importance.

RADIOTHERAPY

One of the first therapeutic regimens which was observed
to influence the biodistribution of skeletal reagents was
radiotherapy (3). Two phenomena have been observed namely,
reduced uptake in mineral bone situated in the radiation
field (fig 1) and diffuse enhanced uptake in soft tissues
which have been exposed to significant radiation. It is,
indeed, often possible to delineate the radiotherapy field on
the basis of soft tissue uptake on the skeletal scintigram
(fig 2).

It has been suggested that an increased cell membrane
permeability is responsible for soft tissue uptake in irradiated areas although this may be coupled with an increased intracellular calcium level. The reduced bone uptake is primarily
related to local fibrotic changes which result in a decreased
vascularity.

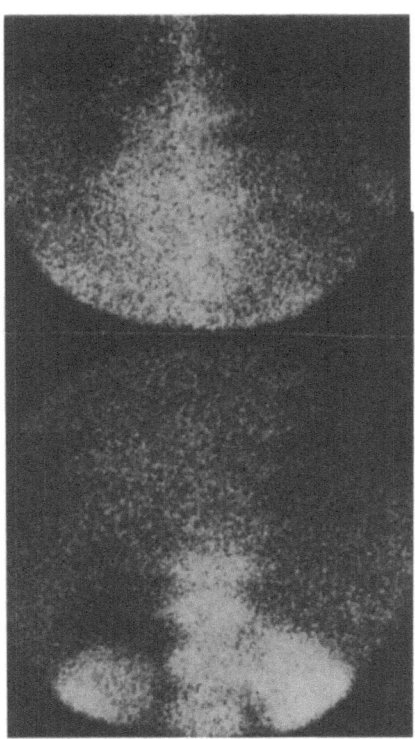
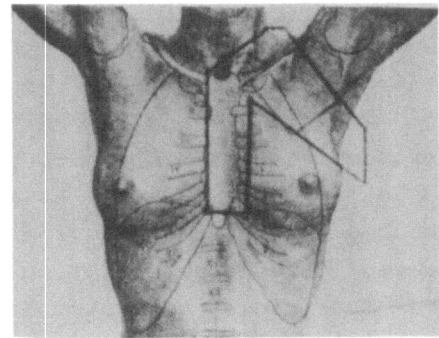

Fig. 1. Reduced uptake in mineral bone situated in the radiation field.

FOCAL UPTAKE IN SOFT TISSUES

A number of pharmaceuticals have been reported as causing enhanced local uptake of bone scanning agents. Probably the best known are intramuscular iron depot injections which are clearly visible on skeletal scintigrams (4). The reaction involved here is probably a combination of chemical binding to the iron complex and local accumulation due to inflammation around the injection site. Steroids (5) used in chemotherapy, particularly of prostate carcinoma, cause gynomastia with focal uptake in the male breast. This treatment may also cause a diffuse uptake in the calvaria of the skull. Cytostatic drugs result in focal renal accumulation of phosphate complexes (6) and regional chemotherapy perfusion with mephalan and actinomycin may result in enhanced bone and soft

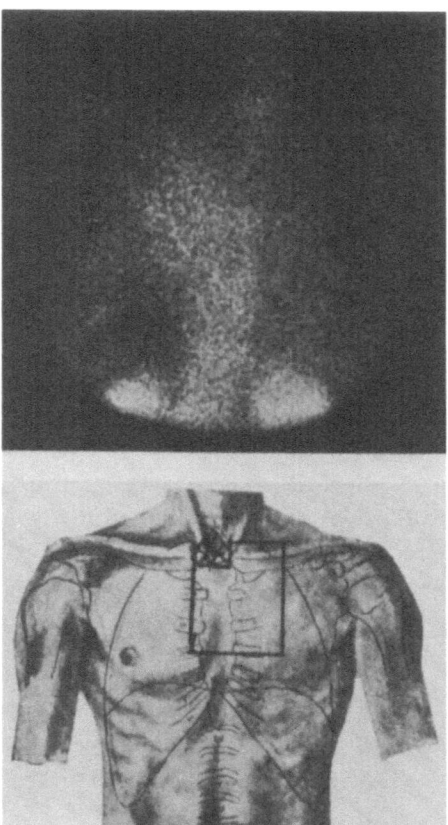

Fig. 2. Diffuse enhanced uptake in soft tissues which have been exposed
to significant radiation.

tissue uptake in the perfused limb (7). This is thought to be
related to hyperemia and erythema induced by the high concentrations of the drug used.

Dextrone infusions in paediatric patients have been observed to cause focal renal accumulation (8) whilst in dialysis
patients gastric uptake may be observed which appears to be
related to calcification of the stomach wall (9).

Hepatic accumulation has been related to aluminium intoxi-
cation (10) which has also been linked with irregular uptake
of phosphate complexes in bone (11). Cardiotoxic drugs such as

234

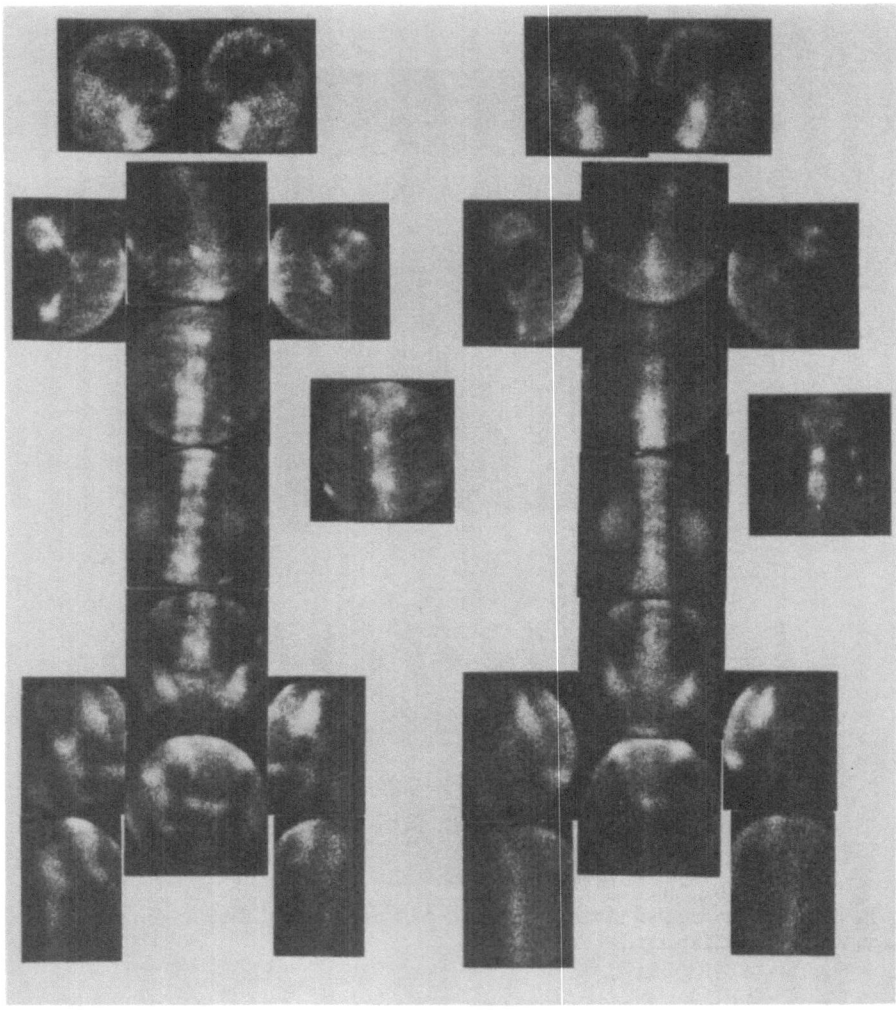

Fig. 3. Skeletal scintigrams of a patient before (left) and after (right) steroid therapy.

adriamycin (12) may cause myocardial activity to be observed on skeletal scintigrams. Rhabdomyolysis due to acute alcohol misuse has been observed to cause a generalised intense muscle uptake (13).

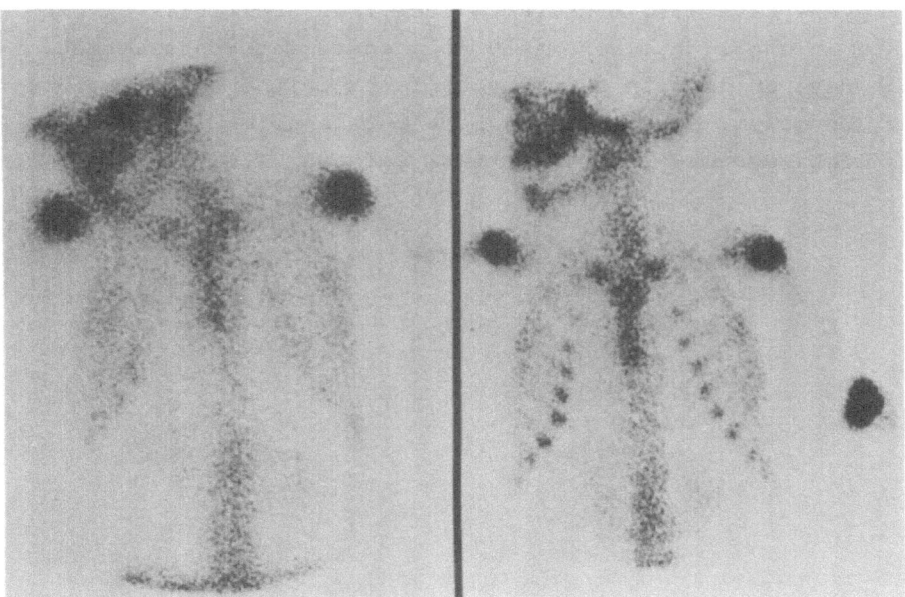

Fig. 4. Scintigram of a child before (right) and after (left) chemo-therapy demonstrating a general suppression of skeletal uptake.

REDUCED BONE UPTAKE

A general depression of skeletal uptake has been observed in patients with iron (14) or phosphorus overload (15). Similar effects can be observed with steroids (16), Vitamin D3 (17) and cytostatic drugs. Fig 3 shows the skeletal scinti-gram of a patient with breast carcinoma metastases before (left) and after (right) steroid treatment. A suppression of uptake in both lesions and normal bone can be seen although progression of the disease is also evident from the visualisa-tion of new lesions in the ribs (far right).

Fig 4 demonstrates the effect of cytostatic drugs in a dramatic manner. The right hand scintigram is that of a child prior to chemotherapy. Normal uptake in bone and in the growth areas of the ribs and humeri are clearly visible. The left hand scintigram is a repeat study made after cessation of cytostatic therapy, a dramatic general depression of skeletal uptake is evident and in particular the normal growth areas are virtually non existent. In children on cytostatic drug therapy we have also observed a localised depression of bone uptake in one limb, presumably related to vasoconstriction, which gave an impression of hyperplasia in the contralateral limb. On cessation of therapy bone uptake normalized and both limbs assumed a normal uptake pattern (18).

237

REFERENCES

1. Pauwels EKJ, Schütte HE, Taconis WK, Bone Scintigraphy, Boerhaave Series, Vol. 20, Leiden University Press, The Hague, The Netherlands, 1981.

2. Cox PH, The pharmacological behaviour of technetium reagents in bone, bone marrow and joints, its significance in relation to the detection of malignant disease. In: Progress in Radiopharmacology, Vol. 1. Cox PH (ed), Elsevier/North-Holland Biomedical Press, Amsterdam, New York, pp 109-128, 1979.

3. Cox PH, Abnormalities in skeletal uptake of 99m Tc-polyphosphate complexes in areas of bone associated with tissues which have been subjected to radiation therapy. Brit. J. Rad. 47:851, 1974.

4. Byun HH, Rodman SG, Chung KE, Soft tissue concentration of 99m Tc phosphates associated with injections of iron dextran complex. J. nucl. Med. 17:374, 1976.

5. MacGillivray I, Hall MH, Obstetric and gynaecological disorders. In: Drug Treatment - Principles and practice of clinical pharmacology and therapeutics. Avery GS (ed), Adis Press, New York, pp 445-492, 1980.

6. Lutrin CL, McDougall IR, Goris ML, Intense accumulation of Tc-99m pyrophosphate in the kidneys of children treated with chemotherapeutic drugs for malignant disease. Radiology 128:165, 1978.

7. Sorkin SJ et al, Augmented activity on bone scan following local chemoperfusion, Clin. Nucl. Med. 2:451, 1977.

8. Samson CB, A study of paediatric radiopharmaceuticals in America. Brit. J. Pharm. Pract. (Jan.) pp 17-25, 1980.

9. De Graaf P, Pauwels EKJ, Schicht IM, Scintigraphic detection of gastric calcification in dialysis patients. J. nucl. Med. 21:197, 1980.

10. Chaudhuri TK, The effect of aluminium and pH on altered body distribution of 99m Tc-EHDP. Int. J. Nucl. Med. Biol. 3:37, 1976.

11. Sebes JI et al, Radiographic manifestations of aluminium induced bone disease. Amer. J. Roentgenol. 142:424, 1984.

12. Landgarden S, Gordon A, Radionuclide demonstrations of adriamycin induced toxicity. Clin. Nucl. Med. 2:429, 1977.

13. Silberstein EA, Bove KE, Visualisation of alcohol induced rhabdomyolysis. J. nucl. Med. 20:127, 1979.

14. Parker JA et al, Reduced uptake of bone seeking radiopharmaceuticals related to iron excess. Clin. Nucl. Med. 1:267, 1976.

15. Saha GB et al, Unusual in vivo distribution of 99m Tc diphosphonate. Clin. Nucl. Med. 2:303, 1977.

16. Powell ML, Bone imaging. In: Handbook of Clinical Nuclear Medicine. Malin P (ed), Medical Examination Publishing Co., Flushing New York, pp 238-262, 1977.

17. Carr EA et al, The use of adjunctive drugs to alter the uptake of 99m Tc-Sn-pyrophosphate by myocardial lesions and bone. Life Sci. 22:1261, 1978.

18. Cox PH, The influence of drugs on the biodistribution of radiopharmaceuticals. In: Yearbook of Radiopharmacy and Radiopharmacology. Cox PH (ed), Vol. 2, (in print) 1985.

INTERACTION BETWEEN SOME DISINFECTANTS AND Tc^{99m}-
RADIOPHARMACEUTICALS

A. VERBRUGGEN, B. CLEYNHENS, M. HOOGMARTENS, M. DE ROO

INTRODUCTION

Radiopharmaceuticals labelled with Tc^{99m} are intended
primarily for parenteral use. For that reason the radio-
pharmacist or the technician have to prepare these radioactive
solutions aseptically and to keep them free of bacterial contamination. One of the precautions taken for this purpose is
disinfecting the rubber closure of the vials used in the preparation (1,2). This disinfecting can be done with the solution
present in the disinfecting swabs that some firms include with
the Tc^{99m}-generator and the labelling kits, or with disinfecting solutions available from the hospital pharmacy or with a
virtually unlimited number of commercial disinfectants.

The often rather abundant use of bactericide solutions
during the manipulation of Tc^{99m}-radiopharmaceuticals involves
the risk of introducing small amounts of the disinfectant into
the vials or the syringes containing the radioactive injection.
This holds true particularly

- at the moment of perforation of the disinfected and still
  wet rubber closure of evacuated vials such as those used
  for the elution of the Tc^{99m}-generator and for some commercial labelling kits;
- when a negative pressure is produced in a multiple-dose
  vial after the withdrawal of a few doses without the use
  of a breather needle;
- during the withdrawal of the needle from the vial while a
  negative pressure is maintained in the syringe to prevent
  recoil of the radioactive solution;
- at the moment of injection when the skin is generously
  disinfected, although the risk of contact is less pronounc-

Table 1. Tested disinfectants with their composition

A. Cationic compounds

chlorhexidine solution — 0.5 % chlorhexidine in 70% alcohol

Hibitane[R] — 0.5 % chlorhexidine in 70% alcohol

H.A.C.[R] — 0.05% chlorhexidine in 70% alcohol / 0.5 % cetrimide

Sterwipe disinfection swab BM[R] — 0.05% chlorhexidine in 70% isopropanol / 0.5 % cetrimide

B. Chlorine compounds

chloramine solution — 2 % chloramine in water

strong sodium hypochlorite solution (Eau de Javelle[R]) — 13 % chlorine in NaOH solution

Neo-Sabenyl[R] — 0.8 % chlorophene in 70% isopropanol

Dettol[R] — 0.25% chloroxylenol in water

C. Iodine compounds

Alcoholic iodine solution — 2 % iodine in 70% alcohol

Isobetadine[R] — 10 % polyvidone iodine in water-glycerol

D. Oxygen releasing compounds

Dilute hydrogen peroxide solution — 3 % w/w H_2O_2 in water

E. Organic solvents

70% w/w ethylalcohol

70% w/w isopropylalcohol

ced in this case.

Contamination of Tc^{99m} sulphur colloid with small amounts
of iodinated antiseptics has been described to result in the
formation of free pertechnetate and excessive blood-pool activity upon injection (3-6). As far as we know similar or other
interactions have not been reported for disinfectants that are
effective by another mechanism than oxidizing activity. The
present study has been set up to investigate the effect of
small amounts of a wide variety of commonly available antiseptics on the radiochemical and biological behaviour of different Tc^{99m} labelled radiopharmaceuticals.

MATERIALS AND METHODS

The disinfectants tested are listed in table 1 according
to their chemical nature or mechanism of action. They were
obtained commercially or from the hospital pharmacy. Tc^{99m}
radiopharmaceuticals were prepared by adding sodium pertechnetate solution from a Mallinckrodt Ultratechnekow generator to
commercial or home made labelling kits.

The content of free pertechnetate was determined by ascend-
ing paper chromatography on Whatman 4 strips using methylethyl-
ketone as the solvent (7). Formation of colloidal Tc^{99m} was
checked by the gel chromatography column scanning method of
Persson (8) on Sephadex G25 medium.

Biodistribution of Tc^{99m} DMSA preparations was investigated
in male Whistar rats. 0.1 ml aliquots of the solutions were
injected by tail vein and animals were killed after 4 hours.
Liver and kidneys were removed and their activity was measured
on an Anger camera.

RESULTS AND DISCUSSION

During the preparation of most Tc^{99m} radiopharmaceuticals
pertechnetate ions are reduced to a lower oxidation state by
stannous ions. As many disinfectants are effective because of
their oxidizing properties, reoxidation of reduced technetium
to pertechnetate may be expected following contamination of
Tc^{99m} injections with one of these compounds.

Table 2.   Formation of pertechnetate in ^{99m}Tc DTPA[1] by 50 μl of different disinfectants.

disinfectant[2]		percentage of pertechnetate	
name	class[3]	after 5 min.	after 2 hours
-	-	0.2	0.3
chlorhexidine solution	A	0.3	0.2
H.A..C.^{R}	A	0.3	0.3
Swab B.M.	A	0.2	0.2
Neo-Sabenyl^R	B	0.3	0.2
Dettol^R	B	0.2	0.2
Ethanol 70%	E	0.2	0.2
Isopropanol 70%	E	0.2	0.2
Isobetadine^R	C	12.6	43.4
Chloramine solution	B	17	51.4
Dilute H_2O_2 solution	D	44.9	98.1
Alcoholic iodine solution	C	56.2	98.2
Strong hypochlorite solution	B	68.2	82.1

(1) Kit composition: Ca Na$_3$DTPA   10 mg

                     $SnCl_2 2H_2O$ 0.25mg

                     pH   5

   Reconstituted with 1.5 ml ^{99m}Tc sodium pertechnetate solution (12 mCi)

(2) Disinfectant added 10 min after reconstitution

(3) See Table 1

Table 3. Formation of pertechnetate by oxidizing disinfectants in
^{99m}Tc DTPA containing 1 mg of SnCl$_2$, 2H$_2$O[1]

| disinfectant | | percentage of pertechnetate | |
name	volume[2]	after 5 min	after 2 hours
Chloramine solution	10 μl	0.2	0.2
	50 μl	0.3	0.4
Isobetadine	10 μl	0.3	0.3
	50 μl	1.2	1
Alcoholic iodine solution	10 μl	0.3	0.6
	50 μl	8.3	94.2
Strong hypochlorite solution	10 μl	0.2	0.2
	50 μl	52.6	87.7
Dilute H$_2$O$_2$ solution	10 μl	23.1	92.7
	50 μl	50.4	99.2

(1) Kit composition: Ca Na$_3$DTPA   15 mg

SnCl$_2$,2H$_2$O   1 mg

pH   5

Reconstituted with 1.5 ml ^{99m}Tc sodium pertechnetate solution (12 mCi)

(2) Disinfectant added 10 min after reconstitution

Table 2 shows the effect of adding 50 μl of different disinfecting solutions on the purity of a Tc^{99m} DTPA preparation,
formulated with a relatively small amount of stannous chloride.
The disinfectants containing a cationic compound, an organic
solvent or a chlorine compound in which chlorine is bound to
an aromatic nucleus (Dettol and Neo-Sabenyl) do not affect

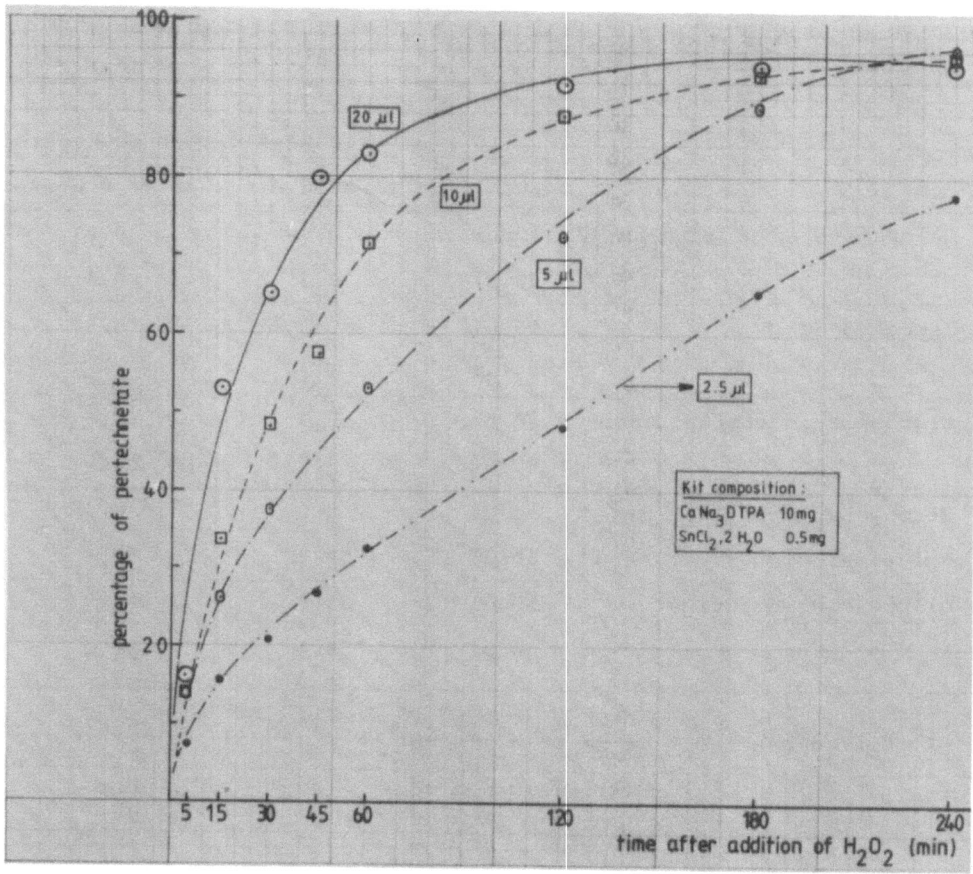

Fig. 1. Formation rate of pertechnetate in Tc^{99m} DTPA after addition of different amounts of dilute H$_2$O$_2$ solution.

the content of free pertechnetate in the preparation. On the other hand, the antiseptics characterized by the liberation of oxygen (H$_2$O$_2$) or other oxidizing substances as hypochlorite (chloramine, Eau de Javelle) and iodine (alcoholic iodine and Isobetadine) cause the formation of significant percentages of pertechnetate almost immediately. As can be seen in table 3, increasing the tin content of the DTPA labelling kit to 1 mg of stannous chloride may efficiently protect the Tc^{99m} preparation against some of these oxidizing compounds. However, the formation rate of pertechnetate remains high in

case of contamination with 50 µl of alcoholic iodine solution
or hypochlorite solution and certainly in presence of even
very small amounts of dilute hydrogen peroxide solution. The
deteriorating properties of the latter with respect to Tc^{99m}
radiopharmaceuticals are also illustrated by fig 1, showing
the content of pertechnetate in a Tc^{99m} DTPA preparation after
contamination with increasing volumes of dilute hydrogen
peroxide solution. The graph demonstrates a distinct correlation between the amount of H_2O_2 added and the percentage of
pertechnetate at each moment. It appears however that the
oxidation rate of reduced Tc^{99m} to pertechnetate is actually
low, as 2.5 µl of dilute H_2O_2 solution is able to generate
about 35 µg or 2.2 µ-atoms of oxygen, whereas the tin content
in the DTPA solution is also 2.2 µmol of stannous chloride.
This observed rather slow reoxidation of reduced technetium
is consistent with the results of other authors (9), who reported that the reduction of Tc^{99m} pertechnetate by stannous ions
is not easily reversible, once it is accomplished.

From the results it is clear that the formation rate of
pertechnetate in Tc^{99m} DTPA by oxidizing disinfectants is
dependent on the nature and the amount of the oxidizing substance and on the amount of stannous ions. Further experiments
have shown however that the nature of the complexing agent
present in the labelling kit also influences the stability of
the Tc^{99m} preparation against reoxidation. After addition of
10 µl of dilute hydrogen peroxide solution to different Tc^{99m}
radiopharmaceuticals, all containing the same amount of
stannous chloride but with respectively MDP, DTPA and pyrophosphate as complexing agents, the formation rate of pertechnetate appeared to be very different (fig 2). As shown by
the graph, Tc^{99m} MDP is much more stable than Tc^{99m} DTPA and,
of the preparations tested, Tc^{99m} pyrophosphate is the most
subject to oxidation. We suggest that this varying stability
may be attributed to the different complexation strength of
these chelating ligands.

A second type of interaction between disinfectants and
Tc^{99m} radiopharmaceuticals that we expected is the possible

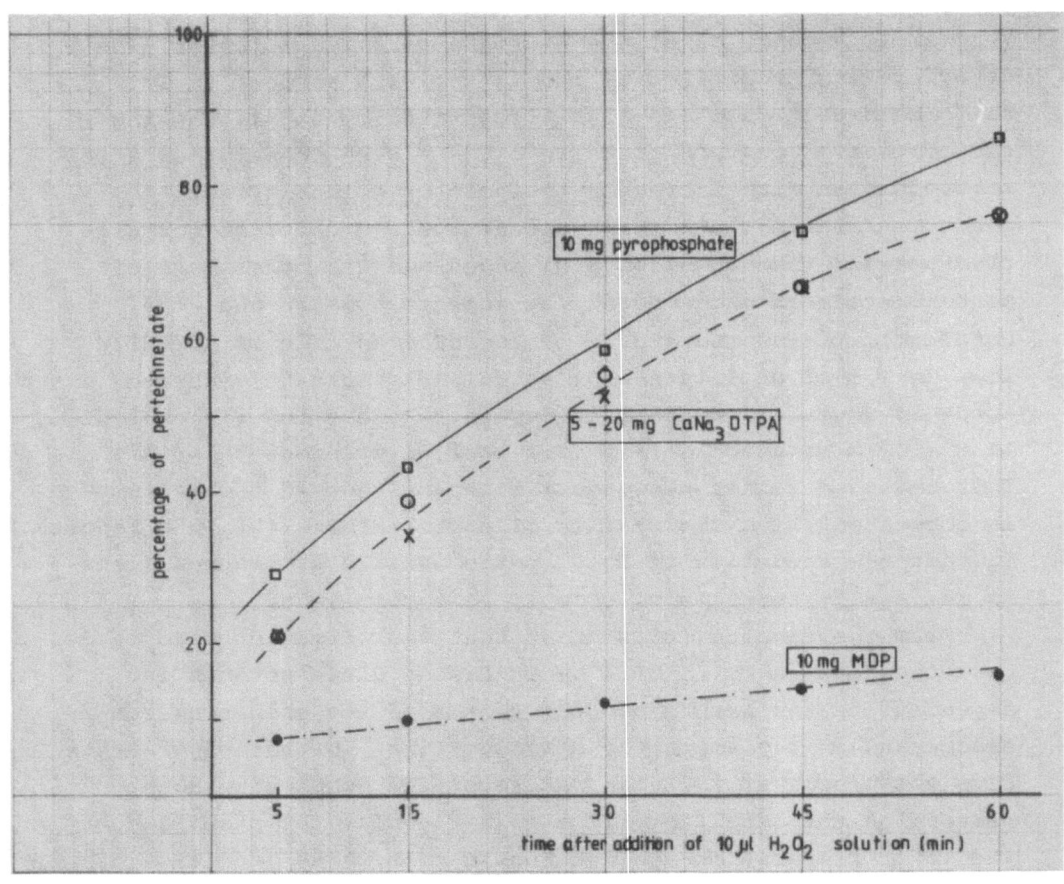

Fig. 2. Influence of nature of complexing agent in labelling kits
containing 0.5 mg $SnCl_2$, $2H_2O$ on formation rate of percentage after
addition of 10 µl of dilute H_2O_2 solution.

denaturation of Tc^{99m} albumin by organic solvents. But, even
after the addition of 0.4 ml of 70% ethanol to a Tc^{99m} HSA
preparation containing about 1.5 mg albumin and 3 µg of
stannous chloride, no colloid or particulate matter formation
was observed.

We found, however, another and rather unexpected type of
interaction between the disinfectants containing chlorhexidine
and Tc^{99m} DMSA. Analysis with gel chromatography on Sephadex
G25 of Tc^{99m} DMSA preparations contaminated with different

247

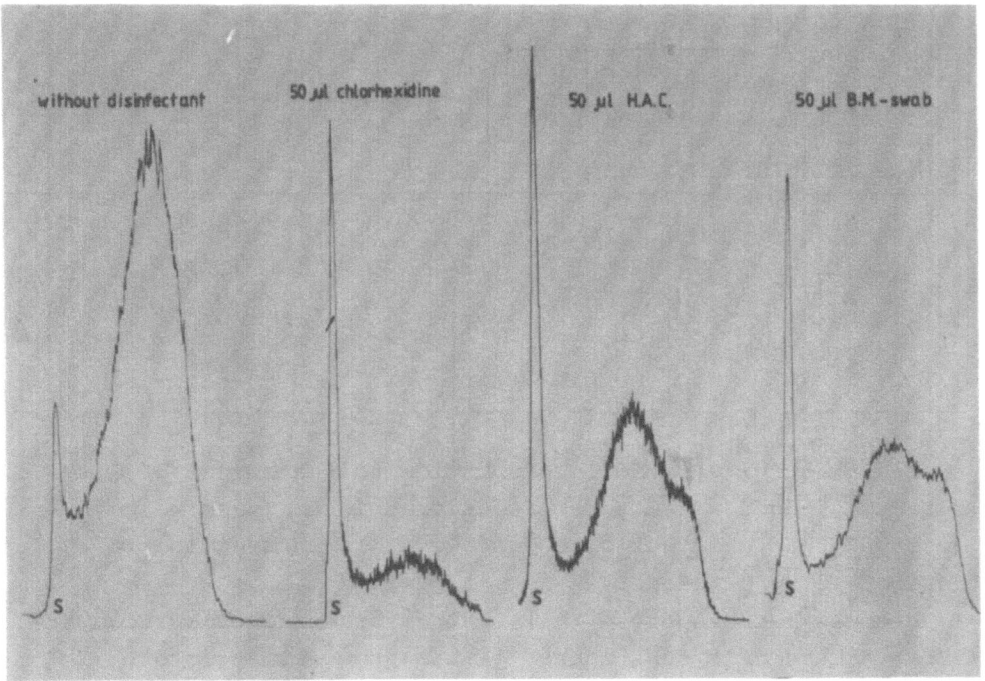

Fig. 3. Radiochromatograms after Sephadex G25 gel chromatography of Tc^{99m} DMSA preparations contaminated with chlorhexidine containing disinfectants.

disinfecting solutions (fig 3) revealed a thoroughly different elution pattern in the chromatograms of the preparations
treated with the chlorhexidine solution, HAC or the disinfection solution in the Sterwipe swab, all of which contain
chlorhexidine. A major fraction of the radioactivity remains
at the application point, which indicates the formation of an
insoluble colloidal or particulate Tc^{99m} compound. This was
confirmed by studying the biodistribution of Tc^{99m} DMSA
preparations contaminated with chlorhexidine in rats (table 4).
Upon injection of preparations treated with 50 μl or 5 μl
chlorhexidine solution a significant amount of the radioactivity was taken up in the liver, resulting in a much lower kidney

Table 4. Alteration of biodistribution of ^{99m}Tc DMSA in rats (n=
         by contamination of injection with chlorhexidine (CH)

amount CH added to ^{99m}Tc DMSA preparation		$\dfrac{\text{activity 2 kidneys}}{\text{activity liver}}$ after 4 hour
µl of CH solution	µg of CH	
0	0	8.9 ± 1.4
1	5	8.1 ± 1.3
5	25	3.8 ± 0.6
50	250	1.6 ± 0.1

to liver activity ratio in proportion to the amount of disinfectant added. From the chromatographic analyses we have
observed that chlorhexidine provokes this interaction in a
dose of 10 µg or higher.

It has been reported (10) that chlorhexidine is incompat-
ible with anionic substances, causing the formation of
insoluble compounds. As most of the commonly used Tc^{99m}
complexes wear a negative charge, we tried to find this kind
of interaction with other Tc^{99m} radiopharmaceuticals as gluco-
heptonate, Hida, DTPA, MDP and pyrophosphate and with other
disinfectants, but we did not succeed. The reaction seems to
be specific to the combination of Tc^{99m} DMSA and chlorhexidine.

CONCLUSIONS

The present study has shown that adverse interactions are
possible between many disinfectants and most of the Tc^{99m}
radiopharmaceuticals, which result in the formation of free
pertechnetate or insoluble colloidal technetium. Contamination
of technetiated preparations with disinfectants may result
from the abundant use of bactericide solutions on evacuated
and multiple-dose vials. It is wise not to use oxidizing

disinfectants during the manipulation of Tc^{99m} preparations as very small amounts of some of them cause significant re-oxidation of reduced Tc^{99m}. On the other hand, organic solvents as 70% ethanol and 70% isopropanol do not seem to interfere with the composition or biodistribution of Tc^{99m} injections, not even with Tc^{99m} albumin, and may thus safely be used. Finally one has to be extremely careful when using solutions containing chlorhexidine for disinfecting vials with Tc^{99m} DMSA.

ACKNOWLEDGEMENTS

The authors wish to thank Mrs. M.J. Vangoetsenhoven for graciously preparing the manuscript.

250

REFERENCES

1. Kristensen K, Good radiopharmacy practice for special radiopharmaceutical procedures. In: Preparation and quality control of radiopharmaceuticals in hospitals. IAEA, Vienna, 1979.

2. Department of Health and Social Security: Good pharmaceutical manufact-
   uring practice applied to the hospital preparation of radiopharmaceuticals. Notes for guidance issued by the Medicines Inspectorate,
   London, 1977.

3. Fisher SM, Brown RG, Greyson RD, Unbinding of Tc^{99m} by iodinated antiseptics. J. nucl. Med. 18:1139, 1977.

4. Lentle BC, Scott JR, Noujaim AA, Jackson FI, Iatrogenic alterations in
   radionuclide biodistributions. Sem. Nucl. Med. 9:131, 1979.

5. Hladik WB, Nigg KK, Rhodes BA, Drug-induced changes in the biologic
   distribution of radiopharmaceuticals. Sem. Nucl. Med. 12 (2):184, 1982.

6. Shaw SS, Faint J, Factors and medications affecting the distribution
   of radiopharmaceuticals in nuclear medicine procedures, West Lafayette,
   Purdue Research Foundation, 1981.

7. Verbruggen AM, Practical considerations on the hospital quality control
   of radiopharmaceuticals. J. Belg. Radiol. 63:701, 1980.

8. Persson BRR, Gel chromatography column scanning: a method for identification and quality control of $Tc99m$ radiopharmaceuticals. In: Radiopharmaceuticals. Subramanian G, Rhodes BA, Cooper JF, Sodd VJ (eds),
   The Society of Nuclear Medicine, New York, pp 228-235, 1975.

9. Owunwanne A, Church LB, Blau M, Effect of oxygen on the reduction of
   pertechnetate by stannous ion. J. nucl. Med. 18:822, 1977.

10. Martindale, The Extra Pharmacopoeia, Wade A (ed), The Pharmaceutical
    Press, London, 1978, 2nd printing, p 508, 1978.

ALTERED UPTAKE OF Tc^{99m}-MDP, Ca^{47} AND Ga^{67} BY MICE OSTEOGENIC SARCOMA AFTER ADMINISTRATION OF A CYTOSTATIC DRUG

R. SENEKOWITSCH, H. KRIEGEL, S. MÖLLENSTÄDT

INTRODUCTION

Tc^{99m}-MDP, the most commonly used radiopharmaceutical for bone imaging, localizes in regions of rapid bone mineral turnover. Thus, bone scanning is useful for screening patients with osteosarcoma because the tumour shows a high uptake of boneseeking agents (1,2). Since chemotherapy is often effective in the treatment of patients with primary osteogenic sarcoma, it has become essential that means for evaluating the response of the tumour to chemotherapy are available. A favorable effect of a preoperative chemotherapy achieving regression of the primary tumour allows a resection of the involved bone instead of amputation and gives a knowledge if it is advisable to continue the regimen of the chemotherapeutic agents postoperatively (3).

The aim of our animal studies was to evaluate the effectiveness of doxorubicin on an osteogenic sarcoma in mice by determination of the distribution pattern of boneseeking agents (Tc^{99m}-MDP, Ca^{47} and Ga^{67}) in osteosarcoma of treated and untreated animals. The effect of the administered drug on tumour growth was studied by determination of the tumour diameter on different days after administration of doxorubicin and was checked by scintigraphic follow-up with Tc^{99m}-MDP and in some cases by autoradiographic studies of cell proliferation with H^3-thymidine.

MATERIAL AND METHODS

A radiation induced osteosarcoma was cut into pieces of 1x1x1 mm size that were injected into the right hind limb of 10 weeks old female C_3Hx101 mice. The animals were used in

252

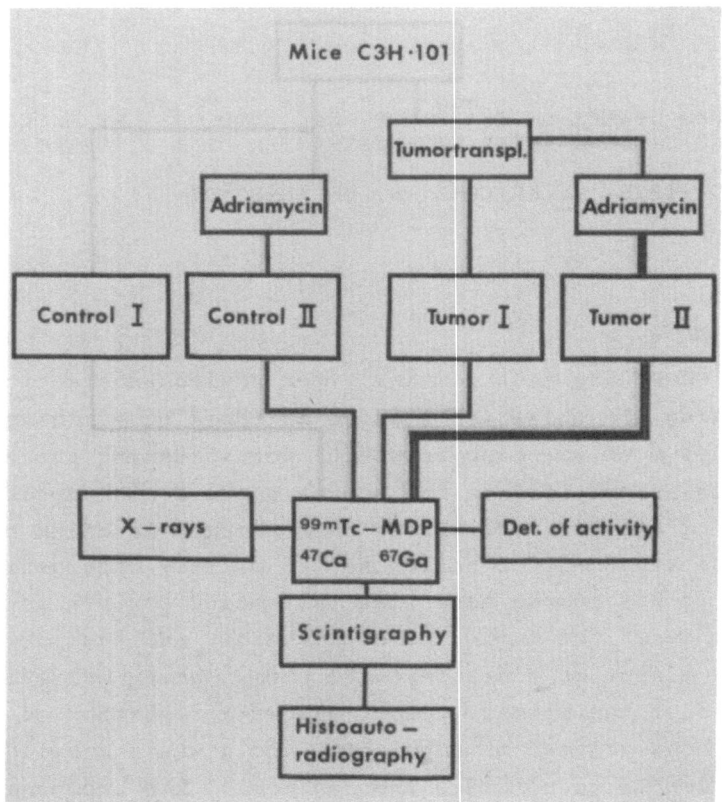

Fig. 1. Experimental design.

the investigation when the tumour reached a mean diameter of
9 mm (approximately 4-5 weeks after implantation).

Adriamycin (doxorubicin), often used for treatment of
bone neoplasm in humans, was administered intraperitoneally
as a single dose of 16 mg/kg body weight.

In our first studies Tc^{99m}-MDP was injected into 4 different animal groups corresponding to the experimental design
shown in fig 1. Animals belonging to the group tumour II were
used for the experiments 2,4,8 and 16 days after adriamycin
administration.

To study the biodistribution and tumour accumulation of
Tc^{99m}-MDP in the different groups all animals were injected
intraperitoneally with an activity of 10 µCi (0.37 MBq). The
animals were killed at 3 h after injection of the radioactivity.

Tab. 1:

Distribution of Tc-99m-MDP in mice 3 hrs p.i. (% inj. activity/g tissue)

Testgroup	Blood	Kidney	Liver	Muscle	Femur right (tumor)	Femur left	Tumor
Osteosarcoma treated	+0.14 −0.06	+0.71 −0.26	+0.20 −0.06	+0.09 −0.03	+14.2 −2.6	+11.0 −1.7	+15.3 −3.3
Osteosarcoma untreated	+0.15 −0.05	+0.65 −0.20	+0.16 −0.05	+0.09 −0.04	+13.7 −2.4	+11.1 −1.5	+7.9 −1.9
Control	+0.27 −0.03	+1.21 −0.26	+0.47 −0.09	+0.10 −0.03	+11.4 −1.2	+11.3 −1.1	—

Blood was taken and kidney, liver, muscle, bone (both femurs) and tumour were dissected, weighed and assayed for radioactivity in a γ-well-counter. The results were expressed as percent of administered radioactivity per gram of tissue.

For scintigraphic follow-up studies 500 μCi (18.5 MBq) of Tc^{99m}-MDP were injected before and on different days after administration of the cytostatic drug. Images of the tumour were obtained from anestetized mice using a gamma-camera and a pinhole-collimator 3 h after injection.

Ca^{47} and Ga^{67} were also injected with an activity of 10 μCi (0.37 MBq) into the 4 animal groups seen in fig 1. The activity, however, was only administered on the 4th day after doxorubicin treatment, because on this day the difference in Tc^{99m}-MDP tumour accumulation between treated and untreated animals revealed to be highest. For determination of the tissue distribution the animals were killed at 2 h and 6 h after Ca^{47} administration, and 24 h and 48 h after Ga^{67} injection. The same organs as in the Tc^{99m}-MDP studies were assayed for radioactivity.

For autoradiographic studies with H^3-thymidine 10 μCi (0.37 MBq) were given i.p. into 5 treated and 5 untreated animals bearing osteosarcoma 2 and 4 days after the treatment with adriamycin. 1 h after the injection the tumours were excised, fixed in 8% formalin and afterwards embedded in paraffin. 6-μ thick sections, cut with a microtome, were dipped into nuclear tracking emulsion (Kodak, D-19). After 3.5 weeks of exposure the microautoradiograms were developed, fixed and stained with hemotoxyline-eosin.

RESULTS AND DISCUSSION

The distribution of Tc^{99m}-MDP in tissues of various groups of animals is shown in table 1. The values represent the means and standard deviations from at least 30 animals in each group. Only one control group is listed in the table, because the differences in the tissue concentrations between the 2 control groups (fig 1) were not significant. Therefore, we can conclude that the administration of doxorubicin does not influence the Tc^{99m}-MDP distribution in animals without tumours. The most striking difference in the accumulation of MDP was found between the tumours of treated and untreated animals (table 1). Four days after the administration of adriamycin the tumour activity concentrations were nearly twice as high in tumours of untreated animals. This elevated tumour uptake caused by the injection of a cytostatic drug could clearly be visualized in scintigrams of the tumours obtained before and 4 days after adriamycin injection (4).

These studies also revealed an increase in Tc^{99m}-MDP uptake in the femur of the osteosarcoma-bearing limb compared to the femur of the opposite extremity. This relative increased activity was also observed in extremities of humans affected by osteosarcoma. The asymmetrical distribution of the radiopharmaceutical is thought to be related to hyperemia that accompanies vascular, malignant bone-forming tumours (5).

The Tc^{99m}-MDP localization within the tumour was highly irregular as shown by scintigraphic and autoradiographic studies (4,6). The highest accumulation, however, clearly corresponded to the areas of ossifications whereas little activity was found in nonossified regions. Since the precise mechanism of MDP-uptake is uncertain, but appears to be related to the osteoblastic activity and osseous metabolism (7), we have also investigated the uptake of other bone-seeking agents such as Ga^{67} and Ca^{47} in osteosarcoma of treated and untreated animals.

Table 2 represents the results from the distribution studies of Ca^{47} 6 hours post-injection. The control group high uptake of this nuclide by the bone was found, being more than 3 times that for MDP; the activity concentration in blood, however, is higher for Ca^{47} by nearly the same factor. In tumour bearing animals the bone-uptake is lower because of the high uptake of the nuclide by the tumour.

The most striking result is the highly significant difference in tumour uptake between treated and untreated animals with activity concentrations of 72.5 and 30.7% of the injected dose per gram tissue respectively. Significant differences in

Tab. 2:

Distribution of Ca-47 in mice 6 hrs p.i. (% inj. activity/g tissue)

Testgroup	Blood	Kidney	Liver	Muscle	Femur right (tumor)	Femur left	Tumor
Osteosarcoma treated	0.67 $+$ $-$0.17	0.69 $+$ $-$0.22	0.50 $+$ $-$0.14	0.80 $+$ $-$0.20	30.5 $+$ $-$5.9	29.1 $+$ $-$6.3	72.5 $+$ $-$19.9
Osteosarcoma untreated	0.58 $+$ $-$0.08	0.62 $+$ $-$0.08	0.39 $+$ $-$0.04	0.88 $+$ $-$0.16	37.9 $+$ $-$2.6	33.4 $+$ $-$4.3	30.7 $+$ $-$6.4
Control	0.64 $+$ $-$0.05	0.64 $+$ $-$0.21	0.41 $+$ $-$0.02	1.12 $+$ $-$0.14	42.3 $+$ $-$1.7	42.7 $+$ $-$2.5	—

Tab. 3:
Distribution of Ga-67 in mice 24 hrs p.i. (% inj. activity/g tissue)

Testgroup	Blood	Kidney	Liver	Muscle	Femur right (tumor)	Femur left	Tumor
Osteosarcoma treated	3.05 ± 0.24	6.31 ± 0.97	4.93 ± 0.36	0.36 ± 0.08	11.6 ± 0.9	9.6 ± 0.7	31.0 ± 7.7
Osteosarcoma untreated	2.97 ± 0.23	4.34 ± 0.50	5.32 ± 0.53	0.37 ± 0.04	14.7 ± 1.8	10.3 ± 1.2	11.0 ± 3.3
Control	3.19 ± 0.76	4.94 ± 0.61	5.80 ± 0.86	0.41 ± 0.08	12.6 ± 1.6	12.5 ± 1.5	—

the tumour uptake between the groups "Tumour I" and "Tumour II" (fig 1) resulted from the distribution studies with Ga^{67}, too (table 3). As in Tc^{99m}-MDP studies we could not find an effect of the treatment with adriamycin on the distribution of Ca^{47} and Ga^{67} in control animals. An alteration of Ga^{67} distribution has been demonstrated in control and tumour bearing mice after administration of methotrexate (MTX) by Chilton et al (8). The altered Ga^{67} distribution following this therapy showed decreased levels in blood and increased uptake in bone. A similar result was recently reported by Bekerman et al (9). In patients who had Ga^{67} scintigrams before and after MTX-therapy they found an increased uptake in bone with suppressed uptake in liver, muscle and tumour.

Comparing the differences between the activity concentrations in treated and untreated tumours for the 3 radiopharmaceuticals investigated, the highest differences were found for Ga^{67} followed by Ca^{47} and Tc^{99m}-MDP. The tumour-to-blood ratios, however, are much higher for MDP and Ca^{47} than for Ga^{67}, because of the known slow blood-clearance of this nuclide. The high Ga^{67} concentration in muscle tissue results in most favourable tumour-to-muscle and bone-to-muscle ratios for Tc^{99m}-MDP.

The presented results for the 3 bone-seeking radiopharmaceuticals indicate a clear elevated osteogenic activity in tumours after treatment with the antitumour antibiotic adriamycin (doxorubicin).

To answer the questions for the mechanism on cellular level for the given results, autoradiographic studies with H-3-thymidine were carried out. The uptake of this substance reflects DNA synthesis and is, therefore, a measure of cell proliferation.

The incorporation of H-3-thymidine in tumour cells of treated and untreated mice is seen on fig 2. A survey demonstrates a regional variability in proliferating cell density especially in untreated tumours (right). In ossified regions, mostly stained with hematoxylin the density of labelled cells is low, while areas of soft tissue (stained with eosin) show

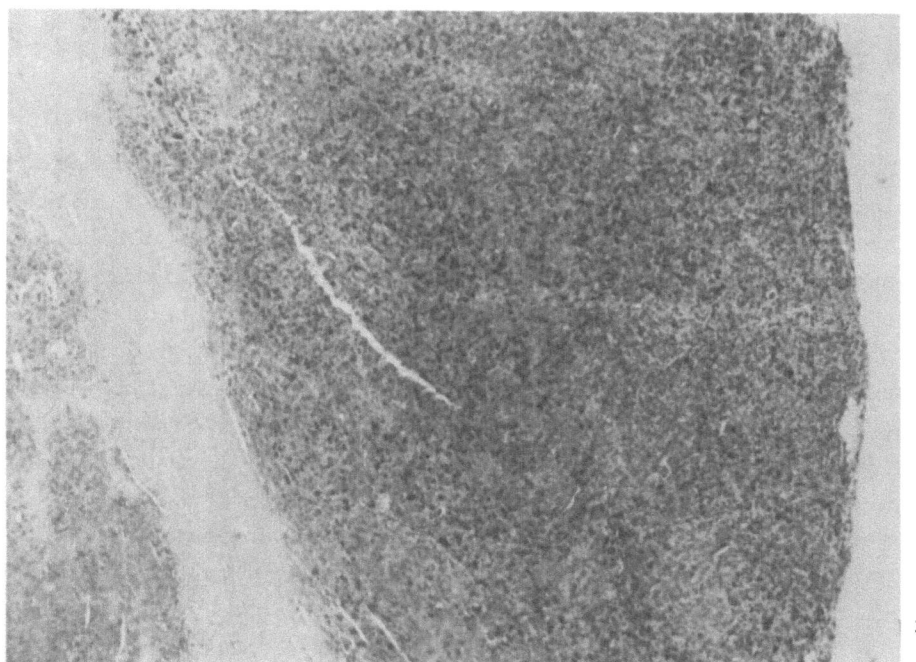

right

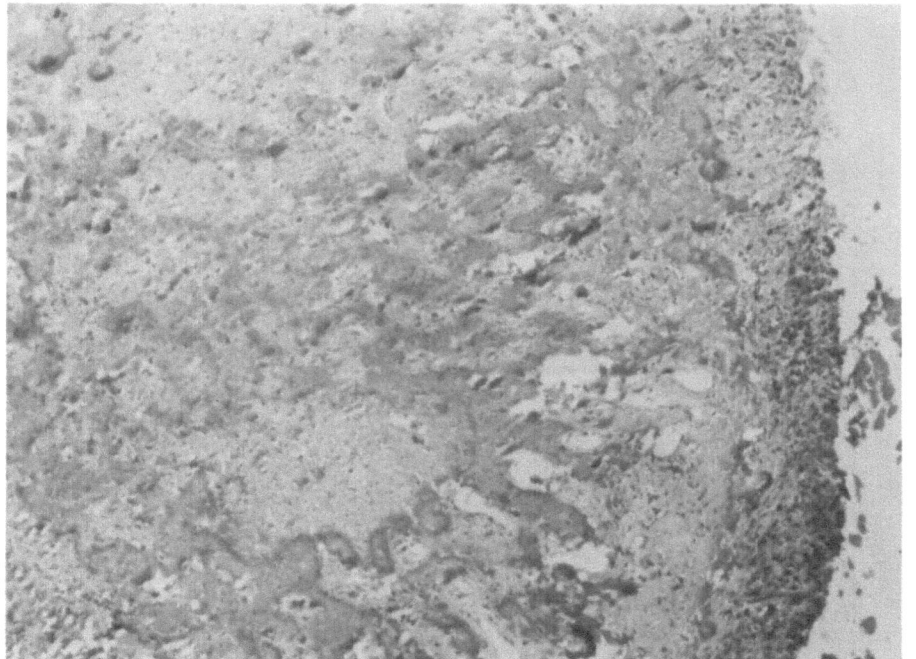

left

fig. 2. H-3-thymidine-autoradiograms of untreated (right) and doxorubicin-treated (left) osteosarcoma.

a high rate of cell proliferation. In treated tumours (left)
the overall density of labelled cells is significantly reduced, but one can clearly recognize new bone formation.

These findings lead to the conclusion that the antitumour
antibiotic adriamycin induces new bone-formation while inhibit-
ing the proliferation of cells. The areas of intense uptake of
bone-seeking substances after treatment can be correlated with
active tumour osteoid formation which is in the process of
mineralization during the time of administration of the radiopharmaceuticals (10-13). The shift to a higher mineralization
of the tumour tissue is the reverse which results in cell
proliferation typical of malignant cells (14).

In summary, it can be stated that an elevated uptake of
bone-seeking radiopharmaceuticals into osteosarcoma tissue
after administration of a cytostatic drug can prove the effectiveness of a preoperative chemotherapy.

REFERENCES

1. Lisbona R, Rosenthall L, Role of radionuclide imaging in osteoid osteoma. Amer. J. Roentgenol. 132:77, 1979.

2. Büll U, et al, Wertigkeit der "Region of Interest". Technik in der skeletszintigraphischen Diagnostik primärer Knochentumoren. Radiology 21:46, 1981.

3. Rosen G, et al, Preoperative chemotherapy for osteogenic sarcoma. Cancer 49:1221, 1982.

4. Senekowitsch R, Kriegel H, Der Einfluss einer Chemotherapie auf die Retention von ^{99m}Tc-Methylendiphosphonat im Osteosarkom der Maus. Nucl. Med. 19:200, 1980.

5. Goldman AB, Braunstein P, Augmented radioactivity in bone scans of limbs bearing osteosarcomas. J. nucl. Med. 16:423, 1975.

6. Nakashima H, et al, Uptake and localization of ^{99m}Tc-MDP in mouse osteosarcoma. Eur. J. Nucl. Med. 7:531, 1982.

7. Francis MD, et al, Comparative evaluation of three diphosphonates. In vitro adsorption (C-14 labeled) and in vivo osteogenic uptake (Tc-99m complexed). J. nucl. Med. 21:1185, 1980.

8. Chilton HM, et al, Alteration of Gallium-67 distribution in tumor-bearing mice following treatment with Methotrexate: Concise communication. J. nucl. Med. 22:1064, 1981.

9. Bekerman C, et al, The effects of inadvertent administration of antineoplastic agent prior to Ga-67 injection. J. nucl. Med. 25:430, 1984.

10. Guillemart A, et al, Bonekinetics of Ca-45 and phyrophosphate labeled with Tc-96: An autoradiographic evaluation. J. nucl. Med. 21:466, 1980.

11. Christensen SB, Krogsgaard OW, Localization of Tc-99m-MDP in epiphyseal growth plates of rats. J. nucl. Med. 22:237, 1981.

12. Gerson BD, et al, Patterns of localization of ^{85}Sr in osteosarcoma. J. Bone Jt. Surg. 54A:817, 1972.

13. King MA, et al, A study of irradiated bone. III. Scintigraphic and radiographic detection of radiation-induced osteosarcoma. J. nucl. Med. 21:426, 1980.

14. Kolber AR, et al, Drug-induced differentiation of a rat glioma in vitro: II. The expression of S-100, a glial specific protein and steroid sulfatase. Brain Res. Rev. 143:513, 1978.

VISUALIZATION OF GALLBLADDER AND GUT ON Tc^{99m} BONE
SCINTISCANS

A. FOUNTOS, J. MALAMITSI

In this paper we report three cases in which activity was
visualized in gallbladder and gut on a Tc^{99m}-MDP bone scan.

Case 1

A 48 years old male was admitted to the Naval Hospital of
Athens with severe cough and dyspnoea. On investigation oat-
cell carcinoma of the lung was diagnosed. His blood-count
values being normal, the patient was started on chemotherapy
(Endoxan, Oncovin, Adriamycin) and radiotherapy. A bone, scan
performed a fortnight after the third course of chemotherapy
showed good bone uptake but also gallbladder and intestinal
visualization (fig 1,2). Chemotherapy was discontinued when
the patient developed agranulocytosis. Soon after that the
patient died.

Case 2

A 73 years old female with a past history of a resected
carcinoma of the stomach presented with dyspeptic symptoms
and slight anaemia. On endoscopy recurrence of the carcinoma
of the oesophageal anastomosis was revealed. The patient
suffered also from mild osteoporosis and osteoarthritis of
the cervical spine. The bone scan was unremarkable apart from
the fact that gallbladder and gut were again visualized
(fig 3).

Case 3

A 26 year old male presented with diffuse arthralgias and
stiffness of the metacarpophalangeal and proximal phalangeal
joints. Ra-test and HLA-B27 were negative. The diagnosis of

264

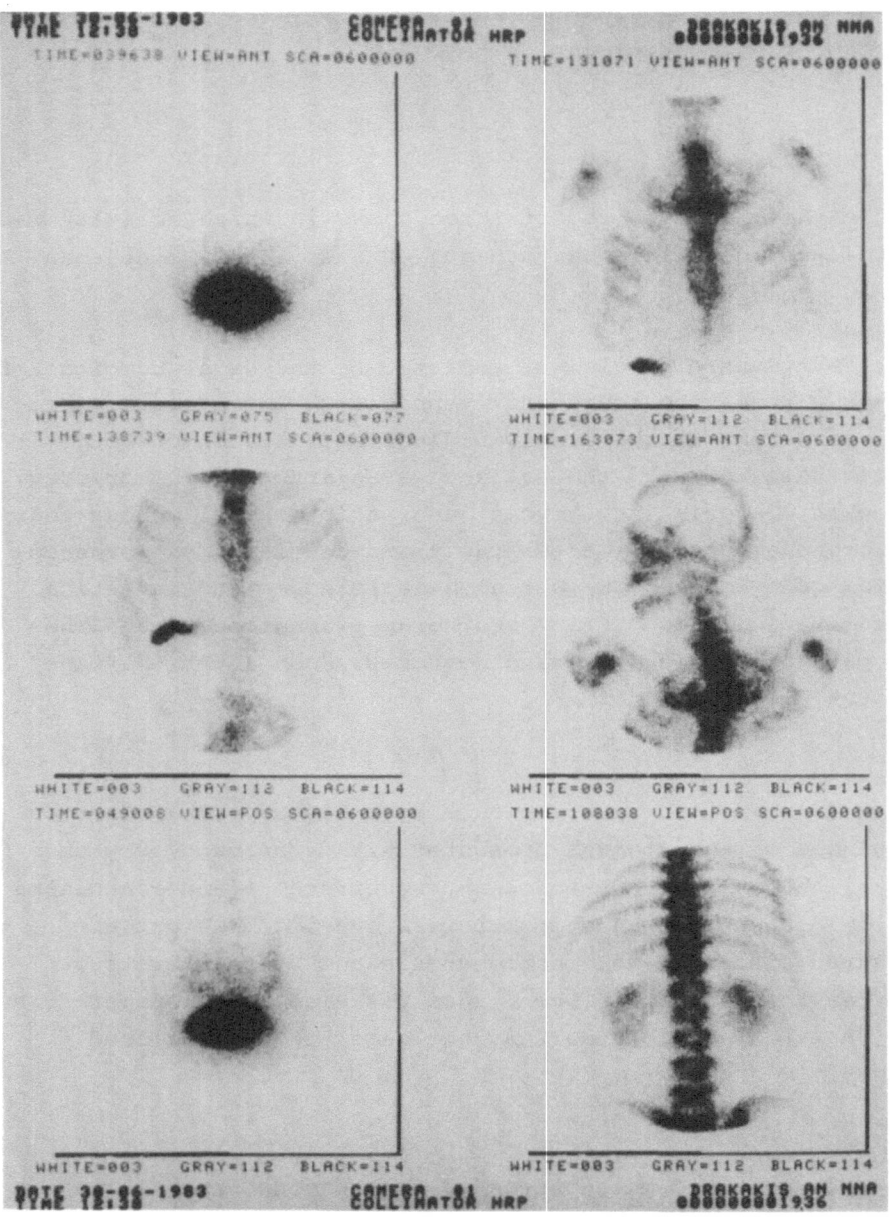

Fig. 1. Normal bone scan with radioactivity in the gallbladder and the gut.

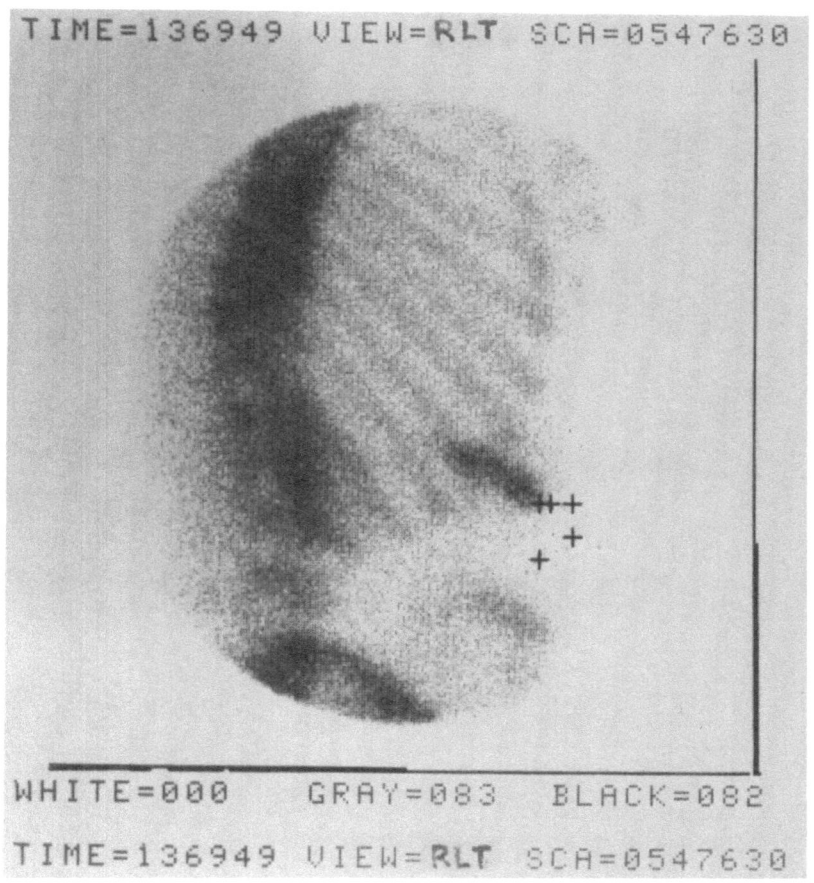

Fig. 2. Right lateral view of the patient of fig 1 in which the gall-bladder is clearly visualized.

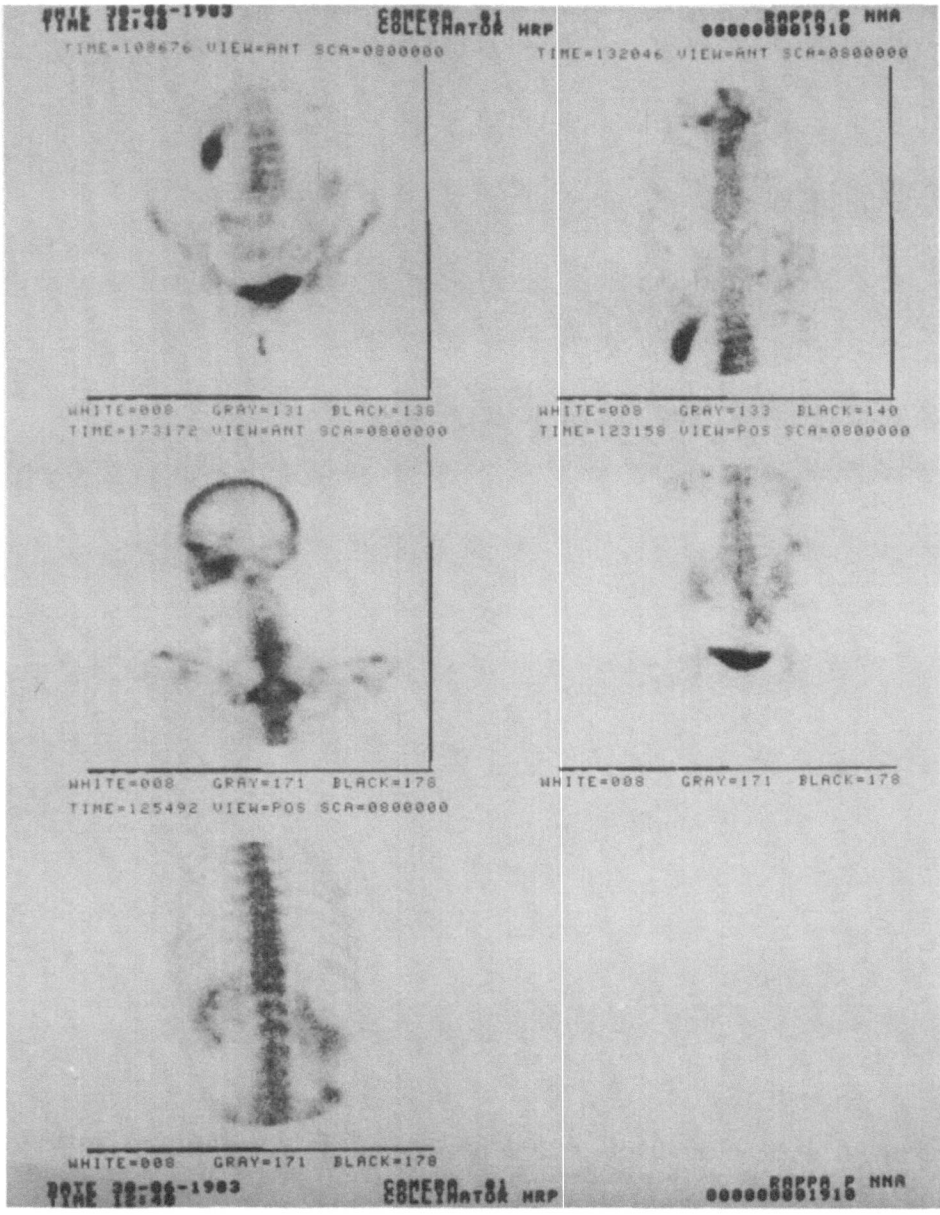

Fig. 3. Normal bone scan with radioactivity in the gallbladder and the gut.

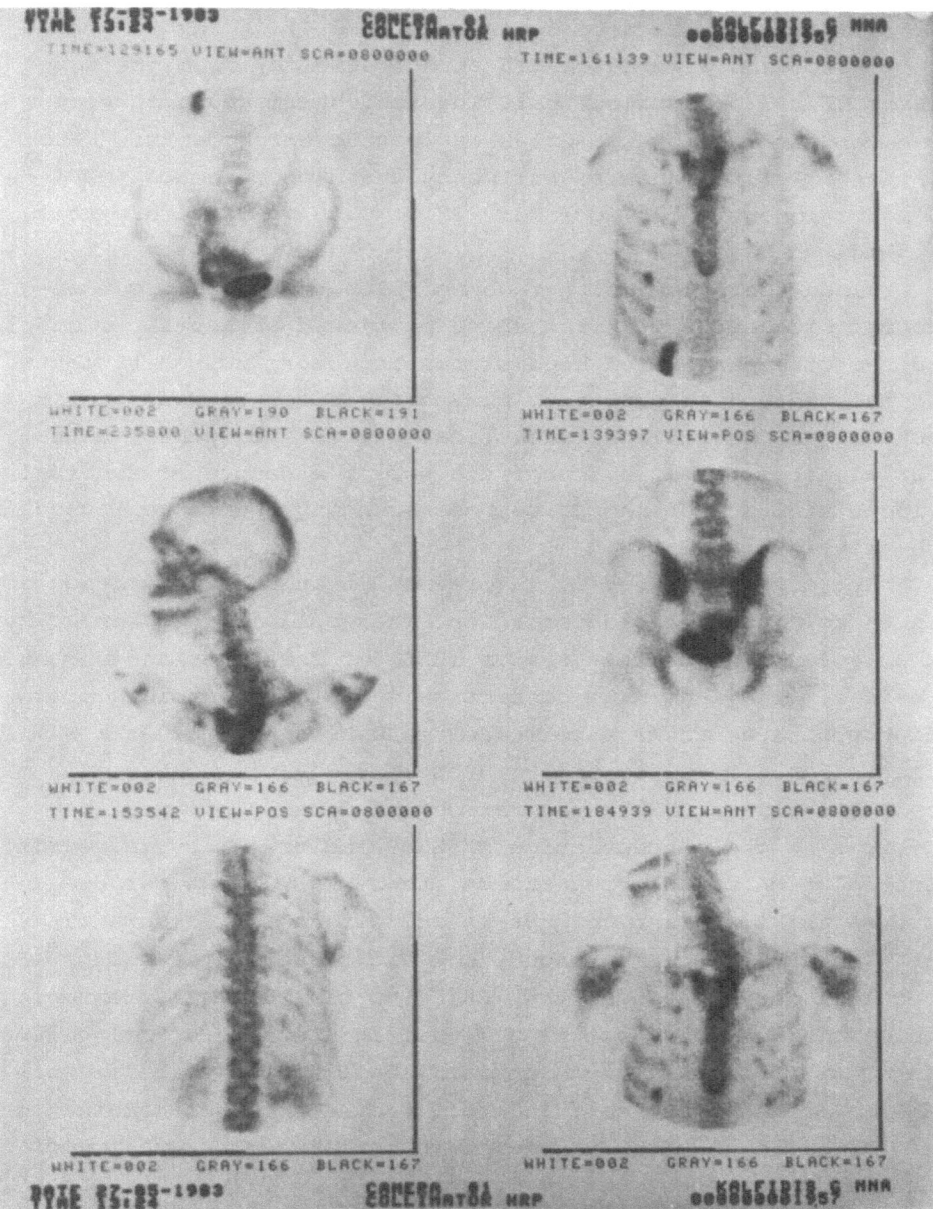

Fig. 4. Bone scan with increased uptake in several ribs as well as in the gallbladder and the gut.

seronegative rheumatoid arthritis was considered and the
patient was started on steroids. On the bone scan performed,
areas of increased uptake were noticed in several ribs and
gallbladder and gut were again seen (fig 4).

Case 1 and 2 were scanned on the same day from the same
stock of radiopharmaceutical. The radiopharmaceutical used
was manufactured by the Greek Nuclear Research Centre "Democritos". It's synthesis was: methylene diphosphonate (MDP)
5 mg; stannous chloride ($SnCl_2-2H_2O$) 0.36 mg; ascorbic acid
1.8 mg.

Since there was neither common pathology nor common abnormal biochemistry in the above mentioned patients, we concluded that the pattern of biodistribution ought to be attributed
to the radiopharmaceutical. Due to technical reasons quality
control of the radiopharmaceutical was not performed; there-
for we attempted a review of the possible causes of abnormal
biodistribution of phosphate bone scanning agents mentioned in
the literature.

Hydrolyzed reduced Tc^{99m} present in an MDP preparation is
known to cause colloid formation. This colloid is taken up by
the reticuloendothelial system (RES) of the liver and spleen.
Besides, high aluminium content in the eluate combining with
diphosphonates forms a colloidal suspension and gives a similar
image. Yano, McRae et al(1) investigated various chemical
parameters in an EHDP preparation and found that by either
decreasing the concentration of EHDP and tin or by increasing
the dilution of the preparation, there was a considerable increase in kidney and gut uptake indicating a breakdown of
Tc^{99m}-Sn EHDP radiopharmaceutical and formation of a Tc^{99m}-Sn-
complex. They concluded that EHDP and tin concentration must
be maintained above a minimum level in a standard 5 ml volume
in order to promote good initial labelling and stability of
the radiopharmaceutical. In addition the order of combination
of EHDP, tin and $Tc^{99m}O4$ seemed to influence the quality of
the radiopharmaceutical. When tin and $Tc^{99m}O4$ were combined
first there was an insoluble Tc^{99m}-Sn-complex formed, probably
as the Tc^{99m} coprecipitated with tin-oxide (SnO) (2). Stability

was enhanced by evacuating the air from reaction vessel and replacing it with nitrogen. Similarly, Eckelman et al (3) observed while testing a pyrophosphate-tin preparation that if, 0,5 ml of air is injected into the nitrogen purged reaction vial, 34% of the stannous ion is oxidized after 4 hours. Furthermore, large amounts of tin and high pH favour formation of tin-oxide rather than tin-PYP, the technetium being absorbed as the tin-oxide. The same authors showed that low concentration of PYP and tin caused dissociation to tin oxide. However, higher amounts of PYP present in the preparation lead to colloid formation and liver-spleen visualization due to low stability and therefore precipitation of the PYP in the high ionic strength of the plasma.

Lastly, Tc^{99m}-diphosphonate skeletal imaging agents are not considered single chemical entities, but complex mixtures of several components, which can exhibit distinct biological distributions. Therefore, Libson, Deutsch, Heineman et al (4) prepared Tc^{99m} (NaBH4) MDP mixtures as a function of pH, of presence or absence of Tc^{99} carrier, and of presence or absence of air. Several HPLC isolated components used as skeletal imaging agents in rats showed different bone and soft tissue uptakes. pH was the most effective factor in controlling the generation of specific components and consequently the biodistribution of the MDP preparation.

We conclude that in our cases gallbladder and intestinal visualization on Tc^{99m}-MDP bone scintiscans was caused by a partial loss of integrity of the radiopharmaceutical, attributable to one or more of the above mentioned reasons.

LITERATURE

1. Yano Y, McRae J, Van Dyke DC, Anger HO, Technetium-99m labelled stannous Ethan-I-Hydroxy-1-Diphosphonate: A new bone scanning agent. J. nucl. Med. 14:73, 1973.

2. Mass R, Alvarez J, Arriaga C, On a new tracer for liver scanning. Int. appl. Radiat. 18:653, 1967.

3. Eckelman WC, Reba RC, Kubota M, Stevenson JS, ^{99m}Tc-PYP for bone imaging. J. nucl. Med. 15:279, 1974.

4. Libson K, Deutsch E, Heineman WR, Tanabe S, Zodda JP, Preperative control, HPLC analysis and in vivo evaluation of components of a technetium MDP radiopharmaceutical mixture. Proc. 30th Annual Meeting SNM. St. Louis, June 1983. J. nucl. Med. 24:23, 1983.

DRUG-FREE HIGH-QUALITY TUMOUR IMAGING WITH ^{67}Ga

S.K. SHUKLA, I. BLOTTA, C. CIPRIANI, G.B. MANNI

In the preface to the book "Therapeutic Use of Artificial Radioisotopes", P.F. Hahn wrote (1) in 1956: "Ideally, one looks for an agent that will seek out and destroy cancer". 13 Years later in 1969, Edwards and Hayes (2) reported "Tumour scanning with ^{67}Ga citrate". In 1971 Hart and co-workers observed antitumour activity of gallium nitrate in rodents and suggested the potential usefulness of gallium for treatment of various solid tumours in man (3,4). During the last 15 years since the report of Edwards and Hayes (2), much effort has been devoted to improve the tumour imaging results with ^{67}Ga and also to get satisfactory treatment of various tumours in rodents with gold gallium (5). Although ^{67}Ga citrate is widely used for tumour (6) and abscess detection (7), a positive finding is often doubtful due to following difficulties still encountered during radionuclidic examinations with this radiopharmaceutical (8,9).

1. Unduely long time of waiting between the injection of the radiopharmaceutical and scintigraphy, which has to be one to three days (10-12) or still longer, due to slow rate of clearance of the radionuclide from blood and of accumulation in the lesion or other tissues which leads to poor lesion-to-background radioactivity ratio (7,9).

2. In vivo uptake of the radionuclide from commercial ^{67}Ga-citrate is unfortunately not tumour specific (13). It concentrates, for example, also in inflammatory lesions and in many healthy organs like liver, spleen, kidneys and bowel (9,14). Because of this ^{67}Ga tumour imaging has so far remained only a confirmatory examination of the radiological or other tumour imaging techniques (9,13).

Table 1. Drugs administered to enhance tumour-to-background
contrast during tumour imaging with commercial gallium-67

Drugs

Cations: Cold gallium (18-21); scandium (15, 22); Fe^{3+} (23,24).

Chelates: Deferoxamine (7,25,26); citrate (9,19-21); tartrate
(9, 19); malate (9, 19); lactate (19); pyruvate
(19); gluconate (19).

Mixture of cations and chelates: Fesin (saccharated ferric
oxide) (19); Jectofer (ferric sorbitol citrate
complex) (27-29); ferric citrate (30,31); iron
dextran (32,33).

Many attempts have been made to improve tumour imaging
with ^{67}Ga or at least to enhance the tumour-to-back-ground
contrast by administering several types of drugs, given in
table 1, either simultaneously with the radiopharmaceutical,
or before and after the injection of the radiopharmaceutical
to the patient. Although some success has been reported in
vitro studies by the use of these drugs, the toxicity of the
drugs and the poor quality of scintigrams as well as irreproduc-
ible results in humans have discouraged the administration of
these drugs in patients (14-17).

Despite the fact that it is the nature of ^{67}Ga species
in the solution injected which mainly determines the in vivo
distribution of the radionuclide and consequently affects also
the quality of the tumour image (9), it is surprising to

Table 2. Commercial gallium-67 formulations

Supplier	Gallium-67 formulation		
	Gallium-67 (mCi/ml)	Sodium citrate (mg/ml)	NaCl (mg/ml)
Japan Abbott Chiba, Japan	1	50	-
Nihon Medi-Physics	1	28	-
Radiochem. Centre Amersham	1	26	1
Radioisotop Intè-zet, Budapest	3	14.9	5
Sorin Biomed. Saluggia or Byk Mallinckrodt	1	1.75	6.87

observe that so far little attention has been paid to the composition of the ^{67}Ga solution used, both by the radiopharmaceutical producers as well as the nuclear medicine physicians (9). This is evident by the formulations of ^{67}Ga commercially available today for tumour imaging (table 2).

Working with ^{67}Ga citrate solution from the Radiochemical Centre, Amersham, containing 26 mg/ml sodium citrate and with that of Sorin Biomedica, Saluggia, or of Byk-Mallinckrodt, containing only 1.75 mg/ml sodium citrate for the same concentration of ^{67}Ga, we found (9) that the radionuclide from the latter source concentrates more rapidly and in higher intensity

than that from the radiopharmaceutical solutions rich in sodium
citrate (9,34). ^{67}Ga distribution in Morris hepatoma-3924A-
bearing rats injected with highly complexed ^{67}Ga malate or
tartrate solutions also led to the same conclusion that strongly bound ^{67}Ga has low affinity for tumours and concentrates
avidly in liver, spleen and kidneys (9,34). ^{67}Ga formation
containing 1 mCi/ml ^{67}Ga, 0.88 mg/ml sodium citrate cleared
rapidly from the blood and gave high contrast tumour image
after only 6 hours, with little activity in the liver, or
other healthy organs. Chromatographic studies on the stability
of this ^{67}Ga formulation showed, however, the radionuclide to
hydrolyse on standing at room temperature. The injection
solution has to be prepared fresh from Sorin Biomedica ^{67}Ga
preparations. In the present article we report our more recent
results on high-quality tumour imaging with drug-free ^{67}Ga.

MATERIALS AND METHODS
^{67}Ga solutions of desired formulation were prepared by
diluting the ^{67}Ga citrate solutions of Radiochemical Centre,
Amersham, or of Sorin Biomedica, Saluggia, by adding physiological saline. The nature of ^{67}Ga species in the solutions was
examined chromatographically or electrophoretically on Whatman
3 MM paper in physiological saline as described earlier (9).
The suitability of ^{67}Ga solutions for tumour imaging was
examined by studying the distribution of the radionuclide in
Morris hepatoma-3924A-bearing rats. For optimal formulation
the activity in each organ and tumour of the rat was also
counted in a well type gamma counter. Scintigrams of the
animals and patients were taken with a rectilinear scanner of
Italeltronica, Rome.

RESULTS AND DISCUSSION
Chromatographic and electrophoretic analysis of different
^{67}Ga solutions showed that the Radiochemical Centre, Amersham,
^{67}Ga solution, containing 26 mg/ml sodium citrate, has more
than 95% of ^{67}Ga in highly complexed citratogallate-67 form,
while that of Sorin Biomedica, with only 1.75 mg/ml, shows
the presence of only 28% in this highly bound form (9). We

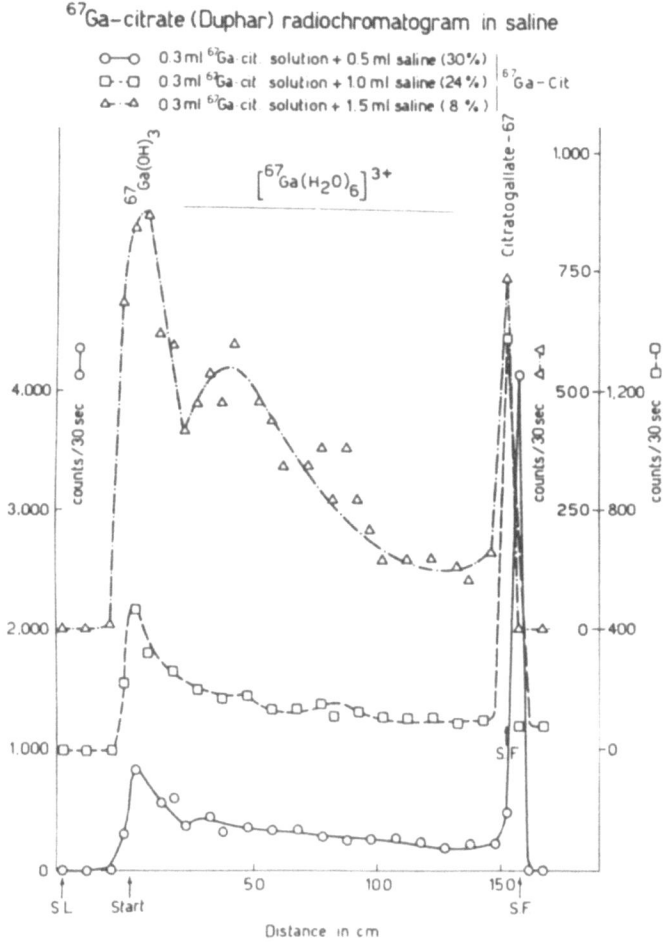

Fig. 1. Variation in the nature of ^{67}Ga species in aqueous solution with dilution of sodium citrate concentration.

further noticed that two samples of ^{67}Ga received on the same or different days from Sorin Biomedica never showed the same chromatographic and electrophoretic behaviour. Each sample from this source had therefore to be first chromatographically analysed before making the dilutions for injection into tumour bearing subjects. Chromatographic prerequisite for the optimal ^{67}Ga composition corresponds to the solution containing 52%

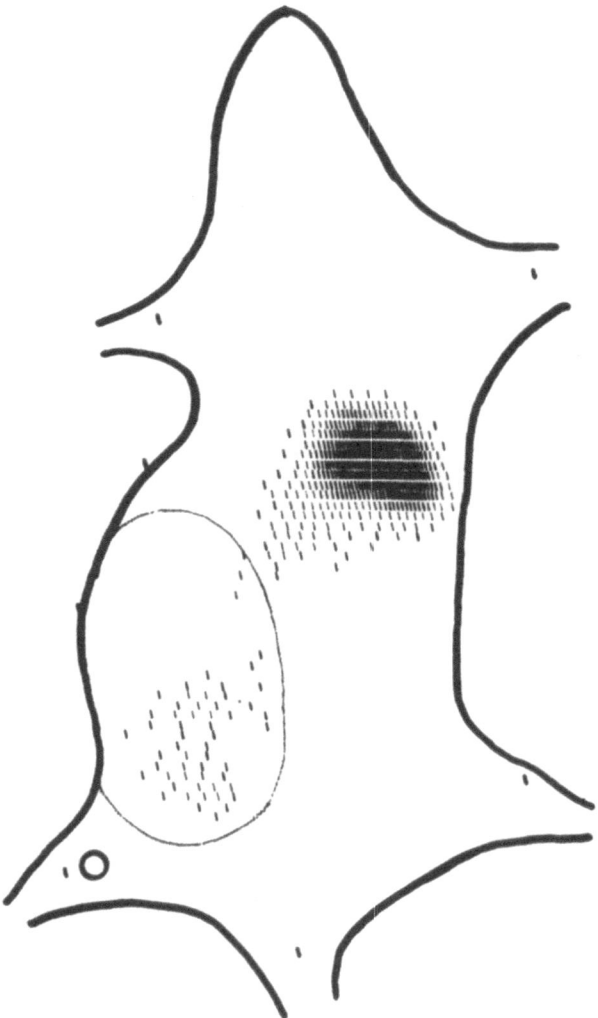

Fig. 2. Scintigram of a Morris hepatoma-3924A-bearing rat injected with the Radiochemical Centre, Amersham, ^{67}Ga-citrate preparation (containing 26 mg/ml sodium citrate).

free ^{67}Ga in equilibrium with strongly bound citrato-gallate-67. This ^{67}Ga solution concentrated uniquely in the tumour and no uptake of the radionuclide in healthy organs was observed. With these preparations we have been imaging routinely different types of tumours in our laboratory.

Highly reactive nature of ^{67}Ga in aqueous solution is

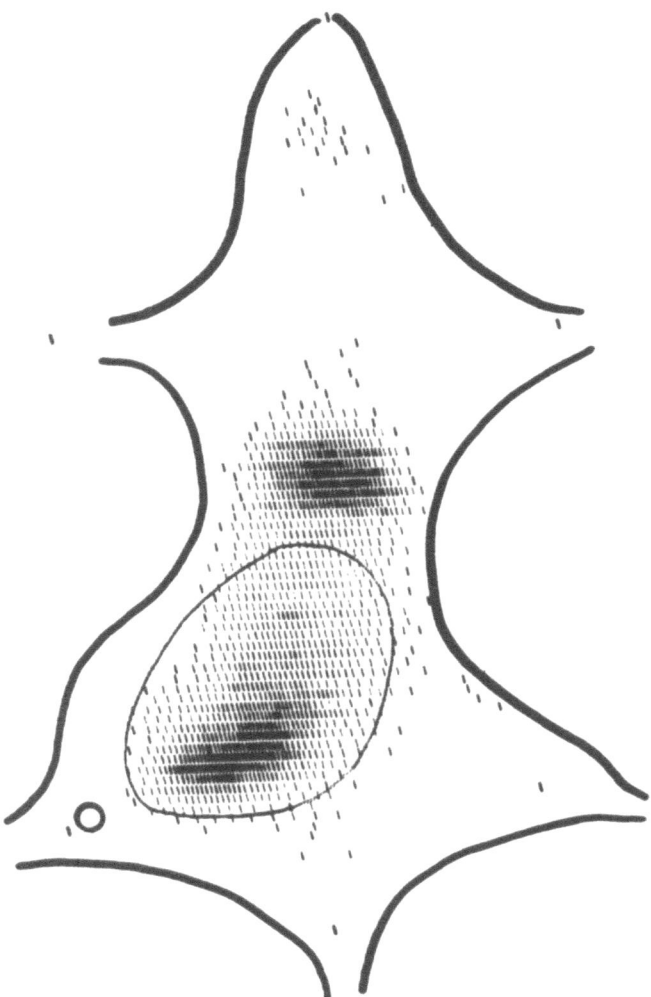

Fig. 3. Scintigram of a Morris hepatoma-3924A-bearing rat injected with Sorin Biomedica 67Ga-citrate preparation (containing 1.75 mg/ml sodium citrate).

shown in fig 1, where the addition of a small amount of physiological saline to the solution shows a change in the chemical nature of the radionuclide in solution.

The effect of sodium citrate concentration in the 67Ga-solution injected for tumour imaging on the distribution of the radionuclide in Morris hepatoma-3924A-bearing rats is shown in figs 2, 3 and 4. Free 67Ga present in the formulation containing 0.88 mg/ml sodium citrate concentrates mainly in

278

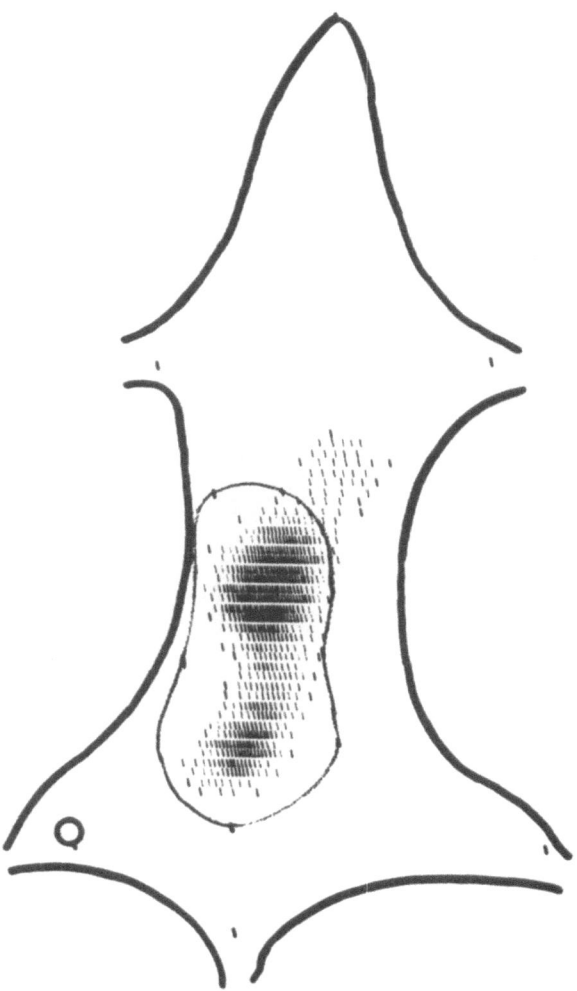

Fig. 4. Scintigram of a Morris hepatoma-3924A-bearing rat injected with ^{67}Ga solution containing 0.88 mg/ml sodium citrate.

the tumour (fig 4).

Fig 5 shows the radiograph and ^{67}Ga scintigram of a lung tumour patient injected with ^{67}Ga solution containing 52% free ^{67}Ga in equilibrium with 48% strongly bound citratogallate-67. With this ^{67}Ga formulation tumour specific uptake of the radionuclide has been obtained in patients with lung, liver tumours, Hodgkin's disease, neuroblastoma. Work is in progress to examine the usefulness of this ^{67}Ga formulation in other types

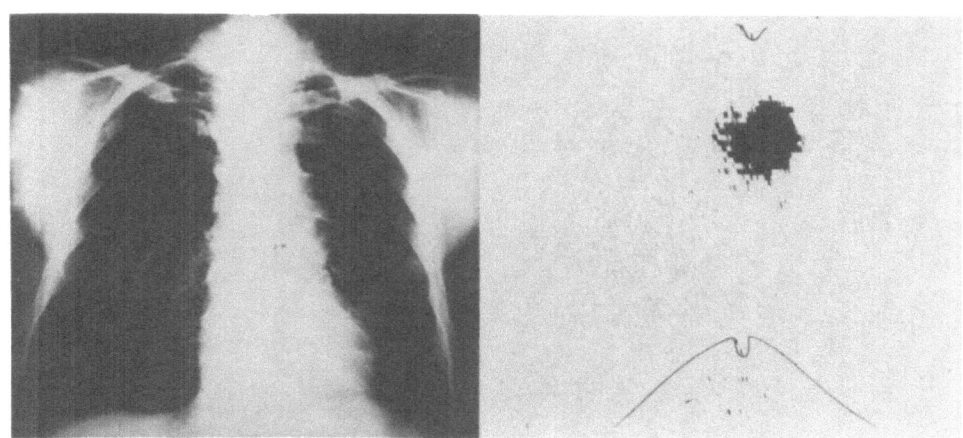

Fig. 5. Radiograph and scintigram of lung tumour patient injected with
67Ga solution containing 52% free 67Ga in equilibrium with 42% strongly
bound citratogallate-67.

of tumours. Four Japanese nuclear medicine centres are using
this formulation ^{67}Ga for tumour imaging. These results will
be published elsewhere.

From the analytical results and from the results on the
biological behaviour of ^{67}Ga published so far we have proposed
a mechanism of ^{67}Ga distribution in healthy and tumour-bearing
subjects which is summarized in the scheme shown in fig 6 (35).

CONCLUSIONS

The nature of ^{67}Ga in solution injected for tumour imaging
is very important to get tumour specific uptake of the radio-

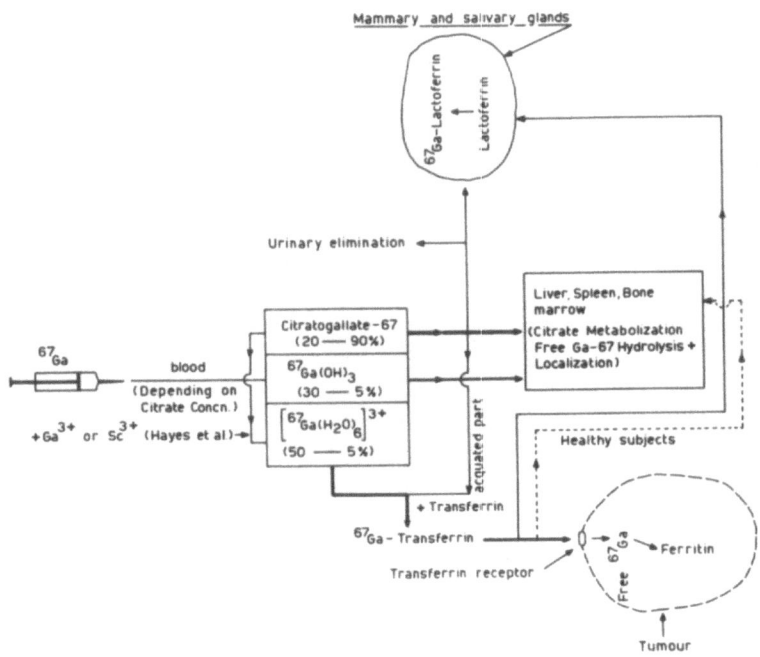

Fig. 6. Scheme of the mechanism of ^{67}Ga-uptake in tumour or normal organ depending on the chemical nature of ^{67}Ga species present in the solution injected for imaging.

nuclide. The solution containing 52% free ^{67}Ga in equilibrium with strongly bound citratogallate-67 gives high-quality tumour scintigram after only 4 hours following the injection of the radiopharmaceutical. Since this formulation of ^{67}Ga contains less than 0.8 mg/ml sodium citrate, it is unstable and cannot be stored at room temperature. This should be prepared at the time of injection by diluting Sorin Biomedica ^{67}Ga solution with physiological saline.

REFERENCES

1. Hahn PF, In: Therapeutic use of artificial radioisotopes, Hahn PF, (ed), John Wiley & Sons, Inc, New York, 1956.

2. Edwards CL, Hayes RL, Tumour imaging with ^{67}Ga citrate. J. nucl. Med. 10:103, 1969.

3. Hart MM, Adamson RH, Antitumour activity and toxicity of salts of inorganic group IIIA metals aluminum, gallium, indium and thallium. Proc. nat. Acad. Sci. USA, 68:1623, 1971.

4. Hart MM, Smith CF, Yancey ST, Adamson RH, Toxicity and antitumour activity of gallium nitrate and periodically related metal salts. J. Nat. Cancer Inst. 47:1121, 1971.

5. Warrel jr, RP, Coonley CJ, Straus DJ, Young CW, Treatment of patients with advanced malignant lymphoma using gallium nitrate administered as a seven day continuous infusion. Cancer 51:1982, 1983.

6. Keller F, Maiga MK, Koeppe P, ^{67}Gallium kinetics in blood of patients with malignant tumours. Nucl. Med. 22:155, 1983.

7. Oberhaensli RD, Mueller RM, Fridrich R, Different actions of deferoxamine and iron on Ga-67 abscess detection in rats. J. nucl. Med. 25:668, 1984.

8. Larson SM, Mechanism of localization of Gallium-67 in tumours. Sem. Nucl. Med. 8:193, 1978.

9. Shukla SK, Castelli L, Cipriani C, Manni GB, What is good in gallium-67 citrate and how to increase its tumour affinity? Radioakt. Isot. Klin. Forsch. 14:179, 1980.

10. Russian LD, Staab EV, Radionuclide imaging of intestinal infarction. Radiology 122:171, 1977.

11. Levitt RG, Riello DR, Sagel SS, Stanley RJ, Aronberg DJ, Robinson ML, Siegel BA, Computed tomography and ^{67}Ga citrate radionuclide imaging for evaluating suspected abdominal abscess. Amer. J. Roentgenol. 132: 529, 1979.

12. Beal WH, Chaudhury TK, One week post-injection gallium-67 scan --- is it of any added advantage? J. nucl. Med. 19:733, 1978.

13. Hoffer PB, The utility of gallium-67 in tumour imaging: A comment on the final reports on the co-operative study group. J. nucl. Med. 19: 1082, 1978.

14. Kaplan HS, Hodgkin's disease: Multidisciplinary contributions to the conquest of a neoplasm. Radiology 123:551, 1977.

15. Hayes RL, Byrd BL, Rafter JJ, Carlton JE, The effect of scandium on the tissue distribution of Ga-67 in normal and tumour-bearing rodents. J. nucl. Med. 21:361, 1980.

16. Hagan PL, Halpern SE, Stern P, Dabbs J, Gordon R, The effect of certain variables on the tumour and tissue distribution of tracers, II. Carrier effect: rapidity of onset and concentrations necessary for initiation and maximum response. Invest. Radiol. 15:496, 1980.

17. Higashi T, (private communication on 6-7-1984).

18. Hayes RL, Byrd BL, Carlton JE, Rafter JJ, Factors affecting the

localization of ^{67}Ga in animal tumours. J. nucl. Med. 11:324, 1970.

19. Higashi T, Nakayama Y, Akiba C, Ito K, Hisada T, Miki T, Kawai K, Diagnosis of malignant tumours with [67]Ca citrate, Japanese. J. nucl. Med. 8:155, 1971.

20. Halpern SE, Hagan PL, Chauncey D, McKegney M, Bernstein K, The effect of certain variables on the tumour and tissue distribution of tracers. Part I. Carrier, Invest. Radiol. 14:482, 1979.

21. Stern PH, Halpern SE, Hagan PL, Chen A, The effect of certain variables on the tumour and tissue distribution of tracers VI. False-carrier effect, Part III, Fe, Invest. Radiol. 17:386, 1982.

22. Hayes RL, Edwards CL, The effect of stable scandium on red blood cells and on the retention and excretion of ^{67}Ga in humans. South Med. 66:1339, 1973.

23. Hill JH, Merz T, Wagner jr, HH, Iron-indiced enhancement of ^{67}Ga uptake in a model human leukocyte culture system. J. nucl. Med. 16:1183, 1975.

24. Muranaka A, Ito Y, Saito J, Otsuka N, Nagai K, Role of $FeCl_3$ in ^{67}Ga uptake by HeLa S3 cells in vitro. Eur. J. Nucl. Med. 8:408, 1983.

25. Hoffer PB, Samuel A, Bushberg JT, Thakur M, Desferoxamine mesylate (desferal): A contrast enhancing agent for gallium-67 imaging. Radiology 131:775, 1979.

26. Oster ZH, Som P, Sacker DF, Atkins HL, The effects of desfroxamine mesylate on gallium-67 distribution in normal and abscess-bearing animals: Concise communication. J. nucl. Med. 21:421, 1980.

27. Sephton RG, Martin JJ, Modification of distribution of gallium-67 in man by administration of iron. Brit. J. Radiol. 53:572, 1980.

28. Smith FW, Dendy PP, Modification of gallium-67 citrate distribution in man following the distribution of iron. Brit. J. Radiol. 54:398, 1981.

29. Sephton RG, De Abrew S, Hodgson, mechanisms of distribution of gallium-67 in mouse tumour hosts. Brit. J. Radiol. 55:134, 1982.

30. Hagan PL, Halpern SE, Stern P, Dabbs J, Gordon R, The effect of certain variables on the tumour and tissue distribution of tracers, IV. False carrier: ferric citrate. Invest. Radiol. 16:229, 1981.

31. Hagan PL, Halpern SE, Stern PH, Gordon RM, Dabbs JE, The effect of certain variables on the tumour and tissue distribution of tracers V. False carrier effect, II, Fe, Invest. Radiol. 17:53, 1982.

32. Oster ZH, Larson SM, Wagner jr, HN, Possible enhancement of ^{67}Ga-citrate imaging by iron dextran. J. nucl. Med. 17:356, 1976.

33. Larson SM, Mahler D, Allen DR, Iron-dextran enhancement of ^{67}Ga-concentration in abscess relative to normal tissue. Nucl. Med. 17:95, 1978.

34. Shukla SK, Cipriani C, Manni GB, Castelli L, Increasing the tumour specificity of ^{67}Ga-radiopharmaceuticals. J. Lab. Comp. Radiopharm. 16:192, 1979.

35. Castelli L, Blotta I, Shukla SK, Cipriani C, Manni GB, Sul meccanismo di captazione des gallio-67 nei tumori. Radiol. Med. 69:103, 1983.

AUTHOR INDEX

Adam,W.E   3

Angelberger,P   73

Bartsch,P   23

Bauer,R   161

Biersack,H.J   123

Blotta,I   271

Bofilias,I   49

Chiotellis,E   131

Cipriani,C   271

Cleynhens,B   239

Cox,P.H   57   231

Dassiou,C   195

Doppelfeld,E   123

Evangelatos,G   131

Fountos,A   263

Fiedler,W   73

Friedrich,G   123

Garzaniti,N   23

Guillaume,M   23

Henze,E   3

Hoogmartens,M   239

Khuc,T   23

Kloster,G   89

Klunenberg,H   123

Knopp,R   123

Kohn,H   73

Kriegel,H   251

Ledda,R   123

Mallamitsi,J   263

Manni,G.B   271

Mollenstadt,S   251

Mostbeck,A   73

Pabst,H.W   161

Pfannenstiel,P   199

Pike,V   141

Pillay,M   57

Roo,M de   239

Roth,J   3

Sawas-Dimopoulou,C   183

Senekowitsch,R   251

Shapiro,B   57

Shukla,S.K   271

Soupli,C   183

Strigl,A   73

Stocklin,G   89

Toubakanis,N   183

Varvarigou,A.D   131

Verbruggen,A   239

Winkler,C   123

Woldring,M.G   219

Zicot,M   23

Zolle,I   73

INDEX

Acetate-1-11C 145
- in myocardium 145
- PET 145
Aerosols 57 et seq
(see also Radioaerosols)
- Clinical studies 76
- Dry 73
- Ham M clinical studies 81
- Inhalator 75
Airway
- Model 57
- obstruction 12
Alveolar clearance
- Of DTPA 66
- Of HIDA 67
Amphetamines 123
- Cerebral uptake 123
- Derivatives 123
Aneurysm 168-171
- False 171
- Traumatic 181
Benzodiazepines 111
Biodistribution
- Extraneous factors affecting 219 et seq
- Effect of drugs on skeletal agents 231
- Iatrogenic effects 228
BMHDA 147
Bullae 54
Cardiac studies isotopes for jD W 2 @ D-glucose analogues 98
Deoxyglucose 2-fluoro 92
- 2-Deoxy-D 96
Diethylida 183
Disinfectants effect on biodistribution 239
DOPA

- 1-11C 109
- 6-fluoro 110
- 18-F-fluoro 109
Dopamine
    - receptors 101
    - Systems 155
F-18 141
Fe-59 citrate 185
Flunitrazepam 111
Fluoro-3-deoxy-D-glucose 98
Gallbladder on bone scans 263
Gallium imaging 271
Generator
    - Krypton 23
    - In process controls 46
    - Produced nuclides 24
D-Glucose 90
Glucose turnover 89
Haloperidol 106
Hepatic cirrhosis of thalassaemia 183
Hyperferremic mice 183
Infarction right heart 175
Inhalator activity balance 80
Iodinated amphetamines 123
Iodine retention 203
Iodine-131 dose formula 203
Iodo-quinuclidinyl benzilate 112
Irradiated tissue volume 200
Jectofer 183
Kentaserin 111
Krypton 81m 23 et seq
    - Angiology 41
    - Availability 35
    - Clinical methodology 34
    - Gas 23
    - Generator characteristics 25

- Intra arterial 45
- Intravenous infusion 41
- Liquid 23
- Production methodology 28
- Perfusion generator 32
- Ventilation technique 50
Lungs
    - Cancer 55
    - Changes in 16
    - Embolism 181
    - Evolution 4
    - Function 4
    - Localised processes 12
    - Model of Wiebel 58
    - Pathophysiology 11
    - Regional function 9,36
    - Vessel obstruction 16
Mean total body radiation 210
    - Haematological response 214
Mesulergin 111
Methyl erythromycin 153
Methyl-D-Glucose 96
Methylheptadecanoate 147
Mitral regurgitation 175
Myocardial blood flow
    - Regional 149
Nebulisers
    - jet 62
    - Systems 62
    - Rotating disc 62
Noble gases 49
Palmitate-1-11C 143
Particle size 61
Pharmacokinetics
    - Diethylida 183
Phytate distribution 195

Pimozide 109
Radiation dose
  - Ham M 85
Radiation hazard from I-131 208
Radioaerosols 57
    - Choice of reagent 63
    - Particle size 61
    - Patient dosimetry 68
    - Study protocol 63
Radiopharmaceuticals
    - Biodistribution 141 et seq
    - Drug effects 224
    - Effect of cytostatic drugs on 251
    - Effect of disinfectants 239
    - For cardiac emergency 161
    - Interaction 222
    - Labelled with 11-C 141
    - Labelled with 18-F 141
    - Metabolism 141 et seq
    - Receptor specific 100 113
    - Secondary drug effects 225
Radiospirometry 5
Receptor density 89
Regional myocardial metabolism 141
Respiratory system
    - Pathophysiology 1
    - Physiology 1
Ro-15-1788 112
RVEF 42

Schiff bases 131
Septal perforation 171
Skeletal reagents effect of drugs on 231
    - Alcohol 234
    - Dextrose 233
    - Effect of radiotherapy 231
    - Gallbladder visualisation 263
    - Dextrose 233
    - Effect of radiotherapy 231
    - Gallbladder visualisation 263
    - Soft tissue uptake 232
SPECT 126
    - Comparison with CT 128
Spiroperidol 107
    - N-methyl 108
    - p-Bromo 108
Technetium
    - Gall bladder on bone scans 263
    - Millimicrospheres 73
    - Effects of disinfectants on 239
Thyroid
    - calculated absorbed dose 204
    - Time factor and absorbed dose 205
    - Treatment 199
Tumour uptake Ga,Tc and Ca
    - Effect of cytostatic drugs 251
Thymidine 258
Wiebel model 58
Xe-133 inhalation 49